T0226640

Pediatric Critical Care

Editor

MARGARET M. PARKER

CRITICAL CARE CLINICS

www.criticalcare.theclinics.com

Consulting Editor
RICHARD W. CARLSON

April 2013 • Volume 29 • Number 2

ELSEVIER

1600 John F. Kennedy Boulevard • Suite 1800 • Philadelphia, Pennsylvania, 19103-2899

http://www.theclinics.com

CRITICAL CARE CLINICS Volume 29, Number 2
April 2013 ISSN 0749-0704, ISBN-13: 978-1-4557-7076-2

Editor: Patrick Manley
Developmental Editor: Donald Mumford

Critical Care Clinics (ISSN: 0749-0704) is published quarterly by Elsevier Inc., 360 Park Avenue South, New York, NY 10010-1710. Months of issue are January, April, July, and October. Business and Editorial Offices: 1600 John F. Kennedy Blvd., Suite 1800, Philadelphia, PA 19103-2899. Customer Service Office: 6277 Sea Harbor Drive, Orlando, FL 32887-4800. Periodicals postage paid at New York, NY and additional mailing offices. Subscription prices are $199.00 per year for US individuals, $482.00 per year for US institution, $97.00 per year for US students and residents, $245.00 per year for Canadian individuals, $597.00 per year for Canadian institutions, $287.00 per year for international individuals, $597.00 per year for international institutions and $141.00 per year for Canadian and foreign students/ residents. To receive student/resident rate, orders must be accompanied by name of affiliated institution, date of term, and the signature of program/residency coordinator on institution letterhead. Orders will be billed at individual rate until proof of status is received. Foreign air speed delivery is included in all Clinics subscription prices. All prices are subject to change without notice. POSTMASTER: Send address changes to Critical Care Clinics, Elsevier Periodicals Customer Service, 11830 Westline Industrial Drive, St. Louis, MO 63146. **Customer Service: 1-800-654-2452 (US). From outside of the US, call 1-314-447-8871. Fax: 1-314-447-8029. E-mail: journalscustomerservice-usa@elsevier.com (for print support) or journalsonlinesupport-usa@elsevier.com (for online support).**

Reprints. For copies of 100 or more of articles in this publication, please contact the Commercial Reprints Department, Elsevier Inc., 360 Park Avenue South, New York, NY 10010-1710. Tel.: 212-633-3813; Fax: 212-462-1935; E-mail: reprints@elsevier.com.

Critical Care Clinics is also published in Spanish by Editorial Inter-Medica, Junin 917, 1er A, 1113, Buenos Aires, Argentina.

Critical Care Clinics is covered in MEDLINE/PubMed (Index Medicus), EMBASE/Excerpta Medica, Current Concepts/ Clinical Medicine, ISI/BIOMED, and Chemical Abstracts.

Printed and bound by CPI Group (UK) Ltd, Croydon, CR0 4YY

Transferred to digital print 2013

Contributors

CONSULTING EDITOR

RICHARD W. CARLSON, MD, PhD
Chairman Emeritus, Director, Medical Intensive Care Unit, Department of Medicine, Maricopa Medical Center; Professor, University of Arizona College of Medicine; Professor, Department of Medicine, Mayo Graduate School of Medicine, Phoenix, Arizona

EDITOR

MARGARET M. PARKER, MD, FCCM
Professor of Pediatrics, Anesthesia, and Medicine, Director of Pediatric Critical Care, Department of Pediatrics, Stony Brook University, Stony Brook Long Island Children's Hospital, Stony Brook, New York

AUTHORS

MICHAEL J. BELL, MD
Associate Professor, Director and Associate Director, Departments of Critical Care Medicine, Neurological Surgery and Pediatrics, Safar Center for Resuscitation Research, University of Pittsburgh, Pittsburgh, Pennsylvania

THOMAS V. BROGAN, MD
Seattle Children's Hospital, University of Washington School of Medicine, Seattle, Washington

TIMOTHY E. BUNCHMAN, MD
Professor and Director, Pediatric Nephrology, Children's Hospital of Richmond, Virginia Commonwealth University, Richmond, Virginia

CHRISTOPHER L. CARROLL, MD, MS
Division of Pediatric Critical Care, Connecticut Children's Medical Center; Associate Professor of Pediatrics, University of Connecticut, Hartford, Connecticut

IRA M. CHEIFETZ, MD, FCCM, FAARC
Director, Pediatric Critical Care Service; Chief and Professor of Pediatrics, Division of Pediatric Critical Care Medicine, Duke University Medical Center, Duke Children's Hospital, Durham, North Carolina

ROBERT S.B. CLARK, MD
Professor and Chief, Pediatric Critical Care Medicine, Departments of Critical Care Medicine and Pediatrics, The Children's Hospital of Pittsburgh of UPMC; Associate Director, Safar Center for Resuscitation Research, University of Pittsburgh School of Medicine, Pittsburgh, Pennsylvania

NANA E. COLEMAN, MD, EdM, FAAP
Assistant Professor of Pediatrics, Weill Cornell Medical College; Quality and Performance Improvement Director, Pediatric Intensive Care Unit, New York-Presbyterian Komansky Center for Children's Health, New York, New York

RODNEY C. DANIELS, MD
Assistant Professor, Pediatric Critical Care, Children's Hospital of Richmond; Assistant Professor, Biomedical Engineering, Virginia Commonwealth University, Richmond, Virginia

YONG SING DA SILVA, MD
Fellow, Department of Critical Care Medicine, The Children's Hospital of Pittsburgh of UPMC, University of Pittsburgh School of Medicine, Pittsburgh, Pennsylvania

REID FARRIS, MD
Seattle Children's Hospital, University of Washington School of Medicine, Seattle, Washington

WILLIAM HANNA, MD
Division of Critical Care Medicine, Cincinnati Children's Hospital Research Foundation, Cincinnati Children's Hospital Medical Center, University of Cincinnati College of Medicine; Department of Pediatrics, University of Cincinnati College of Medicine, Cincinnati, Ohio

PATRICK M. KOCHANEK, MD
Professor and Director, Department of Critical Care Medicine, Safar Center for Resuscitation Research, University of Pittsburgh, Pittsburgh, Pennsylvania

WYNNE E. MORRISON, MD, MBE
Departments of Anesthesiology and Critical Care, The Children's Hospital of Philadelphia; Perelman School of Medicine, University of Pennsylvania, Philadelphia, Pennsylvania

GEORGE OFORI-AMANFO, MBChB, FACC
Associate Professor of Pediatrics, Division of Pediatric Critical Care Medicine, Duke University Medical Center, Duke Children's Hospital, Durham, North Carolina

ALBERTO ORIOLES, MD
Departments of Anesthesiology and Critical Care, The Children's Hospital of Philadelphia, Philadelphia, Pennsylvania

ROBERT I. PARKER, MD
Professor and Vice Chair for Academic Affairs; Director, Pediatric Hematology/Oncology, Stony Brook Long Island Children's Hospital, Stony Brook University School of Medicine, Stony Brook, New York

STEVEN PON, MD, FCCM, FAAP
Associate Professor of Clinical Pediatrics, Weill Cornell Medical College; Medical Director, Pediatric Intensive Care Unit, NewYork-Presbyterian Komansky Center for Children's Health, New York, New York

JOAN S. ROBERTS, MD
Department of Pediatrics, Critical Care Division, Seattle Children's Hospital, University of Washington School of Medicine, Seattle, Washington

KATHLEEN A. SALA, MPH
Division of Pediatric Critical Care, Connecticut Children's Medical Center, Hartford, Connecticut

JAMES SCHNEIDER, MD, FAAP, FCCP
Assistant Professor of Pediatrics, Division of Critical Care Medicine, Hofstra
North Shore-LIJ School of Medicine, Cohen Children's Medical Center of New York,
North Shore Long Island Jewish Health System, New York

DENNIS W. SIMON, MD
Fellow, Department of Critical Care Medicine, The Children's Hospital of Pittsburgh of
UPMC, University of Pittsburgh School of Medicine, Pittsburgh, Pennsylvania

DANIEL SLONIEWSKY, MD
Associate Professor, Division of Pediatric Critical Care Medicine, Department of
Pediatrics, Stony Brook Long Island Children's Hospital, New York

TODD SWEBERG, MD, FAAP
Assistant Professor of Pediatrics, Division of Critical Care Medicine, Hofstra North
Shore-LIJ School of Medicine, Cohen Children's Medical Center of New York,
North Shore Long Island Jewish Health System, New York

ROBERT C. TASKER, MBBS, MD
Professor of Neurology and Anesthesia (Pediatric), Division of Critical Care, Department
of Anesthesia, Pain and Perioperative Medicine, Harvard Medical School; Department of
Neurology, Boston Children's Hospital, Boston, Massachusetts

AMELIE VON SAINT ANDRE-VON ARNIM, MD
Seattle Children's Hospital, University of Washington School of Medicine, Seattle,
Washington

RYAN WILKES, MD
Fellow in Pediatric Critical Care, Division of Critical Care, Department of Anesthesia, Pain
and Perioperative Medicine, Boston Children's Hospital, Boston, Massachusetts

HECTOR R. WONG, MD
Division of Critical Care Medicine, Cincinnati Children's Hospital Research Foundation,
Cincinnati Children's Hospital Medical Center, University of Cincinnati College of
Medicine; Department of Pediatrics, University of Cincinnati College of Medicine,
Cincinnati, Ohio

OFER YANAY, MD
Seattle Children's Hospital, University of Washington School of Medicine, Seattle,
Washington

JERRY J. ZIMMERMAN, MD, PhD, FCCM
Professor of Pediatrics/Anesthesiology, Seattle Children's Hospital, University of
Washington School of Medicine, Seattle, Washington

GIULIO ZUCCOLI, MD
Associate Professor, Department of Radiology, The Children's Hospital of Pittsburgh of
UPMC, University of Pittsburgh School of Medicine, Pittsburgh, Pennsylvania

Contents

> Using the Institute of Medicine framework that outlines the domains of
> quality, this article considers four key aspects of health care delivery which
> have the potential to significantly affect the quality of health care within the
> pediatric intensive care unit. The discussion covers: performance improve-
> ment and how existing methods for reporting, review, and analysis of med-
> ical error relate to patient care; team composition and workflow; and the
> impact of information technologies on clinical practice. Also considered
> is how protocol-driven and standardized practice affects both patients
> and the fiscal interests of the health care system.

> Status asthmaticus is a frequent cause of admission to a pediatric inten-
> sive care unit. Prompt assessment and aggressive treatment are critical.
> First-line or conventional treatment includes supplemental oxygen, aero-
> solized albuterol, and corticosteroids. There are several second-line treat-
> ments available; however, few comparative studies have been performed
> and in the absence of good evidence-based treatments, the use of these
> therapies is highly variable and dependent on local practice and provider
> preference. In this article the pathophysiology and treatment of status
> asthmaticus is discussed, and the literature regarding second-line treat-
> ments is critically assessed to apply an evidence basis to the treatment
> of this severe disease.

> Acute respiratory failure is common in critically ill children, who are at in-
> creased risk of respiratory embarrassment because of the developmental
> variations in the respiratory system. Although multiple etiologies exist,
> pneumonia and bronchiolitis are most common. Respiratory system mon-
> itoring has evolved, with the clinical examination remaining paramount.
> Invasive tests are commonly replaced with noninvasive monitors. Children
> with ALI/ARDS have better overall outcomes than adults, although data
> regarding specific therapies are still lacking. Most children will have
> some degree of long-term physiologic respiratory compromise after re-
> covery from ALI/ARDS. The physiologic basis for respiratory failure and
> its therapeutic options are reviewed here.

Pediatric Postoperative Cardiac Care

George Ofori-Amanfo and Ira M. Cheifetz

Postoperative care of cardiac patients requires a comprehensive and multidisciplinary approach to critically ill patients with cardiac disease whose care requires a clear understanding of cardiovascular physiology. When a patient fails to progress along the projected course or decompensates acutely, prompt evaluation with bedside assessment, laboratory evaluation, and echocardiography is essential. When things do not add up, cardiac catheterization must be seriously considered. With continued advancements in the field of neonatal and pediatric postoperative cardiac care, continued improvements in overall outcomes for this specialized population are anticipated.

William Hanna and Hector R. Wong

Sepsis remains an important challenge in pediatric critical care medicine. This review provides an appraisal of adjunctive therapies for sepsis and highlights opportunities for meeting selected challenges in the field. Future clinical studies should address long-term and functional outcomes as well as acute outcomes. Potential adjunctive therapies such as corticosteroids, hemofiltration, hemoadsorption, and plasmapheresis may have important roles, but still require formal and more rigorous testing by way of clinical trials. Finally, the design of future clinical trials should consider novel approaches for stratifying outcome risks as a means of improving the risk-to-benefit ratio of experimental therapies.

Michael J. Bell and Patrick M. Kochanek

Traumatic brain injury (TBI) remains the leading cause of death of children in the developing world. In 2012, several international efforts were completed to aid clinicians and researchers in advancing the field of pediatric TBI. The second edition of the Guidelines for the Medical Management of Traumatic Brain Injury in Infants, Children and Adolescents updated those published in 2003. This article highlights the processes involved in developing the Guidelines, contrasts the new guidelines with the previous edition, and delineates new research efforts needed to advance knowledge. The impact of common data elements within these potential new research fields is reviewed.

Ryan Wilkes and Robert C. Tasker

The critically ill mechanically ventilated child with ongoing seizures that are refractory to any treatment presents a distinct challenge in pediatric neurocritical care. The evidence base from randomized controlled trials on which anti-epileptic drug (AED) strategy should be used is inadequate. This review of refractory and super-refractory status epilepticus summarizes recent pediatric case series regarding definitions, the second-tier

AED therapies once initial anticonvulsants have failed, and the experience of high-dose midazolam, barbiturate anesthesia, and volatile anesthetics for uncontrolled status epilepticus.

Dennis W. Simon, Yong Sing Da Silva, Giulio Zuccoli, and Robert S.B. Clark

Acute encephalitis remains one of the contemporary challenges of critical care medicine. The diagnosis is difficult and sometimes unconfirmed, and encephalitis remains without clear evidence-based therapies or even therapeutic goals for the prevention of high neurologic sequelae. This article provides a framework for pediatric intensivists to guide the diagnosis and management of patients with suspected encephalitis. It provides an in-depth review of the most common causes of encephalitis in children. The article promotes early recognition, appropriate testing and empiric treatment, and management of the expected complications of acute encephalitis.

Rodney C. Daniels and Timothy E. Bunchman

This article provides the bedside clinician an overview of the unique renal complications that are seen commonly in the pediatric intensive care unit. These sections are purposely succinct to give a quick guide to the clinician for the care of these children. We have identified four major areas that should result in discussion and cooperative care between intensive care physicians and nephrologists for the care of these children: (1) hypertension, (2) chronic kidney failure, (3) acute kidney injury, and (4) renal replacement therapy.

Daniel Sloniewsky

This article describes the incidence and etiology of anemia in critically ill children. In addition, the article details the pathophysiology and clinical ramifications of anemia in this population. The use of transfused packed red blood cells as a therapy for anemia in critically ill patients is also discussed, including the indications for and complications associated with this practice as well as potential reasons for these complications. Finally, the article lists some therapeutic practices that may lessen the risks associated with transfusion, and briefly discusses the use of blood substitutes.

Robert I. Parker

Bleeding in patients in pediatric intensive care units is associated with an increased risk of mortality. Fortunately, most patients with an abnormal coagulation profile do not bleed because this is generally secondary to liver disease or dietary-induced vitamin K deficiency. When the laboratory markers of coagulopathy are the result of disseminated intravascular coagulation, bleeding is common and the risk of mortality extreme.

CRITICAL CARE CLINICS

Preface

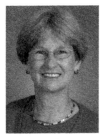

Margaret M. Parker, MD, FCCM
Editor

Pediatric critical care is similar to adult critical care in that a wide variety of clinical problems are encountered. Critically ill children, however, are a distinct and unique population of critically ill patients. This issue of *Critical Care Clinics* looks at some of the most common problems encountered in children in the ICU. The 13 articles cover 10 common medical and surgical problems, including an update on transfusion of red blood cells. These issues are covered by clinical experts in the field and provide a broad overview and practical approach to common problems in pediatric critical care. There is also an article on ethics in pediatric critical care, with an approach to some challenging ethical issues unique to children An article on quality improvement and communication includes information that is generic to critical care but no less essential in the pediatric ICU. The authors for each of these articles have worked to include important diagnostic and management approaches that will be useful to the clinician caring for critically ill children. I hope that you will find them as interesting and useful as I have.

Margaret M. Parker, MD, FCCM
Department of Pediatrics
Stony Brook University
Stony Brook Long Island Children's Hospital
Stony Brook, NY 11794-8111, USA

E-mail address:
Margaret.parker@stonybrookmedicine.edu

Crit Care Clin 29 (2013) xiii
http://dx.doi.org/10.1016/j.ccc.2013.01.004
0749-0704/13/$ – see front matter © 2013 Published by Elsevier Inc.

criticalcare.theclinics.com

Quality

Performance Improvement, Teamwork, Information Technology and Protocols

Nana E. Coleman, MD, EdM[a,b], Steven Pon, MD[a,b],*

KEYWORDS

- Quality • Medical errors • Communication • Teamwork • Workflow
- Information technology • Protocols

KEY POINTS

- Medical errors will occur: how teams deal with mistakes is what matters most.
- Punition does not work, and rather serves to isolate team members and precipitate greater errors as a consequence of the atmosphere of fear, uncertainty, and disempowerment that such an approach breeds.
- A well-structured, highly reliable, and functional team has the potential to significantly affect the patient's experience in the pediatric intensive care unit.
- Handoffs or communications between providers at all phases of care are crucial for accurate, timely, and efficient delivery of care.
- When skilled pediatric providers work closely with patients and their families, the results can be mutually rewarding.
- The specifics of implementing an electronic health records system with attention to alterations of workflow and other unintended consequences could be the decisive factors in determining the success or failure of such a system.
- Health information exchange, a specific implementation of "interoperability," the ability of systems to work with one another, improves quality by increasing the availability of data on patients who have care delivered by different organizations.
- By eliminating unnecessary practice variation, protocols should result in more efficient and effective care with lower overall cost of health care without compromising quality.
- The key feature of an adequately explicit protocol is that it would lead different clinicians to the same decision when faced with the same clinical scenario, allowing the treatment to vary based on patient variability rather than on physician variability.

[a] Division of Critical Care Medicine, Department of Pediatrics, Weill Cornell Medical College, 525 East 68th Street, M-508, New York, NY 10065-4870, USA; [b] Pediatric Intensive Care Unit, NewYork-Presbyterian Komansky Center for Children's Health, 525 East 68th Street, New York, NY 10065, USA
* Corresponding author. 525 East 68th Street, Box 318, New York, NY 10065-4870.
E-mail address: spon@med.cornell.edu

Crit Care Clin 29 (2013) 129–151
http://dx.doi.org/10.1016/j.ccc.2012.11.002
0749-0704/13/$ – see front matter © 2013 Elsevier Inc. All rights reserved.
criticalcare.theclinics.com

QUALITY ANALYSIS AND PERFORMANCE IMPROVEMENT

How quality is defined and measured is at times elusive, and almost always variable (**Table 1**).[1] Although most health environments have in place a systematic method for reporting and reviewing medical errors and disseminating the lessons learned from such analyses, the processes are typically institution-specific and formulated on the needs of a distinct medical environment. The integrity and rigor of such systems are sufficiently different to make a collective assessment of best practice difficult. Nevertheless, we know there is value to acknowledging errors, particularly in real time, and benefit further from designing initiatives to prevent rather than to merely correct similar occurrences. Beyond the formal processes by which medical errors are evaluated, health providers can also benefit from ad hoc debriefing and education, both of which contribute to a unified shared mental model of the goals for care delivery. Together, these initiatives comprise the basis of the quality review process in many pediatric units.

Error Reporting

Recent literature suggests that medical errors are greatly underreported; however, where the culture is perceived as less punitive, self-reporting occurs more frequently.[2] Ideally, reporting of medical errors should be characterized by transparency, consistency, and accuracy, principles that in theory are easily achieved but in reality are difficult to attain. Individuals are reluctant to report errors because they fear retribution, humiliation, or alienation. Failing to do so propagates more mistakes and takes clinicians further from the goals of safe delivery of care.

Even when health care workers strive to provide exemplary care for their patients, there are inevitable system failures that hinder their ability to be at once efficient, and sometimes timely, in their work. Most clinicians working in the pediatric intensive care unit (PICU) can relate to the experience of how a delayed test or procedure for a child can strain a therapeutic relationship with a family or, worse yet, adversely affect the patient's overall care. Yet, consider how often we do (or rather do not) report such

Table 1	
Six aims for health care improvement	
Aims for Health Care Improvement	**Definition**
Safe	Avoid unintentional harm associated with the delivery of health care
Effective	Provide evidence-based health care with observance of best practice balanced with scientific evidence and clinical expertise
Patient-centered	Ensure health care that reflects understanding and awareness of the patient's values, needs and preferences while maintaining compassion and respect
Timely	Minimize delays and waits when possible for those both receiving and providing care to facilitate access to care for patients
Efficient	Avoid waste across all aspects of health care including equipment and personnel resources
Equitable	Provide equal quality and standard of care free from bias related to factors such as gender, race, ethnicity, or socioeconomic status

From Institute of Medicine. Crossing the quality chasm: a new health system for the 21st century. National Academies Press; 2001. Available at: http://www.nap.edu/openbook.php?record_id=10027&page=R1. Accessed September 17, 2012; with permission.

incidents. To many, these situations are a routine part of care; however, when considered and reported as medical errors these "system issues" can both inform and improve clinical practice.[3]

Error-reporting systems have become sophisticated; many are electronic and most allow for retrospective review of data, identification of patterns in types of errors made, and selection of what factors most contribute to the error, that is, human factors or system failures. When used, such tools can help to mitigate the gaps generated by "institutional memory," whereby vague and incomplete recollections of lessons learned from previous events guide initiatives for improvement and move us away from the provision of equitable and effective care. Moreover, when based on reality and fact, remediation for medical errors becomes relevant and sustainable.

Morbidity and Mortality: Review and Analysis

Medical errors will occur: how teams deal with mistakes is what matters most. Despite the efforts to mitigate risk in such susceptible environments, errors do and will occur. No process can be entirely foolproof. When medical mistakes occur, especially in children, several emotions—anger, remorse, disappointment, and mistrust—result among the patient, family, and clinical staff. Errors in care leave the medical team in a position of especial vulnerability and, if not openly addressed, can essentially "paralyze" the subsequent therapeutic relationship with the patient and family. Essential to the successful appraisal of medical mistakes are nonthreatening, secure forums in which providers can openly discuss potential deficiencies in clinical knowledge and understanding that may have contributed to the error; opportunities for experienced providers to discuss clinical alternatives to the choices made when appropriate; and methods of education and training to enhance staff competency and confidence. Punition does not work, and rather serves to isolate team members and precipitate greater errors as a consequence of the atmosphere of fear, uncertainty, and disempowerment that such an approach breeds.

Debriefing and Huddles

Both formal debriefs and ad hoc huddles provide opportunities for informal learning, generation of a shared mental model, and team building.[4] Such elements provide medical teams with the opportunity to evaluate the safety and efficiency of care delivery in an integrated and collaborative way. Unlike formal quality-assurance forums, debriefs often occur in real time, following significant events, and typically include spontaneous and undiluted discussion of key issues, concerns, and patient outcomes. When skillfully moderated, such sessions can provide invaluable insight toward process improvement in that the participants have improved recall of events. Furthermore, the less structured format allows for emotional and nonclinical subject matter to be discussed with greater ease.

Among other disciplines, huddles serve to rally and organize the team; this is no different in medicine. Team huddles in the PICU can be useful for clarifying patient-care objectives, improving workforce morale, and consolidating multiple information sources into a unified plan of care. These "check-ins" can occur at scheduled times or impromptu when specific events prompt their necessity. Both debriefings and huddles help to improve the quality of the delivery of care by adding a measure of (necessary) redundancy and cooperation that underlies patient-centered care.

Postintervention Education

Acknowledging that practice may not make perfect but at least makes better, it is of equal import to consider how to deliver and sustain the lessons learned from quality and performance review. It is known that failures in both provider and system function contribute to medical errors. Although human factors seemingly cannot be modified, enhancing awareness among staff regarding areas of inherent vulnerability, creating modes of redundancy to minimize reliance on human intervention alone, and providing decision-making support are all essential steps in mitigating human error.

While across all aspects of care human factors account for a significant portion of medical errors, system inadequacies can be equally implicated in breakdowns of patient care. System design should therefore account for known risks in performance and implementation and be regularly reevaluated in the context of previous errors, the goals of care delivery, and evidence-based practice. Sustainable modalities that have been used in pediatric settings for performance improvement include Plan-Do-Study-Act and failure modes and effects analysis strategies.[5] Such tools emphasize multidisciplinary collaboration in identifying targeted problems to be addressed by simple, goal-directed initiatives that have measurable outcomes.

Using Quality Analysis to Achieve the Domains of Quality

The process of quality analysis and performance improvement is complex, yet integral to achieving the quality hoped for in the defined domains of our health systems. From the inevitable errors, the lessons learned are invaluable. When grounded with this knowledge and approached with transparency, we are able to provide high-quality patient care.

TEAMWORK AND WORKFLOW

We cannot expect to improve medical outcomes, even in the face of scientific advancement, without a true commitment to the improvement of the function and structure of pediatric medical teams. When asked to identify characteristics of successful teams, even across disciplines, there are several recurring themes. Communication, mutual respect, reliability, cooperation, and creativity are among the qualities that arise most often. Similarly, experience, honesty, patience, and compassion are regarded as necessary attributes of well-performing teams. Cultivating these characteristics requires practice, because although some of these behaviors are innate, if not used they will not develop further. When pediatric teams confront medical illness, they are charged with an exceptional responsibility: to deliver the highest quality of medical care to the patient while balancing the personal and professional challenges such a task can bring. When executed well, however, there is no match for the satisfying and gratifying outcomes that cohesive and productive pediatric teams can bring about.

Why Do Teams Matter?

As already acknowledged, the care of pediatric patients requires special commitment and unique skills. Strong pediatric teams provide a mechanism of support and rejuvenation for their members. The sense of camaraderie and mutual understanding that specialty teams provide for their members is what enables them to survive. Professional teams can also be a source of motivation and self-improvement for their members. By providing a consistent group of individuals with common goals, medical teams serve as a forum for academic enrichment and personal growth. Besides the professional and personal benefits that pediatric teams bring to patients, families, and care providers, their value to health care systems is indisputable. A well-functioning medical team can serve to reduce medical error, increase revenue, improve reputation, and facilitate better health outcomes in almost any medical environment. What distinguishes facilities with strong teams is not their lack of medical errors or inefficiencies; rather, a strong team will promote recognition and acknowledgment of mistakes but also work to devise constructive means of performance improvement. Without organized and efficient teams, health systems become disorganized and unproductive; their performance and reputations suffer. The shared burden of health care is great, but made lesser by the strength of successful medical teams.

Team Composition and Leadership

A well-structured, highly reliable, and functional team has the potential to significantly affect the patient's experience in the PICU. Traditional team structure in the PICU consists of an attending physician, medical trainees such as postgraduate fellows, residents, and students, as well as clinical nurses, pharmacists, respiratory therapists, dieticians, social workers, case managers, and specialty or consultant physicians. In such a team, the attending physician assumes ultimate responsibility for the medical management of the patient while balancing the assessments and opinions of the team at large with his or her experience, expertise, and judgment, to develop a coordinated plan of care for the patient.

Central to the team is the patient and his or her parents and family. Given that no care plan can be executed without the support and consent of patients and parents, patient-centered care remains the clear standard that must be achieved. The value of parents in the care-delivery experience is irrefutable in terms of providing comfort and understanding for their sick children, in the intangible elements of healing they provide, and even in the avoidance of medical errors, given that often no one individual in the medical team can be as attentive to a child's medical needs as a parent. That being said, a careful balance must be achieved to avoid family-centered care from becoming family-dictated care and, perhaps worse, to prevent parents from feeling the burden of having to make medical decisions for their children in areas where they should rather be able to rely on effective medical expertise.

Rounding

A clearly defined shared mental model of care is essential to goal achievement. Foremost among the goals of rounds is the establishment of such a common vision of the key health issues, risks, treatment goals, and plan of care for the patient. As a result of poor system design, workflow interruptions, and unanticipated, but sometimes necessary intrusions, medical team members frequently leave a bedside after making rounds without this unified and clear understanding of the patient.

It is difficult for a pediatric clinical team to achieve its goals without a unified, structured plan of care, often termed a shared mental model. Without such a "road map," individual team members may independently be working toward goals of care without a defined end point or measures of success. Such behaviors place patients at greater risk because the propensity for task duplication and omission increases in the absence of a common goal. The value of shared mental modeling is particularly apparent within the PICU, where the functional efficiency of the office depends on each team member fulfilling his or her role to completion; otherwise, the "downstream" members of the team cannot work at maximum efficiency.

Beyond the clinical team there exists the patient and family. All of these individuals share a common goal: to improve the health of the critically ill patient by providing the highest-quality medical care. The institution of family-centered care and family presence during medical rounds, resuscitation, and procedures in many PICUs provides such opportunities. The direct participation of patients and their families can facilitate understanding, trust, and clarity within the medical team; however, it is not without its challenges. Some team members may feel inhibited by the presence of families; for example, trainees may be reticent to ask questions that may suggest to families that they are insufficiently competent to care for their child. In addition, when there is disagreement among the medical practitioners about the plan of care, long-term outcomes, or disposition, it may be uncomfortable for such discussions to occur in front of parents. Of course, not all members of the team will agree on how to achieve its common goal. It is thereby imperative for the team to have measures in place that promote collaboration and compromise without sacrificing the advancement of medical care for the patient.

What is unique to intensive care unit (ICU) teams is the frequency with which they confront critical illness and the complex, emotional circumstances that the care of acutely ill children raises. For a pediatric clinical team to successfully navigate such issues, it must be prepared to incorporate families directly into its work but also recognize the objective, yet nurturing role it must serve. Pediatric intensive care teams must also devise means for stress release and mutual support because their work is uniquely demanding and psychologically draining. If however, all of these elements function well, pediatric intensive care teams are among the most skilled and proficient at caring for pediatric patients. Optimal team performance in the PICU will be cohesive, yet facilitate a climate in which individual opinions regarding the child's care are readily expressed and valued; where there is a single clearly identified team ultimately responsible for the child's care, despite collaboration with other medical specialists; and in which there is both regard and support for the emotional and professional stresses that uniquely accompany the care of such critically ill children.

Handoffs

Compared with the ICU, few other environments have greater stress, intensity, and propensity for errors. Therefore, handoffs or communications between providers at all phases of care are crucial for accurate, timely, and efficient care delivery.[6] Structured handoffs typically occur during transitions of care, for example, at shift changes, between clinical care units, and when patients are transferred to other sites for care. Less formal handoffs may occur between providers during temporary periods of coverage such as staff breaks or when transient clinical support is needed. Each handoff provides an opportunity for providers to communicate relevant information about the patient and, theoretically, to confirm and validate medical facts about the patient and plan of care.

Unfortunately, the reality is that handoffs are mostly unstandardized, fragmented, and incomplete, so the risk associated with them is high. Factors such as duty-hour limitations, multiple caregivers for individual patients, and unexpected transitions of care result in inefficient handoffs.[7] Partial or sometimes incorrect information may be passed forward across multiple layers of care without recognition, and in the most extreme examples management plans may be based on such information. The goal of handoffs should include transfer of relevant and timely information in a consistent format. The redundancy of such a system would go far in mitigating error and revitalizing the utility of handoff encounters.

Health Care Delivery

Successful teams must strengthen their adaptability and efficiency across clinical situations. Particularly in the pediatric critical care unit, where clinical circumstances change rapidly, teams must remain malleable and competent. Serving patients in the acute setting requires an appreciation of the sadness, anger, frustration, fear, and uncertainty that families often experience with a seriously ill child. Beyond compassion must exist a fundamentally integrative approach to the delivery of patient-centered care.

Patient- and family-centered care represents a practice paradigm designed to involve parents and families more directly in their child's medical care. It is assumed that by providing families with the opportunity to participate directly in their child's care, they will have a more satisfying, cohesive, and safe medical experience. Although this principle holds true in most instances, it can quickly evolve into family-directed care if pediatric practitioners are not careful to maintain the boundaries between practitioner and patient. What may begin as a collaborative, well-intentioned endeavor can degenerate into an antagonistic and uncomfortable practice environment.

When skilled pediatric providers learn to work closely with patients and their families in a mutually rewarding way, the results can be significant. Countless medical errors are averted each year simply by family members who ask for information about medications being administered to their child. Similarly, medical history and information from parents is invaluable, particularly when a patient is unknown to the medical facility and the care team. Families who are engaged with the medical team are typically more satisfied with and less distrusting of the medical experience. Likewise, children thrive in medical environments where their needs are both anticipated and met with the support of their families.

Using Teamwork to Achieve the Domains of Quality

Given the spectrum of unique clinical and environmental circumstances presented, there is no single effort that will completely eliminate the risk of pediatric medical errors; however, high-functioning teams will serve to diminish the risk of errors through several mechanisms. First, teams that are familiar with children have a better understanding of the special clinical considerations that should be observed in the care of children. Such providers are less likely to err simply because of their familiarity and experience with pediatric protocols and specifications.

Teams that work with children must be especially patient, flexible, and understanding not only of the patient but also of parents and families who often are actively involved in their child's care. This process can be demanding for any care provider, but a practiced and efficient team can often derive support and camaraderie through the shared challenges of its practice. As in other work environments, strong teams and leaders can incite energy, passion, and commitment as quickly as they can cultivate frustration, inefficiency, and discord if they are not cohesive and functional. The absolute necessity of dedicated, pediatric specialty care teams in any successful clinical environment that cares for children must be acknowledged and emphasized.

Several models for team composition and structure can be used in pediatric medical settings, but as already emphasized, those models that enable patients, families, and medical personnel to function cooperatively, rather than in parallel, are most likely to succeed. The ideal pediatric medical team model will incorporate the best elements of both vertical and horizontal team dynamics. In vertical teams, there is a defined leader who has primary responsibility for providing the direction, priorities, and goals for the team. The team may create a vision based on a shared mental model; however, the implementation of these goals is often dependent on the leader's initiative and commitment. The team leader is placed in a position of ultimate control for advancing the team's work. By contrast, horizontal-performing teams may also have a team leader; however, the entire team takes ownership for realization of the team's objectives. The team leader does not retain an isolated position of power because hierarchy does not define horizontal teams. Such a team resembles one in which the needs of the pediatric patient is at the core of health care delivery; at various points during the care experience, team members may need to collaborate and compromise to advance the patient's care, but ultimately the medical team bears the responsibility for managing the child's medical needs. In such a system, all participants are invested in success, and there is a means for ensuring accountability in the process, but the roles of the medical providers do not overshadow the value of the contributions of patient and family to the medical care plan.

INFORMATION TECHNOLOGY AND QUALITY

Information technology will rescue health care from inefficiency and waste, and will prevent its practitioners from drowning in an ever-expanding ocean of information and complexity; at least that is the hope of its many proponents. From its 2001 report, *Crossing the Quality Chasm*,[1] to the recently released *Best Care at Lower Cost*,[8] the Institute of Medicine (IOM) documented its faith in information technology in improving quality and efficiency. This conviction helped prompt the federal government to pass the 2009 Health Information Technology for Economic and Clinical Health (HITECH) Act designed to hasten adoption of electronic health records (EHR).[9] There are also technologies beyond EHR that will further improve the quality of care, which include smart pumps, bar codes, telecommunications, and a wide variety of clinical decision-support tools. The possibilities are encouraging.

In the decade between the 2 IOM reports some of the promise has been realized, but much remains to be done. Potential benefits of information technology include providing rapid access to integrated clinical data and extant medical knowledge, eliminating illegibility, improving communication, and issuing applicable reminders and checks for appropriate medical actions, thereby improving adherence to guidelines and decreasing some medical errors.[10] Some of the benefits touted by early research have been criticized for being results of highly customized systems built and designed by a dedicated crew of medical informatics enthusiasts, leaving the remainder of us to struggle with commercial products that may not mesh well with the way we work.[11] Nonetheless, recent data suggest that having an EHR with specific, key functions is associated with high-quality hospitals,[12,13] fewer complications, lower mortality rates, and lower costs.[14]

The benefits of information technologies can be assessed across the 6 domains of quality: that they make health care safe, effective, patient-centered, timely, efficient, and equitable.

Electronic Health Records

EHRs improve efficiency by collating and organizing health information that had previously been scattered on paper, and provide immediate, remote access to information to allow clinicians to better care for patients, particularly those with whom they are not familiar.[8] EHRs can reduce redundant and unnecessary tests and procedures, improve communication among multiple providers about individual patients, and supply data for performance and outcome measures.[15] EHRs can improve safety by potentially increasing the completeness and accuracy of documentation, thus potentially reducing "dropped balls,"[16] and can also improve timeliness through the use of electronic messaging to speed accurate communication among practitioners.[17] This information technology can also enhance patient-centered care that is respectful of and responsive to patient preferences, needs, and values by recording them and appropriately reminding the health care professional.[1]

Trigger-tool methodologies analyze patient records to identify adverse events.[18] For example, the use of naloxone documented in a chart may indicate an opiate overdose. Trigger tools can detect adverse events that might otherwise go unreported. The EHR can be used to automate this process and improve its efficiency.[19] These measurements over time can be used to gauge the success of new safety protocols.

Human factors engineering (HFE) is the multidisciplinary field that studies the interactions between humans and technology. Its principles are increasingly used to help evaluate and refine information technology used in clinical practice. According to these principles, information technology does not directly affect patient safety; it affects the entire system of patient care and only indirectly produces conditions that are safer or more hazardous. Improving safety is contingent on improving the cognitive performance of the health care providers (**Table 2**).[17]

Table 2 Unintended adverse consequences related to CPOE	
Effect	**Examples**
New kinds of errors	Juxtaposition errors in which clinicians mistakenly select an item among a long list of similar items displayed in a small font
	Excessive alerts that interrupt thought processes and result in errors
	Missed doses of phenobarbital or methadone because automatic stop orders are required for controlled substances, a regulation more easily enforced with CPOE
Increased work for clinicians	Requiring physicians to select precise timing schedules for medications, a function formerly performed by nurses
	Prolonged log-in processes or poorly designed interfaces that require complex navigation to commonly used functions
	Loss of notes or orders in progress because of interface crashes or inopportune automatic time-outs and log-offs
Unfavorable alteration of workflow	Medications prepared for patients expected to arrive emergently can no longer be ordered through a CPOE system that requires the patient to be formally admitted to the system
	Computerized orders bypass the nurse who used to "pick up" the order before it was sent to pharmacy and who would know that a medication in pill form could not be administered via a nasogastric tube
Untoward changes in communications patterns	Users assume that the right person will see relevant information just because it went into the system, producing an "illusion of communication"
	Consultants may write a note after seeing a patient but may edit their recommendations after leaving the unit and the primary team may not recognize that the document had been revised
High system demands and frequent changes	Frequent upgrades of hardware and software ensure the system will never be static or stable
	Ongoing changes to the systems require ongoing training to use the new features
Persistence of paper	Increase in paper-towel consumption because it is used as scrap paper to record vital signs to be entered later
Overdependence on technology	Breakdown in the delivery of care as a direct result of EHR downtime
	Overreliance on clinical alerts leading to an erroneous medication order assumed to be correct because no alert was triggered

Abbreviations: CPOE, computerized physician order entry; EHR, electronic health record.
Data from Refs.[20–22]

Besides creating new kinds of errors, there are other unintended consequences that can result from implementing an EHR, including increased work for clinicians, untoward alteration of workflow, changes in communication patterns, increased system demands, persistence of paper use, and potentially fostering overdependence on the technology.[20–22] Information technology has changed the pace of our lives, and the effect is no less apparent in the delivery of health care. It can greatly improve the timeliness of care. The disadvantage of information technology is that it can take over our lives. It has been reported that physicians now spend more time interfacing with the computer than interacting with their colleagues and staff (**Table 3**).[22]

Computerized Physician Order Entry

EHRs with a computerized physician order entry (CPOE) have resulted in documented, significant reductions in the time that it takes to for an order to be written to a medication administered, a radiograph displayed, or a laboratory test to be carried out.[23,24] CPOEs can also rapidly transmit the results of important abnormalities to key clinicians.[25]

Perhaps the greatest benefits to safety offered by information technology lie in CPOE. Numerous studies seem to confirm this benefit, some of which report significant reduction of medication errors,[26,27] and "almost a complete elimination" of medication errors even with commercial products.[28–30] The impact on adverse drug events was less dramatic but still positive.[28–30]

Most of the single-site observational studies cited here suggest a benefit, but many do not distinguish error severity. The minor errors are often reported to decrease the most.[31] Other studies are even less positive, showing either little benefit[16,32] or an unexpected increase in mortality.[33] Although the ultimate conclusions of many studies seem to depend more on the author than on the specific aspects of information technology being studied,[25–27,32,34–36] the discrepant results point to the possibility that the specifics of the implementation process could be a decisive factor that determines success or failure.[30]

Other investigators point out that although electronic prescribing can reduce certain types of medication errors, it can increase the rates of other errors and can also facilitate new types of errors.[34,37,38] Transcription errors are the most commonly cited errors that are eliminated by CPOE.[23] There are reports of increases in the rate of duplicate orders or failure to discontinue medications because of problems with the human interface.[31] Other errors include orders that are written in the open chart of one patient being mistaken for that of another. New types of errors include

Table 3 Ways in which an EHR might affect cognitive performance	
Improve	**Reduce**
Improve legibility and accessibility	Decrease efficiency with poorly designed interfaces, and slow start-up and log-in processes
Increase availability of problem lists or allergy lists that were often lost in the paper record	
Improve completeness of documentation	Bury relevant data among the irrelevant
Reduce delays in receiving results of diagnostic tests	Encourage excessively long notes with copy-and-paste functions
Automatically collate and sort relevant data	Encourage documentation without cognition with automatic data dumps into notes
Reduce fragmentation of the medical record	
Automatically flag abnormal results	Increase work by introducing additional steps that were previously performed by others
Increase availability of references	Increase confusion with distracting alerts

"juxtaposition errors" whereby clinicians intending to select one item select a different but nearby item within a long, dense pick-list displayed in a small font. Inflexible data input can result in misinterpretation of orders because important data can be misplaced or not found. Other aspects of the EHR can contribute to creating other kinds of new errors. Fragmentation of data displays can prevent coherent views of information or might induce physicians to write duplicate orders if the original order is not visible. Interface issues can lead to the misdirection of data to the wrong patient's chart. Transfers of the patient that are not coordinated with the electronic transfer of the chart may result in missed care or care delivered to the wrong patient.[15]

Electronic Medication Administration Record

Implementation of an electronic medication administration record (eMAR) with CPOE improves effectiveness, measuring quality by 11 CMS quality indicators related to medication use that adheres to specific guidelines for acute myocardial infarction, heart failure, pneumonia, and surgical infection prophylaxis. In addition, the duration these technologies have been in use is also correlated with improved quality by these measures.[39]

Decision Support

Decision support is an innovation designed to improve the cognitive performance of practitioners. For example, an automated alert system can warn clinicians of dangerous drug-drug interactions. Safety improvements secondary to CPOE systems are extended with the development and implementation of integrated clinical decision-support systems.[27,40]

Decision-support systems can also help clinicians make better choices of medications[25,41] or laboratory tests,[23,25] and thereby reduce costs.[25] Clinical decision support designed to affect specific aspects of care such as adherence to clinical guidelines for specific diseases,[42] administration of preventive care,[43] or optimizing drug ordering[41,43] have been shown to improve quality and sometimes reduce costs, but few studies show any benefit on patient outcomes.[43] Use of automated reminders based on clinical practice guidelines, computer-assisted diagnosis or management, and evidence-based medicine can improve the effectiveness of medical care.[15]

Implementations of clinical decision support can make care more patient-centered by providing interactive patient-specific guidelines or protocols at the bedside,[44–46] and by tailoring information and disease-management messages to both the patient and physician based on the patient's individual needs.[15]

Although our understanding of the complex interactions of clinical decision-support systems is limited, they seem most effective when reminders are generated automatically rather than by requiring users to ask for advice.[47] Systems that advise users about existing therapies by adjusting the dose or by recommending laboratory testing seem to be particularly effective.[47] Nonetheless, the safety benefits of these tools are not always clear,[31] and at least one study reports that the majority of providers prefer that the drug-interaction alerts be turned off to reduce "alert overload."[48]

A recent survey of commercially available EHRs revealed that not all had the full range of clinical decision-support tools,[49] and careful evaluation of these tools should play a role in deciding which product to purchase and implement.

Barcode Medication Administration

Converging technologies are those positioned between health information technology and medical devices. These technologies include barcode medication administration (BCMA) systems integrated into the eMAR,[50] and were developed to enhance safety.

Although BCMA has been reported to reduce time spent by nurses on medication administration,[51] the benefits of this and other similar technologies can be undermined by workarounds that nurses might develop to save time (paradoxically) or to counter other unintended consequences of altered workflows.[52]

Health Information Exchange

Health information exchange (HIE) allows for sharing of health care information electronically across organizations, and is a specific implementation of interoperability, the ability of systems to work with one another. Formal organizations (governmental or independent) or partnerships (public and private) are emerging to allow for HIE. The 2009 HITECH legislation provided for grants designed to develop Regional Health Information Organizations.[8] The potential benefits of these exchanges include increasing the availability of data on patients who have care delivered by different organizations. Through these exchanges an emergency department can access data from the outpatient health records from the numerous specialists who follow a patient with a complicated medical history, and a rehabilitation facility can access data from a patient's recent hospitalization. There is some evidence that HIE can reduce diagnostic imaging and improve adherence to evidence-based guidelines.[53]

Telemedicine

Telemedicine can improve the timeliness of care. For patients who live in remote locales, it can allow patients to see a consultant without long-distance travel, or even allow pediatric patients to safely receive care in a local adult ICU if they cannot be safely transported to a distant PICU.[54,55] It is also possible for intensivists to remotely monitor patients and participate in emergency care without any delay even if the physician is not on site.[56,57] These solutions have been implemented by fixed cameras and electronic connections in patient rooms, and by mobile robots that can roam from bedside to bedside; they can also be inexpensively implemented by staff members armed with a smartphone or a mobile computer configured with a webcam and wireless connection.

Enhancing equity among patients and across socioeconomic, geographic, race, and ethnic lines can be achieved with communication technologies that can enhance access to clinicians and clinical knowledge. Such improvements depend less on the availability of the health care resources and more on the technology infrastructure.[15,46,58]

Teleconsultations have been shown to reduce the number of diagnostic tests and medical interventions, reduce the number of contacts with the health care system, and improve patient satisfaction, all while saving patients' time and money.[59]

In at least one PICU with an expansive catchment area whose families might live at great distances from the hospital, Web-based communication is made available to patients and their families. This tool allows parents to give access to other family members, friends, and the referring physician, and provides a means of communication between these users and the PICU staff. Although not quite the same as in-person presence, the families reported that this service helped to empower the families during a most difficult time.[60]

The Internet

The Internet gives clinicians ready access to the medical literature[1] including recent studies and current guidelines. It also give patients access to clinical knowledge through a multitude of Web sites, some reliable and understandable, others not.[61] In 2006, 30% of surveyed health professionals reported that 80% of their patients were

Web informed, and 63% of professionals recommended a Web site to their patients for more information.[62] These numbers are most certainly higher now. The Internet can also allow access to online support groups that can reduce the feelings of isolation and can direct patients to resources, of which they would otherwise be unaware.[61]

The Internet can also afford patients access to consumer information on health plans, participating providers, eligibility for procedures, and covered drugs in a formulary.[8,63] Information regarding cost, outcomes, and value associated with hospitals, practices, or individual physicians may be collected and made available through information technology. Access to practical, usable, and transparent information could help improve the value of care as patients approach health care as consumers.[64]

The increasingly frustrated consumer of health care uses the Internet to acquire information to manage his or her own health. Purveyors of electronic health are providing health information, decision support, and Web-based tools to navigate the health care system and insurance plans while perhaps influencing patterns of health care consumption.[63]

Spurred by the HITECH legislation, the development of patient portals gives patients unprecedented access to their medical records. Clinicians consider valuable the patient's ability to review and comment on data in his or her EHR, as it may increase accuracy of that data.[65] For many of these portals, a delay is imposed between test results and release of such data to allow the patient's physician time to review the results and contact the patient to discuss the meaning of those results. Although intended to limit the panic that some patients may experience when the implications of certain results are initially unclear, many programs are reducing this imposed delay, perhaps encouraging physicians to address those results in an even timelier fashion.

Through patient portals connected to their EHRs, patients can communicate with their physician, obtain medical advice, or receive customized information on health education and disease management.[63] These portals can decrease the number of office visits or telephone contacts, readily allow for changes in the medication regimens, and improve adherence to treatment.[66] At least one health care system implemented electronic visits through these portals to substitute for some types of office visits.[67] Personal health records, whether they are independently managed by patients themselves or hosted by insurance companies or the health care systems to which they belong, are empowering patients to control their health information, although there may be some serious concerns over privacy and security.[68]

For those who consider information technology to be a panacea, the Joint Commission issued this warning:

The overall safety and effectiveness of technology in health care ultimately depend on its human users, ideally working in close concert with properly designed and installed electronic systems. Any form of technology may adversely affect the quality and safety of care if it is designed or implemented improperly or is misinterpreted. Not only must the technology or device be designed to be safe, it must also be operated safely within a safe workflow process.[69]

PROTOCOLS

Medicine is faced with many challenges, but the most pressing issue for the system as a whole is the quality of health care. Quality is threatened by the unbridled escalations in health care costs, particularly when those costs do not buy improved outcomes. The explosive pace of the accumulation of medical knowledge has made medical care overwhelmingly complex. Paradoxically, the health care system is slow to gather evidence directly applicable to clinicians and their patients, and even when such evidence exists, the system is slow to incorporate that evidence into practice.[8] These challenges may be even more acute in critical care. Delivering care is increasingly demanding in the ICU, where patients are monitored and supported by devices of increasing number and complexity, and treated with great numbers of medications from a bloated formulary. The expanding therapeutic armamentarium often succeeds in supporting patients who are more ill and more complicated than ever before, and these factors are among the many that contribute to the rising costs of health care.[70,71]

For these and many other reasons, more if not most of medical care should be protocolized. The idea of protocolized care is not new. For example, clinicians have been using protocols to manage cardiopulmonary arrest for decades. Protocolizing this high-acuity, high-stakes treatment has allowed several things to occur. At the most basic level it allows for knowledge, from expert opinion to cutting-edge research, to be transferred to the patient's bedside with relative efficiency. Cadres of medical professionals and lay persons are regularly trained and retrained in resuscitation, ensuring, to the extent reasonably possible, that patients receive the best care even as they lie on the threshold of death. Furthermore, protocolization allows all members of the team caring for the patient to understand their role when it is assigned. Besides improving the efficiency of care, the shared mental model of the team facilitates ready detection of protocol deviations and, thus, application of corrections. Protocolized care also allows outcomes to be measured and compared more consistently. Changes in protocol can be compared with older protocols and medical knowledge can be advanced, even outside formal clinical trials and within the process of routine care. The routine reevaluation of these cardiopulmonary resuscitation protocols also helps identify areas where additional and perhaps more rigorous research is required.

More recently, some sustained success has been gained with improved outcomes by protocolizing the treatment of early septic shock.[72–74] Development and implementation of an evidence-based protocol or "care process model" for febrile infants younger than 90 days of age was shown to decrease practice variation, improve outcomes, and decrease costs.[75] However, the broad transfer of knowledge to clinical practice is a significant challenge, with multiple barriers in knowledge, attitude, and behaviors.[76]

Guidelines or Protocols

The National Guideline Clearinghouse[77] has more than 3000 guidelines from nearly 300 organizations.[64] Some of these guidelines are redundant but also contradictory. There is clearly a need for a trusted means to reconcile the differences and to channel these guidelines into effective use.[64] Furthermore, many guidelines may be flawed because they are inadequately explicit. Adequately explicit protocols contain sufficient detail to lead different clinicians to the same decision when faced with the same clinical scenario.[78] Evidence-based care process models are protocols that are designed to decrease variation, improve quality, and support local preferences.[75,79]

Objections

Although some protocols are fairly well accepted, many physicians would balk at the idea of protocolizing most aspects of care. Many objections concern the threat this would pose to the role of the physician and the need to preserve physician judgment. Some of these concerns are justified, because the clinician must determine whether the protocol truly applies to his or her specific patient. The protocol may be based on a study performed on a very specific study sample, and therefore has insufficient external validity to address the patient at hand. Tight glycemic control may have a significant mortality benefit for adult surgical patients but may not be beneficial to pediatric medical patients. However, the most common reason for rejecting a validated protocol instruction that the clinician opinion expressed is not based on fact, and that physicians are usually overconfident in the correctness of their beliefs and opinions.[78]

The other objections to protocolized care relate to the apparent rigidity in comparison with the inherently flexible physician judgment.[78] Clearly some protocols can be excessively rigid, and this can become unacceptable if a "practice misalignment" occurs whereby the protocol calls for a treatment that is contrary to "usual care."[80] However, protocols need not be excessively rigid. Protocols should be able to account for a broad range of patients' conditions. The key is to allow the treatment to vary based on patient variability rather than on physician variability. If the patient veers into territory not mapped out in the protocol, the care of that patient must be allowed to deviate, and this deviation can be used to modify the protocol so that it can cover more territory.

Practice Variation

One goal of protocolizing care is to reduce practice variation. Unexplained practice variation is associated with significant variations in the cost of medical care, but higher costs are not associated with higher-quality care or better outcomes.[81–87] It is presumed that decreasing practice variation will result in an overall lower cost of health care without compromising other measures of quality. Although this may not necessarily be true in every case, it is hoped that the incremental increase in cost would purchase better outcomes.

Research Benefits

Other reasons for protocolizing care are related to clinical research. Despite all the clinical research in critical care medicine, very few randomized, multicenter studies have shown durable benefits in mortality reduction.[88] Protocolization of care outside of study interventions can decrease the "noise" generated by unnecessary practice variation, making clinical studies more likely to detect the "signal" resulting from the study intervention. Protocolization of care can also enhance the validity of randomized trials in contradistinction to those whereby a study intervention is compared with a control arm of usual care,[89,90] although it is important to avoid "practice misalignments."[80] Certainly such studies would have greater power than those with a third arm consisting of usual care, as has been suggested.[90] Research in most domains of pediatric critical care can little afford such loss of power, given the already small numbers available for study.

Unfortunately, despite the great strides in the practice of evidence-based medicine, the vast majority of care delivered in state-of-the-art ICUs has little or no evidence to support it.[88] Even the things we think we know today will be overthrown tomorrow. Certainly there are too few effectiveness data to verify the external validity of the positive studies that have been conducted. It may be that we are reaching the limits of the randomized controlled trial design, and that we may need to use different research paradigms, particularly in the ICU.[91] In the absence of evidence it does not matter which expert opinion is chosen as the standard, but simply standardizing to one specific practice may yield significant benefits.

Consider the advances in the treatment of childhood cancer. In the span of 40 years, 5-year survival rates are approaching 80%, improved from a baseline of almost uniform fatality.[92] This progress is likely a result of protocolized care and enrollment of most patients in those study protocols with meticulous data collection and analysis.

This research paradigm may be used to further medicine in general, and specifically pediatric critical care, otherwise known as "critical care for rare diseases."[93]

The Future

One vision for the future is to have standard protocols of care in PICUs where information technology is deployed with sufficient interoperability to allow data sharing. As data are captured at the time care is rendered, novel interventions for rare diseases can be assessed across institutions with the noise of unnecessary practice variation damped to extinction. The Pediatric Acute Lung Injury and Sepsis Investigators,[94] the clinical research network for pediatric critical care, has recently embraced the idea of protocolizing "routine" care. The Laura P. and Leland K. Whittier Virtual Pediatric Intensive Care Unit[95] has been working to improve the interoperability of data among PICUs. The path to the future is being mapped. The hard work is yet to come.

SUMMARY

There is no question that we can do better to improve the quality of care delivered to patients. This article reviews the domains of quality outlined by the IOM; examines the current theories and practice of quality assessment, performance improvement, teamwork, and workflow; reviews the promise and current impact of information technologies on the quality of care; and outlines a possible shifting paradigm for the delivery of care and knowledge discovery based on protocols. Although advances exist in the frameworks used to promote quality, with some resulting improvement in outcomes, achieving quality is an elusive goal that requires ceaseless attention and relentless effort.

REFERENCES

1. Institute of Medicine. Crossing the quality chasm: a new health system for the 21st century. National Academies Press; 2001. Available at: http://www.nap.edu/openbook.php?record_id=10027&page=R1. Accessed September 17, 2012.
2. Linthorst GE, Kallimanis-King BL, Douwes Dekker I, et al. What contributes to internists' willingness to disclose medical errors? Neth J Med 2012;70(5):242–8.
3. Chamberlain CJ, Koniaris LG. Disclosure of "nonharmful" medical errors and other events: duty to disclose. Arch Surg 2012;147(3):282–6.
4. de Feijter J, de Grave W, Koopmans R, et al. Informal learning from error in hospitals: what do we learn, how do we learn and how can informal learning be enhanced? A narrative review. Adv Health Sci Educ Theory Pract 2012;17:1–19.
5. Schriefer J, Leonard MS. Patient safety and quality improvement an overview of QI. Pediatr Rev 2012;33(8):353–60.
6. Chen JG, Wright MC, Smith PB, et al. Adaptation of a post-operative handoff communication process for children with heart disease: a quantitative study. Am J Med Qual 2011;26(5):380–6.
7. DeRienzo CM, Frush K, Barfield ME, et al. Handoffs in the era of duty hours reform: a focused review and strategy to address changes in the Accreditation Council for Graduate Medical Education Common Program Requirements. Acad Med 2012;87(4):403–10.
8. Institute of Medicine. Best care at lower cost: the path to continuously learning health care in America. The National Academies Press; 2012. Available at: http://www.nap.edu/openbook.php?record_id=13444. Accessed September 18, 2012.
9. Blumenthal D. Stimulating the adoption of health information technology. N Engl J Med 2009;360(15):1477–9.

10. Dick RS, Steen EB, Detmer DE, Committee on Improving the Patient Record I of M. The computer-based patient record: an essential technology for health care. Revised edition. Washington, DC: The National Academies Press; 1997.
11. Bitton A, Flier LA, Jha AK. Health information technology in the era of care delivery reform: to what end? JAMA 2012;307(24):2593–4.
12. Elnahal SM, Joynt KE, Bristol SJ, et al. Electronic health record functions differ between best and worst hospitals. Am J Manag Care 2011;17(4): e121–47.
13. Restuccia JD, Cohen AB, Horwitt JN, et al. Hospital implementation of health information technology and quality of care: are they related? BMC Med Inform Decis Mak 2012;12(1):109.
14. Amarasingham R, Plantinga L, Diener-West M, et al. Clinical information technologies and inpatient outcomes: a multiple hospital study. Arch Intern Med 2009; 169(2):108–14.
15. Pon S, Markovitz B, Weigle C, et al. Information technology in critical care. In: Fuhrman BP, Zimmerman JJ, editors. Pediatric critical care: expert consult premium. 4th edition. Philadelphia: Elsevier; 2011. p. 75–91.
16. Weir CR, Staggers N, Phansalkar S. The state of the evidence for computerized provider order entry: a systematic review and analysis of the quality of the literature. Int J Med Inform 2009;78(6):365–74.
17. Holden RJ. Cognitive performance-altering effects of electronic medical records: an application of the human factors paradigm for patient safety. Cogn Technol Work 2011;13(1):11–29.
18. Naessens JM, O'Byrne TJ, Johnson MG, et al. Measuring hospital adverse events: assessing inter-rater reliability and trigger performance of the Global Trigger Tool. Int J Qual Health Care 2010;22(4):266–74.
19. Doupi P. Using EHR data for monitoring and promoting patient safety: reviewing the evidence on trigger tools. Stud Health Technol Inform 2012;180: 786–90.
20. Ash JS, Sittig DF, Dykstra R, et al. The unintended consequences of computerized provider order entry: findings from a mixed methods exploration. Int J Med Inform 2009;78:S69–76.
21. Ash JS, Berg M, Coiera E. Some unintended consequences of information technology in health care: the nature of patient care information system-related errors. J Am Med Inform Assoc 2004;11(2):104–12.
22. Ash JS, Sittig DF, Dykstra RH, et al. Categorizing the unintended sociotechnical consequences of computerized provider order entry. Int J Med Inform 2007; 76(Suppl 1):S21–7.
23. Mekhjian HS, Kumar RR, Kuehn L, et al. Immediate benefits realized following implementation of physician order entry at an academic medical center. J Am Med Inform Assoc 2002;9(5):529–39.
24. Niazkhani Z, Pirnejad H, Berg M, et al. The impact of computerized provider order entry systems on inpatient clinical workflow: a literature review. J Am Med Inform Assoc 2009;16(4):539–49.
25. Bates DW, Pappius EM, Kuperman GJ, et al. Measuring and improving quality using information systems. Stud Health Technol Inform 1998;52(Pt 2):814–8.
26. Bates DW, Leape LL, Cullen DJ, et al. Effect of computerized physician order entry and a team intervention on prevention of serious medication errors. JAMA 1998;280(15):1311–6.
27. Bates DW, Teich JM, Lee J, et al. The impact of computerized physician order entry on medication error prevention. J Am Med Inform Assoc 1999;6(4):313–21.

28. King WJ, Paice N, Rangrej J, et al. The effect of computerized physician order entry on medication errors and adverse drug events in pediatric inpatients. Pediatrics 2003;112(3 Pt 1):506–9.

29. Potts AL, Barr FE, Gregory DF, et al. Computerized physician order entry and medication errors in a pediatric critical care unit. Pediatrics 2004;113(1 Pt 1): 59–63.

30. van Rosse F, Maat B, Rademaker CM, et al. The effect of computerized physician order entry on medication prescription errors and clinical outcome in pediatric and intensive care: a systematic review. Pediatrics 2009;123(4):1184–90.

31. Reckmann MH, Westbrook JI, Koh Y, et al. Does computerized provider order entry reduce prescribing errors for hospital inpatients? A systematic review. J Am Med Inform Assoc 2009;16(5):613–23.

32. Walsh KE, Landrigan CP, Adams WG, et al. Effect of computer order entry on prevention of serious medication errors in hospitalized children. Pediatrics 2008;121(3):e421–7.

33. Han YY, Carcillo JA, Venkataraman ST, et al. Unexpected increased mortality after implementation of a commercially sold computerized physician order entry system. Pediatrics 2005;116(6):1506–12.

34. Walsh KE, Adams WG, Bauchner H, et al. Medication errors related to computerized order entry for children. Pediatrics 2006;118(5):1872–9.

35. Karsh BT, Weinger MB, Abbott PA, et al. Health information technology: fallacies and sober realities. J Am Med Inform Assoc 2010;17(6):617–23.

36. Karsh BT, Holden RJ, Alper SJ, et al. A human factors engineering paradigm for patient safety: designing to support the performance of the healthcare professional. Qual Saf Health Care 2006;15(Suppl 1):i59–65.

37. Koppel R, Metlay JP, Cohen A, et al. Role of computerized physician order entry systems in facilitating medication errors. JAMA 2005;293(10):1197–203.

38. Turchin A, Shubina M, Goldberg S. Unexpected effects of unintended consequences: EMR prescription discrepancies and hemorrhage in patients on warfarin. AMIA Annu Symp Proc 2011;2011:1412–7.

39. Appari A, Carian EK, Johnson ME, et al. Medication administration quality and health information technology: a national study of US hospitals. J Am Med Inform Assoc 2012;19(3):360–7.

40. Kaushal R, Shojania KG, Bates DW. Effects of computerized physician order entry and clinical decision support systems on medication safety: a systematic review. Arch Intern Med 2003;163(12):1409–16.

41. Evans RS, Pestotnik SL, Classen DC, et al. A computer-assisted management program for antibiotics and other antiinfective agents. N Engl J Med 1998; 338(4):232–8.

42. Durieux P, Nizard R, Ravaud P, et al. A clinical decision support system for prevention of venous thromboembolism: effect on physician behavior. JAMA 2000;283(21):2816–21.

43. Jaspers MW, Smeulers M, Vermeulen H, et al. Effects of clinical decision-support systems on practitioner performance and patient outcomes: a synthesis of high-quality systematic review findings. J Am Med Inform Assoc 2011;18(3):327–34.

44. Blagev DP, Hirshberg EL, Sward K, et al. The evolution of eProtocols that enable reproducible clinical research and care methods. J Clin Monit Comput 2012; 26(4):305–17.

45. Garibaldi RA. Computers and the quality of care—a clinician's perspective. N Engl J Med 1998;338(4):259–60.

46. Vincent JL, Singer M, Marini JJ, et al. Thirty years of critical care medicine. Crit Care 2010;14(3):311.

47. Pearson SA, Moxey A, Robertson J, et al. Do computerised clinical decision support systems for prescribing change practice? A systematic review of the literature (1990-2007). BMC Health Serv Res 2009;9:154.

48. van der Sijs H, Aarts J, van Gelder T, et al. Turning off frequently overridden drug alerts: limited opportunities for doing it safely. J Am Med Inform Assoc 2008; 15(4):439–48.

49. Wright A, Sittig DF, Ash JS, et al. Clinical decision support capabilities of commercially-available clinical information systems. J Am Med Inform Assoc 2009;16(5):637–44.

50. Poon EG, Keohane CA, Yoon CS, et al. Effect of bar-code technology on the safety of medication administration. N Engl J Med 2010;362(18):1698–707.

51. Dwibedi N, Sansgiry SS, Frost CP, et al. Effect of bar-code-assisted medication administration on nurses' activities in an intensive care unit: a time-motion study. Am J Health Syst Pharm 2011;68(11):1026–31.

52. Wulff K, Cummings GG, Marck P, et al. Medication administration technologies and patient safety: a mixed-method systematic review. J Adv Nurs 2011; 67(10):2080–95.

53. Bailey JE, Wan JY, Mabry LM, et al. Does health information exchange reduce unnecessary neuroimaging and improve quality of headache care in the Emergency Department? J Gen Intern Med 2012. Available at: http://www.ncbi.nlm. nih.gov/pubmed/22648609. Accessed September 21, 2012.

54. Marcin JP, Nesbitt TS, Kallas HJ, et al. Use of telemedicine to provide pediatric critical care inpatient consultations to underserved rural Northern California. J Pediatr 2004;144(3):375–80.

55. Marcin JP, Schepps DE, Page KA, et al. The use of telemedicine to provide pediatric critical care consultations to pediatric trauma patients admitted to a remote trauma intensive care unit: a preliminary report. Pediatr Crit Care Med 2004;5(3):251–6.

56. Rosenfeld BA, Dorman T, Breslow MJ, et al. Intensive care unit telemedicine: alternate paradigm for providing continuous intensivist care. Crit Care Med 2000;28(12):3925–31.

57. Wetzel RC. Telemedicine and intensive care: are we ready and willing? J Intensive Care Med 2004;19(2):117–8.

58. Science Panel on Interactive Communication and Health, Eng TR, Gustafson DH. Wired for health and well-being: the emergence of interactive health communication. Washington, DC: U.S. Department of Health and Human Services, U.S. Government Printing Office; 1999.

59. Wallace P, Barber J, Clayton W, et al. Virtual outreach: a randomised controlled trial and economic evaluation of joint teleconferenced medical consultations. Health Technol Assess 2004;8(50):1–106, iii–iv.

60. Braner DA, Lai S, Hodo R, et al. Interactive Web sites for families and physicians of pediatric intensive care unit patients: a preliminary report. Pediatr Crit Care Med 2004;5(5):434–9.

61. Cain MM, Sarasohn-Kahn J, Wayne JC. Health e-people: the online consumer experience. California HealthCare Foundation; 2000. Available at: http://www.chcf.org/ publications/2000/08/health-epeople-the-online-consumer-experience. Accessed September 20, 2012.

62. Podichetty VK, Booher J, Whitfield M, et al. Assessment of internet use and effects among healthcare professionals: a cross sectional survey. Postgrad Med J 2006;82(966):274–9.

63. Goldsmith J. The Internet and managed care: a new wave of innovation. Health Aff (Millwood) 2000;19(6):42–56.
64. Young PL, Olsen L. Roundtable on evidence-based medicine, institute of medicine. The healthcare imperative: lowering costs and improving outcomes: workshop series summary. The National Academies Press; 2010. Available at: http://www.nap.edu/openbook.php?record_id=12750. Accessed September 19, 2012.
65. Siteman E, Businger A, Gandhi T, et al. Clinicians recognize value of patient review of their electronic health record data. AMIA Annu Symp Proc 2006;2006:1101.
66. Ammenwerth E, Schnell-Inderst P, Hoerbst A. Patient empowerment by electronic health records: first results of a systematic review on the benefit of patient portals. Stud Health Technol Inform 2011;165:63–7.
67. Walters B, Barnard D, Paris S. Patient portals and e-visits. J Ambul Care Manage 2006;29(3):222–4.
68. Paton C, Hansen M, Fernandez-Luque L, et al. Self-tracking, social media and personal health records for patient empowered self-care. Contribution of the IMIA Social Media Working Group. Yearb Med Inform 2012;7(1):16–24.
69. The Joint Commission. Sentinel Event Alert, Issue 42: Safely implementing health information and converging technologies. 2008. Available at: http://www.jointcommission.org/sentinel_event_alert_issue_42_safely_implementing_health_information_and_converging_technologies/. Accessed September 16, 2012.
70. Wunsch H, Gershengorn H, Scales DC. Economics of ICU organization and management. Crit Care Clin 2012;28(1):25–37.
71. Dorman T, Pauldine R. Economic stress and misaligned incentives in critical care medicine in the United States. Crit Care Med 2007;35(Suppl 2):S36–43.
72. Rivers E, Nguyen B, Havstad S, et al. Early goal-directed therapy in the treatment of severe sepsis and septic shock. N Engl J Med 2001;345(19):1368–77.
73. Dellinger RP, Levy MM, Carlet JM, et al. Surviving Sepsis Campaign: international guidelines for management of severe sepsis and septic shock: 2008. Crit Care Med 2008;36(1):296–327.
74. Puskarich MA, Marchick MR, Kline JA, et al. One year mortality of patients treated with an emergency department based early goal directed therapy protocol for severe sepsis and septic shock: a before and after study. Crit Care 2009;13(5):R167.
75. Byington CL, Reynolds CC, Korgenski K, et al. Costs and infant outcomes after implementation of a care process model for febrile infants. Pediatrics 2012;130(1):e16–24.
76. Kahn JM. Disseminating clinical trial results in critical care. Crit Care Med 2009;37(Suppl 1):S147–53.
77. Agency for Healthcare Research and Quality. National guideline clearinghouse. Available at: http://guideline.gov. Accessed October 19, 2012.
78. Morris AH. Treatment algorithms and protocolized care. Curr Opin Crit Care 2003;9(3):236–40.
79. May C, Finch T, Mair F, et al. Understanding the implementation of complex interventions in health care: the normalization process model. BMC Health Serv Res 2007;7(1):148.
80. Takala J. Better conduct of clinical trials: the control group in critical care trials. Crit Care Med 2009;37(Suppl 1):S80–90.
81. Willson DF, Horn SD, Hendley JO, et al. Effect of practice variation on resource utilization in infants hospitalized for viral lower respiratory illness. Pediatrics 2001;108(4):851–5.

82. Pham C, Caffrey O, Karnon J, et al. Evaluating the effects of variation in clinical practice: a risk adjusted cost-effectiveness (RAC-E) analysis of acute stroke services. BMC Health Serv Res 2012;12(1):266.

83. Keating NL, Landrum MB, Lamont EB, et al. Area-level variations in cancer care and outcomes. Med Care 2012;50(5):366–73.

84. Zuckerman S, Waidmann T, Berenson R, et al. Clarifying sources of geographic differences in Medicare spending. N Engl J Med 2010;363(1):54–62.

85. Song Y, Skinner J, Bynum J, et al. Regional variations in diagnostic practices. N Engl J Med 2010;363(1):45–53.

86. Mercuri M, Gafni A. Medical practice variations: what the literature tells us (or does not) about what are warranted and unwarranted variations. J Eval Clin Pract 2011;17(4):671–7.

87. Long MJ. An explanatory model of medical practice variation: a physician resource demand perspective. J Eval Clin Pract 2002;8(2):167–74.

88. Ospina-Tascón GA, Büchele GL, Vincent JL. Multicenter, randomized, controlled trials evaluating mortality in intensive care: doomed to fail? Crit Care Med 2008; 36(4):1311–22.

89. Thompson BT, Schoenfeld D. Usual care as the control group in clinical trials of nonpharmacologic interventions. Proc Am Thorac Soc 2007;4(7):577–82.

90. Silverman HJ, Miller FG. Control group selection in critical care randomized controlled trials evaluating interventional strategies: an ethical assessment. Crit Care Med 2004;32(3):852–7.

91. Vincent JL. We should abandon randomized controlled trials in the intensive care unit. Crit Care Med 2010;38:S534–8.

92. Robison LL, Armstrong GT, Boice JD, et al. The Childhood Cancer Survivor study: a National Cancer Institute-supported resource for outcome and intervention research. J Clin Oncol 2009;27(14):2308–18.

93. Fackler JC, Wetzel RC. Critical care for rare diseases. Pediatr Crit Care Med 2002;3(1):89–90.

94. Pediatric Acute Lung Injury and Sepsis Investigators. PALISI. 2011. Available at: http://www.palisi.org. Accessed October 21, 2012.

95. Virtual Pediatric Intensive Care Unit. VPICU. Available at: http://vpicu.org/. Accessed October 21, 2012.

SUGGESTED READINGS

Anon. Health care spending in the United states & Selected OECD Countries. Kaiser Family Foundation 2011; Available at: http://www.kff.org/insurance/snapshot/oecd042111.cfm. Accessed September 17, 2012.

Backes CH, Reber KM, Trittmann JK, et al. Fellows as teachers: a model to enhance pediatric resident education. Med Educ Online 2011;16. Available at: http://www.ncbi.nlm.nih.gov/pmc/articles/PMC3169169/. Accessed September 26, 2012.

Chamberlain CJ, Koniaris LG. Disclosure of "nonharmful" medical errors and other events: duty to disclose. Arch Surg 2012;147(3):282–6.

Chen JG, Wright MC, Smith PB, et al. Adaptation of a post-operative handoff communication process for children with heart disease: a quantitative study. Am J Med Qual 2011;26(5):380–6.

Cypress BS. Family presence on rounds. Dimens Crit Care Nurs 2012;31(1):53–64.

de Feijter J, de Grave W, Koopmans R, et al. Informal learning from error in hospitals: what do we learn, how do we learn and how can informal learning be enhanced? A narrative review. Adv Health Sci Educ Theory Pract 2012;1–19.

Dentzer S. Still crossing the quality chasm—or suspended over it? Health Aff (Mill-wood) 2011;30(4):554–5.

Doherty C, Mc Donnell C. Tenfold medication errors: 5 years' experience at a university-affiliated pediatric hospital. Pediatrics 2012;129(5):916–24.

Donn S, McDonnell W. When bad things happen: adverse event reporting and disclosure as patient safety and risk management tools in the neonatal intensive care unit. Am J Perinatol 2011;29(01):65–70.

Duncan EM, Francis JJ, Johnston M, et al. Learning curves, taking instructions, and patient safety: using a theoretical domains framework in an interview study to investigate prescribing errors among trainee doctors. Implement Sci 2012; 7(1):86.

Eggly S, Meert KL. Parental inclusion in pediatric intensive care rounds: how does it fit with patient- and family-centered care? Pediatr Crit Care Med 2011;12(6):684–5.

Homer CJ, Kleinman LC, Goldman DA. Improving the quality of care for children in health systems. Health Serv Res 1998;33(4 Pt 2):1091–109.

Institute of Medicine. Best care at lower cost: the path to continuously learning health care in America. The National Academies Press; 2012. Available at: http://www.nap.edu/openbook.php?record_id=13444. Accessed September 18, 2012.

Institute of Medicine. Crossing the quality chasm: a new health system for the 21st Century. National Academies Press; 2001. Available at: http://www.nap.edu/openbook.php?record_id=10027&page=R1. Accessed September 18, 2012.

Implementation Science. Learning curves, taking instructions, and patient safety: using a theoretical domains framework in an interview study to investigate prescribing errors among trainee doctors [abstract]. Available at: http://www.implementationscience.com/content/7/1/86/abstract. Accessed October 8, 2012.

Joy BF, Elliott E, Hardy C, et al. Standardized multidisciplinary protocol improves handover of cardiac surgery patients to the intensive care unit. Pediatric Crit Care Med 2011;12(3):304–8.

Koffuor GA, Anto BP, Abaitey AK. Error-provoking conditions in the medication use process. J Patient Saf 2012;8(1):22–5.

Landry MA, Lafrenaye S, Roy MC, et al. A randomized, controlled trial of bedside versus conference-room case presentation in a pediatric intensive care unit. Pediatrics 2007;120(2):275–80.

Linthorst GE, Kallimanis-King BL, Douwes Dekker I, et al. What contributes to internists' willingness to disclose medical errors? Neth J Med 2012;70(5):242–8.

McPherson G, Jefferson R, Kissoon N, et al. Toward the inclusion of parents on pediatric critical care unit rounds. Pediatric Crit Care Med 2011;12(6):e255–61.

Morag I, Gopher D, Spillinger A, et al. Human factors-focused reporting system for improving care quality and safety in hospital wards. Hum Factors 2012;54(2): 195–213.

Myers JS, Jaeger J. Faculty development in quality improvement: crossing the educational chasm. Am J Med Qual 2012;27(2):96–7.

Palma JP, Sharek PJ, Longhurst CA. Impact of electronic medical record integration of a handoff tool on sign-out in a newborn intensive care unit. J Perinatol 2011; 31(5):311–7.

Phipps LM, Bartke CN, Spear DA, et al. Assessment of parental presence during bedside pediatric intensive care unit rounds: effect on duration, teaching, and privacy. Pediatr Crit Care Med 2007;8(3):220–4.

Rehder KJ, Uhl TL, Meliones JN, et al. Targeted interventions improve shared agreement of daily goals in the pediatric intensive care unit. Pediatr Crit Care Med 2012;13(1):6–10.

Schriefer J, Leonard MS. Patient safety and quality improvement an overview of QI. Pediatr Rev 2012;33(8):353–60.

Singh H, Thomas EJ. Medical errors involving trainees: a study of closed malpractice claims from 5 insurers. Arch Intern Med 2007;167(19):2030–6.

Snapshots: Health Care Costs. Health care spending in the United States, & Selected OECD Countries—Kaiser Family Foundation. Available at: http://www.kff.org/insurance/snapshot/oecd042111.cfm. Accessed September 17, 2012.

Stockwell DC, Slonim AD, Pollack MM. Physician team management affects goal achievement in the intensive care unit. Pediatr Crit Care Med 2007;8(6):540–5.

Typpo KV, Tcharmtchi MH, Thomas EJ, et al. Impact of resident duty hour limits on safety in the intensive care unit. Pediatr Crit Care Med 2012;13(5):578–82.

Van Cleave J, Dougherty D, Perrin JM. Strategies for addressing barriers to publishing pediatric quality improvement research. Pediatrics 2011;128(3): e678–86.

Vats A, Goin KH, Villarreal MC, et al. The impact of a lean rounding process in a pediatric intensive care unit. Crit Care Med 2012;40(2):608–17.

Young PL, Olsen L. Roundtable on evidence-based medicine, institute of medicine. The healthcare imperative: lowering costs and improving outcomes: workshop series summary. The National Academies Press; 2010. Available at: http://www.nap.edu/openbook.php?record_id=12750. Accessed September 19, 2012.

Pediatric Status Asthmaticus

Christopher L. Carroll, MD, MS[a,b,]*, Kathleen A. Sala, MPH[a]

KEYWORDS

- Asthma • Status asthmaticus • Pediatrics • Critical care

KEY POINTS

- Status asthmaticus is a frequent cause of admission to a pediatric intensive care unit. Prompt assessment and aggressive treatment are critical.
- First-line or conventional treatment includes supplemental oxygen, aerosolized albuterol, and corticosteroids.
- There are several second-line treatments available; however, few comparative studies have been performed and in the absence of good evidence-based treatments, the use of these therapies is highly variable and dependent on local practice and provider preference.

INTRODUCTION

Status asthmaticus is a major cause of acute illness in children and one of the top indications for admission to a pediatric intensive care unit (ICU).[1–5] Mortality is rare after a child arrives at medical attention, but morbidity can be high with some children requiring days or weeks of hospitalization and recovery. Additionally, even children with mild or intermittent baseline asthma can have severe exacerbations requiring ICU admission,[6] so predicting who will progress to a more severe exacerbation is challenging. Several risk factors have been identified, but no combination can sufficiently predict the likelihood of a particular child developing a more severe exacerbation (**Box 1**).

PATHOPHYSIOLOGY

Bronchial smooth muscle spasm, airway inflammation, and increased mucous production are the key components of acute asthma.[1–3] This pathophysiology results in increased pulmonary resistance, small airway collapse, and dynamic hyperinflation. Unlike during normal breathing, in status asthmaticus a child's inspiratory muscle activity can persist through exhalation, significantly increasing respiratory muscle workload and

[a] Division of Pediatric Critical Care, Department of Pediatrics, Connecticut Children's Medical Center, 282 Washington Street, Hartford, CT 06106, USA; [b] University of Connecticut, Hartford, CT 06117, USA
* Corresponding author.
E-mail address: ccarrol@ccmckids.org

Crit Care Clin 29 (2013) 153–166
http://dx.doi.org/10.1016/j.ccc.2012.12.001
0749-0704/13/$ – see front matter © 2013 Elsevier Inc. All rights reserved.

> **Box 1**
> **Risk factors for life-threatening deterioration during status asthmaticus**
>
> Prior history of life-threatening exacerbation
>
> > Previous ICU admission
> >
> > Previous endotracheal intubation
>
> Older age
>
> Inability to recognize airflow obstruction
>
> Poor asthma control
>
> *Data from* Soroksky A, Stav D, Shpirer I. A pilot prospective, randomized, placebo-controlled trial of bilevel positive airway pressure in acute asthmatic attack. Chest 2003;123:1018–25; and Echeverria Zudaire L, Tomico Del Rio M, Bracamonte Bermejo T, et al. Status asthmaticus: is respiratory physiotherapy necessary? Allergol Immunopathol (Madr) 2000;28:290–1.

fatigue.[1–3] Additionally, because of heterogeneous areas of premature closure and obstruction, there can be significant ventilation-perfusion mismatching and hypoxemia.

Cardiopulmonary interactions can also be an important factor during status asthmaticus. Dynamic hyperinflation and hypoxic pulmonary vasoconstriction contribute to a decrease in right ventricular preload and increase in biventricular afterload. These changes can be observed clinically in pulsus paradoxus, which is an exaggeration of the normal decrease in arterial pressure that occurs during inspiration.[1–3] In addition, tachycardia caused by bronchodilators further reduces ventricular filling time and can have a net effect of reducing overall cardiac output. This can manifest clinically as a need for additional intravascular volume and low diastolic blood pressures, but does not typically require inotropic support in the absence of impaired end-organ perfusion and in children with appropriate urine output and mental status.

Underlying components of the acute exacerbation are treated in different manners and at different times or phases of a child's illness (**Fig. 1**). In the initial phase of an acute exacerbation, treatment of bronchospasm is paramount. Bronchodilator therapy has the potential to most rapidly improve clinical status. Corticosteroid therapy should also be initiated promptly, because although the peak action is later than bronchodilators, early administration of corticosteroids has been associated with improved outcomes.[7] After this acute bronchospastic phase begins to resolve, simple airway clearance techniques may be helpful in augmenting mucous clearance.

EVALUATION

Prompt assessment and rapid evaluation of clinical status are needed to determine the appropriate treatments and levels of monitoring in children with status asthmaticus.[8] Assessment of observed signs and symptoms can be helpful in determining degree of distress (**Table 1**). Whenever possible, this evaluation should be done without increasing patient anxiety, because crying increases turbulent airflow and work of breathing, and can make clinical assessment more challenging. To determine the appropriate types and levels of care, other testing and assessment may also be useful in certain situations.

Quantifying Disease Severity

Quantifying disease severity is an important tool in the clinical care of children with status asthmaticus. However, obtaining reliable and reproducible measures of pulmonary

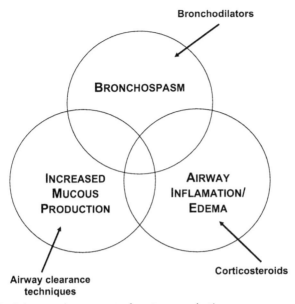

Fig. 1. Pathophysiology and treatment of acute exacerbation.

function or mechanics is difficult in sick children.[9,10] Often, because of age-related or developmental factors, sick children cannot perform the peak flow or spirometry that is routinely used in adults with acute asthma.[9,10] As a result, a variety of clinical asthma scores have been developed to quantify a child's degree of respiratory distress.[9,10] These scores are used to communicate illness severity between providers, to determine types and levels of care, and to determine patient disposition. Clinical asthma scores use a combination of subjective and objective variables that are found in children with severe disease and then rank the degree of distress for each variable to determine a total numerical value. None of these clinical asthma scores have been shown to be superior to any other. However, when choosing a clinical asthma score, providers should use one that has a high degree of interobserver reliability and has been linked to clinical outcomes.

Blood Gases

Blood gases are frequently obtained on children with status asthmaticus and are used to predict impending respiratory failure in this population. However, blood gas findings

Table 1	
Signs and symptoms of severe disease	
Subjective	**Objective**
Shortness of breath	Respiratory rate
Work of breathing and accessory muscle use	Heart rate
Diminished or absent breath sounds	Pulse oximetry
Degree and timing of wheezing	
Ability to speak in sentences or count to 10	
Level of alertness	
Anxiety or diaphoresis	

should not be used to supersede a provider's clinical judgment.[1,5,11] Children with acute asthma most commonly have hypocarbia or normocarbia on their blood gases.[1,5,11] A rising P_{CO_2} may indicate impending respiratory failure, although modest degrees of hypercarbia can be well tolerated in nonintubated children with status asthmaticus.[8] Clinical decision-making in this population should be dependent on a combination of factors, and not primarily dictated by blood gas findings. Additionally, a provider should not be reassured by the absence of respiratory acidosis. Even in the absence of respiratory acidosis, a somnolent child struggling to breathe should be endotracheally intubated. Similarly, in an awake and alert child with tachypnea, increased work of breathing and respiratory acidosis does not typically require intubation. Importantly, if blood gases or other laboratory studies are ordered, they must not delay initiation of asthma treatment.[8]

Chest Radiography

Routine chest radiography is not indicated for all children with status asthmaticus. Generally, these radiographs do not add to the clinical care of this population and only rarely reveal findings that are useful in the treatment of children with status asthmaticus.[12,13] However, there are certain clinical situations where radiography might be helpful. Specifically, a chest radiograph should be obtained when the cause of wheezing is unclear; when there are localizing findings on examination; or when there is suspected pneumonia or barotrauma (pneumothorax or pneumomediastinum).[4,12,13]

FIRST-LINE TREATMENTS
General

First-line or conventional treatment of status asthmaticus consists of supplemental oxygen for hypoxemia, aerosolized albuterol for bronchodilation, and corticosteroids for airway inflammation and edema (**Table 2**).[1–5] Typically, these are given in the emergency department setting. Therapies should be titrated according to clinical asthma score and using an asthma pathway or guidelines. The use of asthma guidelines and clinical asthma scoring systems to titrate these guidelines has been linked to improved outcomes including decreased length of stay and decreased hospital costs.[14–17] However, no specific guideline has been shown to be superior to any other. The mechanism behind these improved outcomes may be a more aggressive titration of therapy and a more efficient weaning process,[15] rather than any specific drug effect per se.

Oxygen

Children with status asthmaticus have a greater frequency of hypoxemia than adults. These children are at a higher risk of ventilation-perfusion mismatch because of age-related differences in pulmonary mechanics including lower functional residual capacity/total lung capacity ratio, increased chest wall compliance, and higher peripheral airways resistance.[1] This mismatch may be exacerbated initially by bronchodilators and can cause desaturation during the early stages of therapy. Pulse oximetry should be obtained and humidified oxygen should be delivered to relieve dyspnea.[1–5] Decreased oxygen saturation on room air is associated with the need for hospitalization in this population.[4] In children with chronic lung disease, supplemental oxygen may be associated with hypoventilation because of suppression of hypoxemic respiratory drive; however, this consideration is not a factor in an otherwise healthy child with asthma.[1]

Table 2 Ranking of status asthmaticus treatment	
	Dosage/Type/Goal
Conventional or first-line therapies	
Continuous albuterol nebulization	10–25 mg/h
Corticosteroids (prednisone or methylprednisolone)	2–4 mg/kg/d divided q 6–12 h
Supplemental oxygen	To maintain saturations >92%
Early supplemental therapies	
Intravenous magnesium	25–75 mg/kg (up to total of 2 g total) over 20 min
Ipratropium nebulization	0.25–0.5 mg every 20 min for 3 doses
Second-line therapies	
Noninvasive positive pressure	Titrated to comfort and tidal volume
Intravenous terbutaline	0.5–4 μg/kg/min
Rescue therapies	
Intubation	Pressure-limited ventilation or pressure-regulated volume control modes
Intravenous ketamine	Load of 2 mg/kg followed by infusion of 0.5–2 mg/kg/h
Intravenous aminophylline	Load of 6 mg/kg followed by infusion of 1 mg/kg/h with goal serum levels 10–20 μg/mL
Inhaled anesthetics	Halothane or isoflurane
Helium-oxygen	60%–80% helium/20%–40% oxygen
Extracorporeal support	Extracorporeal life support or Extracorporeal carbon dioxide clearance

Albuterol

β-Adrenergic agonists, such as albuterol, are the most effective and commonly used bronchodilators in the United States and form the foundation of treatment of acute asthma. These medications bind to β_2-adrenergic receptors in the airway smooth muscle to produce bronchodilation by smooth muscle relaxation. Albuterol is initially delivered by intermittent nebulization, and changed to continuous nebulization in children with inadequate response. Continuously administered albuterol has been shown to improve outcomes and to be more cost effective than continued intermittent therapy.[18] High doses (as much as 20–30 mg/hour) are generally well tolerated and have been used for days in this population.[1,7,19] Differences in tidal volume, airflow turbulence, and nebulizer gas flow all significantly impact the amount of drug delivered; therefore, weight adjusting of albuterol aerosol dosages is not necessary.[1] These agents can also cause tachycardia and hypertension through binding of other systemic β-adrenergic receptors, although when delivered by aerosol, these systemic effects are reduced. Orally administered β-adrenergic agents are not indicated for status asthmaticus.

Titrating albuterol aerosol therapy using a clinical asthma score may be helpful in reducing length of stay and duration of therapy in children with status asthmaticus. As a child improves, this continuously administered aerosol can be weaned in dosage, then changed to intermittent dosing, which can also be weaned in frequency as clinical status improves. No specific guideline has been shown to be superior to any other.

Levalbuterol, which contains only the single active (R)-enantiomer of typically delivered racemic albuterol, is a potentially attractive selective bronchodilator in the treatment of status asthmaticus, because previous authors have suggested that repeated doses of the racemic albuterol mixture may be related to more severe bronchospasm.[2] However, a recent negative randomized controlled trial of racemic albuterol versus levalbuterol in children with status asthmaticus adds to the literature that levalbuterol does not convey additional benefit and does not lead to reduced side effects.[20] Considering the increased cost and the lack of improvement in outcomes, the routine use of this medication cannot be recommended in this population.

Corticosteroids

Corticosteroids are used to treat airway inflammation and edema in children with acute asthma.[7,21,22] These medications have been shown to improve outcomes by reducing inflammatory cellular mediators and proinflammatory cytokines and by decreasing mucous production. Short-term usage is usually not associated with significant side effects. However, hyperglycemia, hypertension, and behavioral changes have been reported, and neuromyopathies can occur in children treated with corticosteroids and neuromuscular blocking agents.[23]

There is little published evidence regarding the duration and dosage of corticosteroids for the treatment of status asthmaticus in children. Duration of therapy is typically driven by the severity of the exacerbation and the rapidity of response to therapy.[1,5,8] If corticosteroid treatment is longer than 7 days, a slow dosage taper is recommended.[22]

Currently, National Heart, Lung and Blood Institute guidelines recommend administration of corticosteroids systemically rather than by an inhaled route.[8] Orally administered medications may be used if a child can tolerate oral medication, but if not, intravenous (IV) medication is preferred. Children receiving high-dose β-adrenergic agonist therapy may develop impaired gastric absorption and vomiting, so in these children IV administration may be preferable. Early administration of systemic corticosteroids is key and has been shown to improve outcomes. In one study, children treated within 75 minutes of triage had significantly reduced hospitalization rates and lengths of treatment.[7]

The National Heart, Lung and Blood Institute guidelines suggest that 2 mg/kg/d of systemic prednisone or methylprednisolone be used for acute asthma, but offer no recommendations for children in impending respiratory failure.[8] In this population of children with more severe disease, some authors have suggested using dosages as high as 4 mg/kg/d. There is no evidence that this increased dosage is superior; however, the practice of using this higher dosage seems to be widespread. In a recent national survey of pediatric intensivists, almost a third reported using a starting dosage of 4 mg/kg/d and most cited clinical experience as their rationale for this dosage.[24] Research is needed to determine the appropriate dosage and duration of therapy in this population.

Hydration Status

The need for IV fluid boluses should not be overlooked in children with status asthmaticus.[1,3] Several pathophysiologic mechanisms contribute to the need for robust intravascular volume in these children. Specifically, an increased intrathoracic pressure from air-trapping can lead to decreased venous return, which coupled with bronchodilator-induced tachycardia can reduce filling time and also potentially decrease cardiac output. Additionally, children with acute disease frequently present somewhat dehydrated because of decreased oral intake and elevated respiratory rate. This dehydration can also be exacerbated by the nausea and vomiting associated with β-adrenergic agonist therapy. All of these factors contribute to the need to restore euvolemia in this population. However, previous authors have identified a syndrome of inappropriate antidiuretic hormone in children with status asthmaticus, so fluid balance should be monitored carefully.[25]

SECOND-LINE TREATMENTS

Any child who does not sufficiently respond to first-line treatment of status asthmaticus should be strongly considered for admission to an ICU setting. These children require close monitoring of their clinical status including continuous cardiorespiratory monitoring. Second-line therapies should be considered, but these should be additive and not replace the first-line therapies. There are several second-line treatments available; however, few comparative studies have been performed, and none have been shown to be superior to any of the others.[1–5] In the absence of good evidence-based treatments, the use of these therapies is highly variable and dependent on local practice and provider preference.[26–28] Nonetheless, it is possible to determine a broad-based ranking of therapies in this population when examining the literature (see **Table 2**). For example, magnesium and ipratropium therapy have been shown to be effective early in the course of a child's disease and not in the later stages of illness, whereas such therapies as terbutaline and noninvasive positive pressure have been shown to be effective during the whole course of a child's illness. Other therapies with a weaker evidence basis, however, such as ketamine, inhaled anesthesia, and helium-oxygen mixtures, should be used solely as rescue therapies.

Magnesium

Magnesium causes bronchodilation by inhibiting smooth muscle contraction, and by decreasing cholinergic stimulation and histamine release.[29,30] Studies conflict on the use of magnesium therapy, but IV magnesium has been shown to reduce hospitalization when added to conventional therapy in children with status asthmaticus.[29,30] Toxicity, which includes weakness, respiratory depression, and cardiac arrhythmias, is rare in children with asthma.[1]

Anticholinergics

Anticholinergic medications, such as ipratropium, cause bronchodilation through bronchial smooth muscle relaxation mediated by the parasympathetic nervous system. Additionally, the cardiovascular side effects of ipratropium, which is not absorbed into the bloodstream when delivered by inhalation, are minimal. In children with status asthmaticus, the addition of ipratropium nebulizations to albuterol therapy has been shown to significantly reduce hospitalizations.[31–33] This therapy was most effective in moderate to severely ill children.[32,33] However, the continuation of anticholinergic medications after this initial period is not routinely recommended.[1–5]

Terbutaline

The use of IV β-adrenergic agonist therapy, such as terbutaline, is frequently considered as a second-line treatment of acute asthma.[1,14,34,35] Some children, including those with severe obstruction and small effective tidal volumes, may have ineffective delivery of nebulized medications, such as albuterol. In these children, IV β-adrenergic receptor agonists may be used despite the risk of systemic side effects. IV terbutaline has been shown to acutely improve pulmonary function and gas exchange, and to shorten hospital and ICU length of stay when delivered according to a nurse-driven protocol in children with status asthmaticus.[15,35] The one randomized placebo-controlled trial of IV terbutaline versus placebo showed no statistically signif-icant improvement when terbutaline was added to standard therapy. However, there was a trend toward decreased ICU length of stay and improved clinical asthma score in the first 24 hours.[34]

There is some evidence that certain children are better responders to β-adrenergic agonist therapy than others.[19] Previous investigators have linked obesity and ethnicity to a slower response to therapy during severe asthma exacerbations. Some of this decreased response may be caused by genetics; however, these studies are prelim-inary and require replication.[36,37]

When receiving IV β-adrenergic agonist therapy, a child requires close monitoring for systemic side effects. Although tachyarrhythmias are rare, children receiving IV terbutaline should have continuous cardiac monitoring. Several authors have found a low and transient incidence of cardiotoxicity, as measured by elevated serum tropo-nins, in children treated with IV terbutaline.[38,39] However, tachyarrythmias, such as supraventricular tachycardia, have also been reported. Other common side effects include hypertension, electrolyte disturbances, nausea and vomiting, and agitation.

Noninvasive Positive Pressure Ventilation

Noninvasive positive pressure ventilation (NPPV) is used increasingly in the care of children with status asthmaticus. Early intervention has been shown to improve out-comes and potentially avoid endotracheal intubation in this population.[40–45] NPPV improves the condition of children with asthma by preventing airway collapse during exhalation and thereby unloading fatigued respiratory muscles. During an acute asthma exacerbation, inflammation of small airways leads to increased airways resis-tance and expiratory time constants.[41] This results in premature airway closure during exhalation and dynamic hyperinflation.[41] Positive pressure can maintain small airway patency and reduce the change in alveolar pressure needed to initiate inspiration by providing a continuous expiratory pressure.[41] Adding inspiratory pressure further improves dyspnea and gas exchange by augmenting spontaneous tidal volumes. NPPV has the additional benefit of preserving the child's natural airway and thereby potentially avoiding some of the complications of the more invasive endotracheal intubation.[41–43]

However, the use of NPPV requires close monitoring by trained providers. One of the primary predictors of success with the use of NPPV is the involvement of providers who are trained and comfortable with the care of children receiving NPPV.[40] The initi-ation of this therapy must be performed gradually, with attention paid to avoiding any increase in anxiety in the child from either the mask itself or the airflow. Finding an appropriate sized mask can be challenging because of the great variation in size and shape of children's faces. Sedation should be used sparingly and cautiously, because sedation can potentially reduce a child's already taxed respiratory drive. Providers should also observe children closely for potential complications of therapy including skin breakdown, gastric distention, and the development of barotrauma.[40–45]

RESCUE THERAPIES
Intubation

Intubation should be a last resort therapy for children with status asthmaticus. The presence of a tracheal foreign body can aggravate bronchospasm, children can require significant amounts of sedation to facilitate this therapy, and gas exchange immediately after intubation is frequently worse than before intubation. Clearly, how-ever, there are children who require intubation for impending respiratory failure, but weighing the risks and benefits can be challenging a priori. After the decision to intubate has been made, this procedure should be performed by an experienced clinician because these children are frequently unstable.

Several authors have found that children intubated outside the ICU setting are intubated for shorter durations than children intubated in the ICU setting.[23,46] Some have suggested that these children may represent an acute asphyxia asthma phenotype of children that progress to respiratory failure rapidly and then resolve quickly.[47] However, there is mounting evidence that nonclinical factors, such as provider practice and local geography, may play a larger role than patient characteristics in the decision to intubate a child with status asthmaticus.[23]

Once intubated, the management of children with status asthmaticus is challenging and requires close monitoring of gas exchange and hemodynamic parameters. Permissive hypercapnea and lung protective strategies should be used while allowing for sufficient exhalation to minimize the amount of dynamic hyperinflation. A ventilator mode with a decelerating flow pattern, such as pressure-limited ventilation or pressure-regulated volume control, results in a lower peak airway pressure and a higher mean airway pressure than a volume control mode, and theoretically provides better ventilation in children with status asthmaticus.[48,49] Sufficient positive end-expiratory pressure should be provided to surpass the lower inflection point of alveolar collapse duration exhalation.[1] Sedation and sometimes muscle relaxation are needed to facilitate mechanical ventilation in children, although the duration and depth of muscle relaxation should be limited when possible to reduce the risk of myopathies.

Ketamine

Ketamine is a dissociative anesthetic with sympathomimetic and bronchodilator properties.[50] Unfortunately, the usefulness of ketamine is somewhat mitigated by its potential to increase bronchial secretions and its dissociate properties including a frightening emergence phenomenon in older children. However, ketamine is a potentially attractive agent in children intubated and mechanically ventilated for status asthmaticus.[1–5]

Methylxanthines

Once the primary treatment of status asthmaticus, methylxanthines, such as theophylline and aminophylline, have recently fallen out of favor. This is caused in part by decreased bronchodilator effectiveness compared with β-adrenergic agonists and the small therapeutic window and their unfavorable side effect profile. However, they still may have a role in select patients with refractory status asthmaticus.[51,52]

Inhaled Anesthetics

Inhalational anesthetics, such as halothane and isoflurane, can cause bronchodilation through smooth muscle relaxation and have been used anecdotally to treat status asthmaticus in children refractory to conventional therapies.[53–55] Unfortunately, the use of these medications requires intubation and mechanical ventilation and a scavenging system typically found only in the operating room of many institutions, thereby limiting the usefulness of this therapy. Additionally, there is also sometimes a reduced ability to provide effective mechanical ventilation in these children, because the ventilatory equipment needed to provide the medication may not be as sophisticated as the ventilators in the ICU.

Helium-oxygen

The use of a helium-oxygen gas mixture is another potentially attractive therapy for the treatment of status asthmaticus in children. Because of its lower density and higher viscosity, a mixture of helium and oxygen flows through small and obstructed airways with less turbulence and resistance than the nitrogen and oxygen mixture of gases found in atmospheric air. Theoretically, the use of helium-oxygen–driven aerosolized therapy might also be expected to increase drug delivery by improving gas exchange to the distal airways. Unfortunately, the literature regarding the effectiveness of this therapy in children with acute asthma has been mixed.[56–59] Randomized controlled studies of helium-oxygen therapy in this population have been contradictory and have not demonstrated efficacy in terms of shortening durations of exacerbation or improving outcomes.[56–59] Furthermore, to significantly reduce airways resistance, 60% to 80% helium is needed in the gas mixture. This limits the use of helium-oxygen mixtures in hypoxemic children with status asthmaticus. In the literature, most of the benefit of a helium-oxygen mixture has been found early in the acute phase of illness,[57,58] but it may also be useful as a rescue therapy in certain children with lower oxygen requirements and refractory status asthmaticus.

Extracorporeal Support

Extracorporeal life support and extracorporeal carbon dioxide clearance have been advocated in extreme cases of status asthmaticus.[60–62] A recent review of the extracorporeal life support registry found that 71 children with status asthmaticus were treated with extracorporeal life support and survival in this population was 83%.[60] Clearly, however, this therapy is associated with a significant risk of adverse events, and should only be undertaken as a rescue technique. The use of extracorporeal carbon dioxide clearance is experimental at this time.[62]

AIRWAY CLEARANCE TECHNIQUES

Theoretically, airway clearance techniques can be helpful in improving the speed of resolution of status asthmaticus.[63–65] Mucous production is increased during acute asthma, and several mechanisms, such as respiratory muscle fatigue and bedrest, may contribute to ineffective airway clearance by children during acute exacerbations. Aggressive airway clearance techniques, such as chest percussion, vibration, and postural drainage, have been found to improve airway clearance in children with other types of chronic lung disease.[63] In children with asthma, reducing mucous plugging could, in theory, improve gas exchange through improvement in ventilation-perfusion mismatch, and potentially also shorten the duration of illness.

However, despite the use of these therapies clinically, there is little evidence in the literature supporting the effectiveness of these techniques.[64] Additionally, these techniques are often bundled into the term "chest physiotherapy," which obscures the potentially significant variation in the types and performance of these techniques by a variety of practitioners.[64] A more specific description of the type and method of each technique and how they are performed in children with asthma might aid in investigating whether these techniques improve outcomes.

Frequently in pediatrics, augmenting mucous clearance can be accomplished by getting a child upright, out of bed, and ambulating. Often, a child needs little encouragement to perform these simple techniques. Anecdotally, these techniques can sometimes dramatically improve mucous plugging and speed recovery, but importantly should only be performed as bronchospasm starts to improve. However, until there is more literature exploring the use of more aggressive airway clearance techniques in children with status asthmaticus, the routine use of these more vigorous techniques is not recommended, and providers need to balance the risks and benefits in specific children.

SUMMARY

Despite a plateau in the incidence of asthma and a decreasing incidence of hospital admissions for asthma, status asthmaticus is a frequent cause of admission to the ICU. Prompt assessment and aggressive treatment are crucial steps toward improving outcomes in this population. Fortunately, most children with status asthmaticus improve rapidly, but there is a cohort of difficult-to-treat children who are challenging to study and who have significant variations in terms of response to treatment. As a result, therapies are used in a trial-and-error format, without a clear evidence-based rationale to therapy. A broad-based ranking of therapies is possible to develop when examining the literature, but more research is needed into the small but significant population of children with status asthmaticus.

REFERENCES

1. Werner HA. Status asthmaticus in children. Chest 2001;119:1913–29.
2. Chipps BE, Murphy KR. Assessment and treatment of acute asthma in children. J Pediatr 2005;147:288–94.
3. Mannix R, Bachur R. Status asthmaticus in children. Curr Opin Pediatr 2007;19: 281–7.
4. Kercsmar CM. Acute inpatient care of status asthmaticus. Respir Care Clin N Am 2000;6:155–70.
5. Smith SR, Strunk RC. Acute asthma in the pediatric emergency department. Pediatr Clin North Am 1999;46:1145–65.
6. Carroll CL, Schramm CM, Zucker AR. Severe exacerbations in children with mild asthma. J Asthma 2008;45:513–7.
7. Bhogal SK, McGillivray D, Bourbeau J, et al. Early administration of systemic corticosteroids reduces hospital admission rates for children with moderate and severe asthma exacerbation. Ann Emerg Med 2012;60:84–91.
8. U.S. Department of Health and Human Services. National Heart, Lung and Blood Institute. National asthma education and prevention program expert panel report 3: guidelines for the diagnosis and management of asthma. Publication 08–4051. Bethesda, MD: U.S. Department of Health and Human Services; 2007. Available at: http://www.nhlbi.nih.gov/guidelines/asthma/asthgdln.pdf.
9. van der Windt DA, Nagelkerke AF, Bouter LM, et al. Clinical scores for acute asthma in pre-school children. J Clin Epidemiol 1994;47:635–46.
10. Keogh KA, Macarthur C, Parkin PC, et al. Predictors of hospitalization in children with acute asthma. J Pediatr 2001;139:273–7.
11. Qureshi F. Management of children with acute asthma in the emergency department. Pediatr Emerg Care 1999;15:206–14.
12. Brooks LJ, Cloutier MM, Afshani D. Significance of reoentgenographic abnormalities in children hospitalized for asthma. Chest 1982;82:315–8.
13. Hederos CA, Janson S, Andersson H, et al. Chest X-ray investigation in newly discovered asthma. Pediatr Allergy Immunol 2004;15:163–5.
14. Norton SP, Pusic MV, Taha F, et al. Effect of a clinical pathway on the hospitalisation rates of children with asthma: a prospective study. Arch Dis Child 2007;92:60–6.
15. Carroll CL, Schramm CM. Protocol-based titration of intravenous terbutaline decreases length of stay in pediatric status asthmaticus. Pediatr Pulmonol 2006; 41:350–6.
16. Kelly CS, Andersen CL, Pestian JP, et al. Improved outcomes for hospitalized asthmatic children using a clinical pathway. Ann Allergy Asthma Immunol 2000; 84:509–16.

17. McDowell KM, Chatburn RL, Myers TR, et al. A cost-saving algorithm for children hospitalized for status asthmaticus. Arch Pediatr Adolesc Med 1998;152: 977–84.
18. Papo MC, Frank J, Thompson AE. A prospective, randomized study of continuous versus intermittent nebulized albuterol for severe status asthmaticus in children. Crit Care Med 1993;21:1479–86.
19. Carroll CL, Schramm CM, Zucker AR. Slow responders to IV β2-adrenergic receptor agonist therapy: defining a novel phenotype in pediatric asthma. Pediatr Pulmonol 2008;43:627–33.
20. Andrews T, McGintee E, Mittal MK, et al. High-dose continuous nebulized levalbuterol for pediatric status asthmaticus: a randomized trial. J Pediatr 2009;155: 205–10.
21. Smith M, Iqbal S, Rowe BH, et al. Corticosteroids for hospitalized children with acute asthma. Cochrane Database Syst Rev 2003;(2):CD002886.
22. Warner JO, Naspitz CK. Third international pediatric consensus statement on the management of childhood asthma: international pediatric asthma consensus group. Pediatr Pulmonol 1998;25:1–7.
23. Newth CJ, Meert KL, Clark AE, et al. Fatal and near-fatal asthma in children: the critical care perspective. J Pediatr 2012;161:214–21.
24. Giuliano JS, Faustino EV, Li S, et al. Corticosteroid therapy in critically ill pediatric asthmatic patients. Pediatric Academic Societies 2012. 3844.504. Available at: http://www.abstracts2view.com/pas/view.php?nu=PAS12L1_367.
25. Baker JW, Yerger S, Segar WE. Elevated plasma antidiuretic hormone levels in status asthmaticus. Mayo Clin Proc 1976;51:31–4.
26. Bratton SL, Odetola FO, McCollegan J, et al. Regional variation in ICU care for pediatric patients with asthma. J Pediatr 2005;147:355–61.
27. Roberts JS, Bratton SL, Brogan TV. Acute severe asthma: differences in therapies and outcomes among pediatric intensive care units. Crit Care Med 2002;30: 581–5.
28. Bratton SL, Newth CJ, Zuppa AF, et al. Critical care for pediatric asthma: wide care variability and challenges for study. Pediatr Crit Care Med 2012;13:407–14.
29. Markovitz B. Does magnesium sulphate have a role in the management of paediatric status asthmaticus? Arch Dis Child 2002;86:381–2.
30. Cheuk DK, Chau TC, Lee SL. A meta-analysis on intravenous magnesium sulphate for treating acute asthma. Arch Dis Child 2005;90:74–7.
31. Crave D, Kercsmar CM, Myers TR, et al. Ipratropium bromide plus nebulized albuterol for the treatment of hospitalized children with acute asthma. J Pediatr 2001;138:51–8.
32. Schuh S, Johnson DW, Callahan S, et al. Efficacy of frequent nebulized ipratropium bromide added to frequent high-dose albuterol therapy in severe childhood asthma. J Pediatr 1995;126:639–45.
33. Qureshi F, Pestian J, Davis P, et al. Effect of nebulized ipratropium on the hospitalization rates of children with asthma. N Engl J Med 1998;133:479–85.
34. Bogie AL, Towne D, Luckett PM, et al. Comparison of intravenous terbutaline versus normal saline in pediatric patients on continuous high-dose nebulized albuterol for status asthmaticus. Pediatr Emerg Care 2007;23:355–61.
35. Stephanopoulos DE, Monge R, Schell KH, et al. Continuous intravenous terbutaline for pediatric status asthmaticus. Crit Care Med 1998;26:1744–8.
36. Carroll CL, Sala K, Zucker AR, et al. Beta-adrenergic receptor polymorphisms and response to therapy in pediatric status asthmaticus: a prospective cohort study. Pediatr Pulmonol 2012;47:233–9.

37. Carroll CL, Stoltz P, Schramm CM, et al. β2-adrenergic receptor polymorphisms affect response to treatment in near fatal asthma exacerbations in children. Chest 2009;135:1186–92.

38. Chiang VW, Burns JP, Rifai N, et al. Cardiac toxicity of intravenous terbutaline for the treatment of severe asthma in children: a prospective assessment. J Pediatr 2000;137:73–7.

39. Carroll CL, Coro M, Cowl A, et al. Occult cardiotoxicity in children receiving continuous beta-agonist therapy. Chest 2009;136(4_MeetingAbstracts):18S-e-18S.

40. Carroll CL, Schramm CM. Non-invasive ventilation for the treatment of status asthmaticus in children. Ann Allergy Asthma Immunol 2006;96:454–9.

41. Meduri GU, Cook TR, Turner RE, et al. Noninvasive positive pressure ventilation in status asthmaticus. Chest 1996;110:767–74.

42. Hill NS. Noninvasive positive pressure ventilation for non chronic obstructive pulmonary disease causes of acute respiratory failure. In: Hill NS, editor. Noninvasive positive pressure ventilation: principles and applications. Armonk (NY): Futura Publishing Company; 2001. p. 85–104.

43. Pollack CV, Fleisch KB, Dowsey K. Treatment of acute bronchospasm with ß-adrenergic agonist aerosols delivered by a nasal bilevel positive airway circuit. Ann Emerg Med 1995;26:552–7.

44. Soroksky A, Stav D, Shpirer I. A pilot prospective, randomized, placebo-controlled trial of bilevel positive airway pressure in acute asthmatic attack. Chest 2003;123:1018–25.

45. Basnet S, Mander G, Andoh J, et al. Safety, efficacy and tolerability of early initiation of noninvasive positive pressure ventilation in pediatric patients admitted with status asthmaticus: a pilot study. Pediatr Crit Care Med 2012;13:393–8.

46. Carroll CL, Smith SR, Collins M, et al. Endotracheal intubation and pediatric status asthmaticus: site of original care affects treatment. Pediatr Crit Care Med 2007;8:91–5.

47. Maffei FA, van der Jagt EW, Powers KS, et al. Duration of mechanical ventilation in life-threatening pediatric asthma: description of an acute asphyxial subgroup. Pediatrics 2004;14:762–7.

48. Sarnaik AP, Daphtary KM, Meert KL, et al. Pressure-controlled ventilation in children with severe status asthmaticus. Pediatr Crit Care Med 2004;5:133–8.

49. Sabato K, Hanson JH. Mechanical ventilation for children with status asthmaticus. Respir Care Clin N Am 2000;6:171–88.

50. Petrillo TM, Fortenberry JD, Linzer JF, et al. Emergency department use of ketamine in pediatric status asthmaticus. J Asthma 2001;38:657–64.

51. Ream RS, Loftis LL, Albers GM, et al. Efficacy of IV theophylline in children with severe status asthmaticus. Chest 2001;119:1480–8.

52. Self TH, Redmond AM, Nguyen WT. Reassessment of theophylline use for severe asthma exacerbation. J Asthma 2002;39:677–86.

53. Shankar V, Churchwell KB, Deshpande JK. Isoflurane therapy for severe refractory status asthmaticus in children. Intensive Care Med 2006;32:927–33.

54. Restrepo RD, Pettignano R, DeMeuse P. Halothane, an effective infrequently used drug, in the treatment of pediatric status asthmaticus: a case report. J Asthma 2005;42:649–51.

55. Tobias JD. Therapeutic applications and uses of inhalational anesthesia in the pediatric intensive care unit. Pediatr Crit Care Med 2008;9:169–79.

56. Rivera ML, Kim TY, Stewart GM, et al. Albuterol nebulized in heliox in the initial ED treatment of pediatric asthma: a blinded, randomized controlled trial. Am J Emerg Med 2006;24:38–42.

57. Kudukis TM, Manthous CA, Schmidt GA, et al. Inhaled helium-oxygen revisited: effect of inhaled helium-oxygen during the treatment of status asthmaticus in children. J Pediatr 1997;130:217–24.

58. Kim IK, Phrampus E, Venkataraman S, et al. Helium/oxygen-driven albuterol nebulization in the treatment of children with moderate to severe asthma exacerbations: a randomized, controlled trial. Pediatrics 2005;116:1127–33.

59. Bigham MT, Jacobs BR, Monaco MA, et al. Helium/oxygen-driven albuterol nebulization in the management of children with status asthmaticus: a randomized, placebo-controlled trial. Pediatr Crit Care Med 2010;11:356–61.

60. Zabrocki LA, Brogan TV, Statler KD, et al. Extracorporeal membrane oxygenation for pediatric respiratory failure: survival and predictors of mortality. Pediatr Crit Care Med 2011;39:364–70.

61. Hebbar KB, Petrillo-Albarano T, Coto-Puckett W, et al. Experience with the use of extracorporeal life support for severe refractory status asthmaticus in children. Crit Care 2009;13:R29.

62. Elliot SC, Paramasivam K, Oram J, et al. Pumpless extracorporeal carbon dioxide removal for life-threatening asthma. Crit Care Med 2007;35:945–8.

63. Echeverria Zudaire L, Tomico Del Rio M, Bracamonte Bermejo T, et al. Status asthmaticus: is respiratory physiotherapy necessary? Allergol Immunopathol (Madr) 2000;28:290–1.

64. De Boeck K, Vermeulen F, Vreys M, et al. Airway clearance techniques to treat acute respiratory disorders in previously healthy children: where is the evidence? Eur J Pediatr 2008;167:607–12.

65. Malmstrom K, Kaila M, Korhonen K, et al. Mechanical ventilation in children with severe asthma. Pediatr Pulmonol 2011;31:405–11.

Acute Respiratory Failure

James Schneider, MD*, Todd Sweberg, MD

KEYWORDS

- Acute respiratory failure • Pediatrics • Acute lung injury • Monitoring
- Respiratory physiology

KEY POINTS

- Acute respiratory failure is common in critically ill children.
- Monitoring for respiratory failure includes commonly used invasive tests, such as blood gas analysis, but noninvasive monitoring has recently grown in importance and proven reliable.
- Recent advancements in therapeutic options for respiratory failure have improved the overall outcome of critically ill children, but much more rigorous investigation is still needed.

INTRODUCTION

Acute respiratory failure is a common dilemma faced by pediatric critical care practitioners. As many as two-thirds of pediatric intensive care unit (PICU) patients will be admitted with a diagnosis of respiratory failure,[1] which represents a common end point to multiple pathologic processes, categorized as hypoxemic, hypercapnic, or mixed. Common causes are listed in **Table 1**. In 2012, primary infections of the lung were responsible for 2% of all mortalities in children younger than 5 years in the United States and 18% worldwide.[2] Developmental variations contribute to the diverse etiologies and higher incidence of acute respiratory failure in children compared with adults. Infants have more compliant chest walls than adults, making it more difficult to generate the negative intrathoracic pressure required to inspire sufficient tidal volumes in conditions of decreased lung compliance (ie, pneumonia, hyaline membrane disease). The infant chest wall also has less elastic recoil. Further, collateral ventilation through pores of Kohn or Lambert are not well developed in early life. These characteristics make young children more susceptible to alveolar collapse. Childhood airways lack the more rigid cartilaginous supports that strengthen into

The authors do not have any financial conflict of interest to disclose.

Division of Critical Care Medicine, Hofstra North Shore-LIJ School of Medicine, Cohen Children's Medical Center of New York, North Shore Long Island Jewish Health System, 269-01 76th Avenue, New Hyde Park, NY 11040, USA

* Corresponding author.

E-mail address: jschneide2@nshs.edu

Crit Care Clin 29 (2013) 167–183

http://dx.doi.org/10.1016/j.ccc.2012.12.004

0749-0704/13/$ – see front matter © 2013 Elsevier Inc. All rights reserved.

criticalcare.theclinics.com

Table 1 Etiologies of acute respiratory failure in children	
Location	**Example**
Upper airway obstruction	• Infection (croup, epiglottitis, bacterial tracheitis) • Laryngotracheomalacia • Foreign body • Anaphylaxis
Lower airway obstruction	• Asthma • Bronchiolitis • Cystic fibrosis
Restrictive lung disease	• Acute respiratory distress syndrome • Pleural effusion • Pneumonia • Pulmonary edema • Abdominal compartment syndrome
Central nervous system disorder	• Intracranial injury (hemorrhage, ischemia) • Medication (sedatives) • Metabolic encephalopathy
Peripheral nervous system and muscle disorders	• Guillian Barré syndrome • Muscular dystrophy • Scoliosis • Spinal cord injury • Botulism • Intoxications (ie, organophosphates)

Adapted from Ghuman AK, Newth CJ, Khemani RG. Respiratory support in children. Paediatr Child Health 2011;21(4):163–9; with permission.

adulthood, making them more susceptible to dynamic compression and subsequent airway obstruction in disease states associated with increased airway resistance (ie, bronchiolitis, asthma). Last, the pediatric airways are naturally smaller in diameter than in adults. Because the resistance to airflow is inversely proportional to the fourth power of the radius ($R = 8NL/\pi r^4$), any narrowing of the pediatric airway will have a much greater impact on the resistance. This will lead to a more profound decrease in airflow, as laminar flow transitions to turbulent flow, as described by Reynolds number ($Re = 2 rV\rho/N$, where r is the radius of the airway, V is the velocity of the gas flow, ρ is the density of the gas, and N is the viscosity of the gas). In the adult, the peripheral airways contribute about 20% of the total airway resistance. In infants and young children, they contribute about 50%, explaining why diseases affecting the peripheral airways (ie, bronchiolitis) have such a profound clinical impact. It is clear that the management of acute respiratory failure in children requires a thorough understanding of these physiologic differences, reminding the clinician that children are, in fact, not little adults.

Acute respiratory failure occurs when embarrassment of the respiratory system results in the inability to properly transfer oxygen (O_2) from the atmosphere to the blood or remove carbon dioxide (CO_2) from the blood and eliminate it to the atmosphere. Hypoxic respiratory failure is defined by a partial pressure of arterial O_2 (PaO_2) that is less than 60 mm Hg on room air at sea level, and hypercapnic respiratory failure occurs when the partial pressure of CO_2 ($PaCO_2$) is greater than 50 mm Hg (with a concomitant respiratory acidosis) under the same conditions. To better understand these, it is first important to examine the mechanisms of oxygenation and ventilation.

Oxygenation

Ideally, oxygen that is contained within the alveolus at inspiration will equilibrate with arterial blood, as described by the alveolar gas equation:

$$P_{AO_2} = P_{IO_2} - (P_{ACO_2}/R),$$

then $P_{AO_2} = F_{IO_2} (P_B - P_{H2O}) - P_{ACO_2}/R,$

where P_{AO_2} = partial pressure of alveolar oxygen; P_{IO_2} = partial pressure of inspired oxygen; P_{ACO_2} = partial pressure of alveolar CO_2 (substituted by arterial [$PaCO_2$] due to the highly efficient manner that CO_2 crosses cell membranes); R = respiratory quotient: ratio of CO_2 production (VCO_2) to O_2 consumption (VO_2) (R = VCO_2/VO_2), averages 0.8 on a normal, mixed adult diet; P_B = barometric pressure; and P_{H2O} = water vapor pressure.

Adequate gas exchange also requires that the inspired alveolar gas matches blood distribution in the pulmonary capillaries. There is a normal gradient between alveolar and arterial P_{O_2}, known as the A-a gradient, which is less than 10 mm Hg. The alveolar gas equation also helps to understand some of the mechanisms behind hypoxemia (**Box 1**).[3] Nonpulmonary causes, such as decreased cardiac output, increased extraction of O_2, and abnormal hemoglobin, can also contribute to abnormal gas exchange.[4]

The most common etiology for hypoxemia in critically ill children is inequality in the relationship between ventilation and perfusion (V/Q). Regional differences in ventilation and blood flow, owing to regional differences in intrapleural pressures and gravitational forces, cause ventilation and perfusion to decrease from the base to the apex of the lung, although perfusion does so much more rapidly. This leads to an abnormally high V/Q ratio at the apex of the lung (in an upright position) and a much lower one at the base.[3] Atelectasis from various pathologic states (ie, pneumonia, mucous plug) exaggerates the mismatching of V/Q, causing well-oxygenated blood from high V/Q regions to mix with poorly oxygenated blood from low V/Q regions, leading to worsening hypoxia with an increased A-a gradient. Pulmonary edema (ie, cardiac failure, systemic inflammatory response syndrome, acute respiratory distress syndrome [ARDS]) will lead to worsening V/Q mismatching, compromised diffusion, and atelectasis. Hypoxemia caused by V/Q inequality can be corrected by inspiring a higher concentration of oxygen, as well as the provision of positive pressure ventilation, which may recruit consolidated or collapsed lung units and improve V/Q matching.

When alveolar ventilation is decreased, insufficiently replenishing alveolar oxygen, the alveolar P_{O_2} falls as the P_{CO_2} rises, not altering the normal A-a gradient. Elevation of $PaCO_2$ that occurs with airway obstruction will not result in hypoxemia until severe obstruction is present, with forced expiratory volume in 1 second less than

Box 1
Causes of hypoxemia
Hypoventilation
Shunt
Ventilation-perfusion inequality
Diffusion limitation
Low inspired fraction of oxygen

approximately 15% predicted.[5] The hypoxia that results from CO_2 retention is easily overcome with the addition of increased inspired oxygen.

Shunting describes the direct mixing of deoxygenated venous blood that has not undergone gas exchange in the lungs with arterial blood. Normal anatomic shunting occurs as venous blood from the bronchial veins and Thebesian veins collects in the left-sided circulation. Pathologically, patients may have abnormal vascular connections (ie, arterial-venous fistula) or intracardiac communications allowing blood to traverse the heart from the right to the left without undergoing gas exchange at the level of the lungs. Intrapulmonary shunting most commonly occurs as blood perfuses regions of the lung that are not well ventilated. The addition of mixed venous blood (with depressed Po_2) to oxygenated capillary blood results in decreased PaO_2, increasing the A-a gradient. The amount of shunted blood that would need to be mixed with arterial blood to account for the A-a gradient can be calculated by the shunt equation:

$$Q_S/Q_T = (CcO_2 - CaO_2)/(CcO_2 - CvO_2),$$

where Q_S is shunt flow to unventilated lung units; Q_T is total pulmonary blood flow; and CaO_2, CcO_2, and CvO_2 is the content of oxygen in arterial, end-capillary, and mixed venous blood, respectively.[3] In healthy individuals, normal physiologic shunting accounts for less than 5% of cardiac output.[6] The addition of supplemental oxygen, increasing the PAO_2, has minimal effect on improving the hypoxemia, as the shunted blood is not exposed to the high alveolar Po_2.

Diffusion of oxygen between the alveolus and capillary blood can be altered by thickening of the alveolar-capillary barrier, by decreased alveolar capillary volume, or increased oxygen extraction. Further, decreasing the PAO_2 at high altitude decreases the alveolar-capillary Po_2 pressure gradient, limiting diffusion. Diffusion impairment is a rare primary cause of hypoxemia in children, although it can contribute to the hypoxemia associated with shunt and V/Q mismatching. More than 50% of the diffusion capacity of the lung must be compromised to develop hypoxemia from primary diffusion limitation. Supplemental oxygen can rapidly overcome hypoxemia associated with diffusion limitations.

Ventilation

Exchange of CO_2 follows similar physiologic principles to O_2. Because of differences in the solubility, dissociation curves of CO_2 and O_2, as well as the way each gas effects central ventilatory control, CO_2 exchange (and invariably $PaCO_2$) is ultimately determined by alveolar minute ventilation and the degree of dead space present. $PaCO_2$ is related to the balance between the production of CO_2 (VCO_2), which is a function of the metabolic conditions of the patient, and the alveolar minute ventilation (V_A), as described by the equation:

$$P_{ACO_2} = VCO_2 * K/V_A$$

Minute ventilation is determined by the product of the respiratory frequency (f) and the tidal volume (V_t). Dead space gas, both anatomic (in the conducting airways) and physiologic (areas of ventilation lung units that are poorly perfused; V>Q), does not participate in CO_2 elimination. Therefore, total alveolar ventilation is determined by the difference between total minute ventilation (V_E) and the degree of dead space ventilation (V_D):

$$V_A = V_E - V_D$$

As a result, elevations in $PaCO_2$ will result from conditions of decreased tidal volume or increased physiologic dead space (**Table 2**). Ventilatory muscles generally can maintain adequate tidal volumes with only 50% of normal strength.[7] Hyperinflation further compromises respiratory muscle function. Diseases associated with airway obstruction increase the end expiratory lung volume greater than functional residual capacity (FRC), decreasing muscle fiber length below what is optimal. Muscle fibers generate less force at these shorter lengths.[8] Similarly, hyperinflation causes a flattening of the diaphragm, putting it at a mechanical disadvantage.

V/Q mismatching generally does not cause a direct increase in P_{CO_2} because elevated CO2 from low V/Q units is a potent stimulator of the central respiratory centers, increasing alveolar minute ventilation.[3]

EPIDEMIOLOGY

As a common end point to multiple clinical conditions, the incidence of respiratory failure in the pediatric population is difficult to ascertain. In one study, 17.1% of patients admitted to a PICU at several large children's hospitals required mechanical ventilation, with acute respiratory conditions as the culprit in 62.4% of these patients. In this cohort of patients, bronchiolitis (26.7%) and pneumonia (15.8%) were the leading etiologies for respiratory failure.[9]

Acute lung injury (ALI) accounts for 12.8 cases per 100,000 person years, with an in-hospital mortality rate of 18% to 22%[10,11]; 10% of intubated children admitted to a European PICU had ALI, with a mortality rate of 27%. Of the patients with ALI, 54% had ARDS at presentation and 80% progressed to ARDS at some point during their hospitalization.[12]

Bronchiolitis, both respiratory syncytial virus (RSV) and non-RSV, accounts for up to 16% of all hospital admissions, with RSV bearing responsibility for 1 of every 334 hospitalizations.[13,14] From 7.4% to 28.0% of children with bronchiolitis require mechanical ventilation. The burden of RSV is more severe at younger age and in patients with chronic disease. Of all RSV admissions, for both bronchiolitis and pneumonia, 4% require intubation and mechanical ventilation.[15]

Table 2
Causes of hypercarbia

Decreased Tidal Volume	Increased Dead Space

Sedative overdose:
• Opioid
• Benzodiazepine
	Hyperinflation
	• Obstructive airway disease
	  ○ Asthma
	  ○ Bronchiolitis
	  ○ Cystic fibrosis
	• Excessive PEEP on mechanical ventilator

Neuromuscular weakness • Central nervous system disease • Spinal cord injury/inflammation • Peripheral nerve disorder • Neuromuscular junction disease • Myopathy • Metabolic derangements	Decreased cardiac output • Dehydration • Dysrhythmia • Myocarditis/cardiomyopathy • Post cardiopulmonary bypass
Flail chest (post trauma)	Increased pulmonary vascular resistance
	Pulmonary embolism

Respiratory failure in asthmatic individuals has declined over time, as novel therapies have emerged. Current intubation rates vary widely for asthmatic patients, from 5% to 17% based on presentation to a community hospital or tertiary care center, with a higher rate for those presenting to community hospitals.[16]

MONITORING

Monitoring respiratory function appropriately will help identify the development of respiratory failure as well as guide therapy based on response, and can predict outcome.[17] The fundamental and most important assessment of respiratory function is the clinical examination. Respiratory rate and pattern are indicative of the physiologic status of the respiratory system. Tachypnea is often the first sign of respiratory compromise.[18,19] Dys-coordinate, paradoxic movement of the chest during breathing is evidence of impending respiratory failure and requires immediate attention.[20] Infants and young children may present with grunting in an attempt to increase their positive end-expiratory pressure and maintain functional residual capacity, indicating the presence of restrictive lung disease.[21] Cyanosis is evident when greater than 3 to 5 g/dL of deoxygenated hemoglobin is present in arterial blood. This correlates with an arterial saturation of 80% in healthy individuals, but is unreliable in conditions of anemia, or in the presence of abnormal forms of hemoglobin, such as methemoglobin or carboxyhemoglobin.

Traditionally, adequacy of gas exchange has been monitored by invasive means, in particular blood gas analysis. The arterial blood gas (ABG) is the gold standard for Po_2 determination, as it reliably measures Po_2 directly. The percent oxyhemoglobin saturation from a blood gas is highly unreliable, as it is a calculated value based on temperature, $PaCO_2$, pH, and PaO_2. Free-flowing capillary blood can accurately assess pH and $PaCO_2$.[22–25] Peripheral venous samples are unreliable for estimating pH or $PaCO_2$,[22,26,27] and should be avoided for clinical decisions regarding ventilation.

Since the 1980s, noninvasive monitoring of oxygenation has been available in the form of pulse oximetry (SpO_2). Pulse oximeters are accurate when oxyhemoglobin concentrations are greater than 60%, but may not be reliable in conditions of poor perfusion (ie, septic shock), peripheral vasoconstriction (ie, norepinephrine), hypothermia, peripheral edema, significant extremity movement, or in the presence of methemoglobin or carboxyhemoglobin. Other important clinical data can be interpreted by the pulse oximeter as well, such as heart rate, rhythm, and peripheral perfusion.[28,29] The presence of pulsus paradoxus, indicated by respiratory variability in the pulse oximeter plethysmography tracing, correlates with important upper airway obstruction (eg, croup), as well as degree of lower airway obstruction (eg, asthma), and offers a continuous and accurate evaluation of response to therapy (**Fig. 1**).[30,31] Pediatric intensivists frequently substitute pulse oximetry for arterial catheters while caring for critically ill children with respiratory failure, with management decisions and outcomes remaining equal.[32]

Similarly, ventilation can be monitored continuously and noninvasively. Capnography monitors detect CO_2 levels, determined by its unique infrared light absorption characteristics. Capnography can be used at the end of the endotracheal tube in intubated patients or in nonintubated patients by nasal cannula during procedural sedation to assess the quality of ventilation.[33–35] **Table 3** lists the many clinical uses of capnography waveforms (**Fig. 2**). Generally, end-tidal CO_2 (ETCO2) is about 1 to 3 mm Hg lower than $PaCO_2$ in healthy individuals owing to physiologic dead space ventilation. In fact, the difference between the ETCO2 and $PaCO_2$ directly correlates

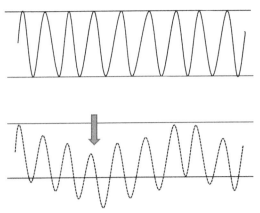

Fig. 1. Pulse oximeter waveforms. *Solid line*: normal. *Broken line*: evidence of pulsus para-doxus. Arrow indicates inspiration and concordant decrease in peak of plethysmography tracing, indicating cardiovascular consequence of increased work of breathing, generating a more negative intrapleural pressure. This can be seen in upper airway obstruction (ie, infectious croup, postextubation) or lower airway obstruction (ie, asthma) and improves with appropriate therapy.

with the degree of dead space present, and can be used to estimate dead space ventilation according to the Bohr equation:

$$V_D/V_T = (P_{ACO_2} - P_ECO_2)/P_{ACO_2}$$

Therefore, continuous capnography can be used to detect alterations in dead space ventilation and response to therapeutic interventions.

Severe respiratory illness, such as ALI or ARDS, has traditionally been monitored and defined based on the severity of hypoxemia according to invasive measurements of PaO_2.[36] See **Box 2** for diagnostic criteria for ALI/ARDS. The severity of hypoxemia has been determined by the ratio of PaO_2 to the fraction of inspired oxygen (PaO_2/Fio_2). The oxygenation index (OI) is commonly used as a superior indication of oxygenation impairment, as it takes into account the level of ventilatory support provided ($[OI = Fio_2 *$ mean airway pressure]$/PaO_2$). Unlike in adults, the degree of hypoxemia in children is associated with mortality,[1,11,37–40] length of mechanical ventilation,[38,39] and the

Table 3	
Clinical conditions determined by use of capnography	
Increase in ETCO2	**Decrease in ETCO2**
Hypoventilation	Unplanned extubation
Administration of sodium bicarbonate	Endotracheal tube obstruction
Increase in cardiac output	Ventilator disconnection
	Increased dead space
	Pulmonary embolism
	Decreased cardiac output

Continuous capnography also allows for accurate evaluation of respiratory rate, rhythm, and patient-ventilator asynchrony.
Abbreviation: ETCO2, end-tidal carbon dioxide.

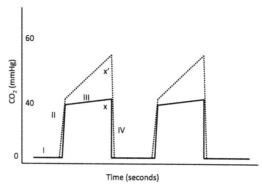

Time (seconds)

Fig. 2. Capnograph (time-based). *Solid line*: normal. Phase I: dead space (anatomic) gas exhaled from conducing airways; CO_2 content near zero. Phase II: mixing of alveolar gas, which contains CO_2. Phase III: plateau phase corresponds to pure alveolar gas. Phase IV: rapid fall due to inspiration, with negligible CO_2. x and x': ETCO2. *Dotted line*: obstructed airway disease. Phase III slopes upward because of delay in emptying of alveolar gas from different lung units owing to increased airway resistance. The upsloping directly correlates with degree of obstruction, and improves with response to bronchodilator therapy. (*Data from* Krauss B, Deykin A, Lam A, et al. Capnogram shape in obstructive lung disease. Anesth Analg 2005;100(3):884–8; and Yaron M, Padyk P, Hutsinpiller M, et al. Utility of the expiratory capnogram in the assessment of bronchospasm. Ann Emerg Med 1996;28(4):403–7.)

development of chronic lung disease in neonates.[41] A significant proportion of children with acute hypoxemic respiratory failure are managed without arterial lines, and therefore cannot be classified as ALI/ARDS.[32] Noninvasive correlates of severity of hypoxemia have now been established, as the definition of ALI/ARDS is being reconsidered. The SpO_2/FiO_2 ratio (substituting SpO_2 for PaO_2), as well as the OSI (oxygen saturation index, substituting SpO_2 for PaO_2) are gaining specific attention as validated measures of hypoxemia.[42–44] Further, with the use of noninvasive measures, up to 35% more patients could be captured for pediatric studies of ALI.[32]

THERAPY

Specific aspects of the therapy for respiratory failure vary depending on the underlying cause. In all cases, however, the goal of therapy is to supplement the patient's

---

Box 2
Consensus criteria for definition of acute lung injury or acute respiratory distress syndrome

Acute onset

Bilateral infiltrates on chest radiograph

Severe hypoxemia resistant to oxygen therapy

- PaO_2/FiO_2 ratio ≤ 200 torr (≤ 26.6 kPa) for ARDS
- PaO_2/FiO_2 ratio ≤ 300 torr (≤ 40 kPa) for ALI

No evidence of left atrial hypertension

- Pulmonary artery occlusion pressure <18

Data from Bernard GR, Artigas A, Brigham KL et al. The American-European Consensus Conference on ARDS. Definitions, mechanisms, relevant outcomes, and clinical trial coordination. Am J Respir Crit Care Med 1994;149(3):818–24.

gas exchange. Initial measures should include steps to ensure airway patency and clearance. Supplemental oxygen may be administered via facemask or nasal cannula.

The use of noninvasive positive pressure ventilation (NPPV), in the form of continuous positive airway pressure (CPAP) or bilevel positive airway pressure (BiPAP), has gained widespread acceptance as a therapy for respiratory failure from a variety of etiologies.[45–50] NPPV may supplement respiratory mechanics by unloading the respiratory musculature, stabilizing the chest wall, and improving minute ventilation. The recruitment of atelectatic alveolar units and improved clearance of intra-alveolar fluid augment end expiratory lung volume, approaching FRC, and decrease the A-a gradient.[47]

A number of disadvantages are intrinsic to NPPV that limit its utility. The risk of aspiration is significant; therefore, enteral feeding is generally avoided, and gastric decompression may be considered prophylactically. Patients, particularly those with developmental or cognitive impairments, may experience substantial anxiety with the placement of the BiPAP mask, risking proper positioning and function. Although small doses of anxiolytics may be administered, caution must be taken when providing respiratory depressants to patients with a native airway and impaired pulmonary function.[47]

ALI/ARDS

The mainstay of therapy in the most severe forms of acute hypoxemic respiratory failure is intubation and mechanical ventilation. The goal of mechanical ventilation in this group of patients is to provide adequate gas exchange while avoiding ventilator-associated secondary lung injury (VILI). Ventilation with high volumes and pressures, cyclic opening and closing of alveoli, and delivery of high Fio_2 result in a proinflammatory cascade causing lung injury and pulmonary edema.[51] By using a "lung-protective" strategy using low tidal volumes of 6 to 8 mL/kg and limiting plateau pressure to 30 or less, secondary lung injury may be curtailed. This approach necessitates decrease in minute ventilation, with a concomitant respiratory acidosis. Usual targets include a pH of 7.25 or higher, with a Pco_2 of 60 to 80 torr, and oxygen saturation goals of 88% or greater. Adult data have demonstrated significant improvement in mortality with this approach.[51] Although no large-scale pediatric studies have been performed to date, this approach has gained widespread acceptance,[4,52] with similar benefit noted in retrospective studies.[53]

Another approach to "lung protective ventilation," or "'open lung strategy," is high-frequency oscillatory ventilation (HFOV). HFOV allows for increased mean airway pressure with decreased peak airway pressure, facilitating recruitment of atelectatic lung segments, while avoiding the cyclic shearing open and subsequent alveolar collapse, decreasing the risk of VILI. Over the past 20 years, HFOV has been used extensively in the pediatric population; however, definitive data demonstrating clear clinical benefit versus low tidal volume conventional ventilation are lacking.[54]

Prone positioning has been suggested as an adjunctive therapy to ventilator management. The prone position improves recruitment and clearance of alveolar debris in dependent lung segments. Studies have documented an improvement in oxygenation in the prone position, but have failed to demonstrate improvements in ventilator-free days or survival.[55–57] A recent meta-analysis found that prone positioning may reduce the relative risk of mortality in patients with PaO_2/Fio_2 ratios of less than 100 mm Hg by 16%, although it was associated with increased risk of pressure ulcers, endotracheal tube obstruction, and chest tube dislodgement.[58] As such, prone positioning may be considered in those patients with the most severe ARDS, although careful consideration of the risks and benefits must be taken.

Another adjunctive therapy used in ARDS is inhaled nitric oxide (iNO). A potent, locally acting pulmonary vasodilator, the aim of therapy is to overcome regional hypoxic vasoconstriction and improve V/Q matching and oxygenation. Studies have demonstrated an initial, albeit transient, improvement in oxygenation; however, no improvement in clinically relevant outcomes, such as ventilator-free days or survival,[59] has been identified.

Qualitative and quantitative surfactant deficiencies occur in ARDS because of intra-alveolar edema and inflammatory mediators, as well as impaired production, resulting in impaired pulmonary compliance.[60] Replacement of surfactant in neonates with meconium aspiration syndrome is well documented to result in improved pulmonary mechanics and survival, and serves as the rational basis for studies in pediatrics.[61] Pediatric studies have demonstrated an improvement in oxygenation, ventilator-free days, and survival.[60,62] Specifically, benefit was identified in patients with ARDS secondary to direct lung injury,[60] although power was lacking to make definitive recommendations for its use. Ongoing clinical trials are further exploring the utility of this therapy.

Corticosteroids have been used for ARDS in an attempt to attenuate the inflammatory process responsible for the syndrome. Although some studies have documented an improvement in survival, others have failed to show benefit, with the indication that steroids started after 14 days of the disease process may worsen survival.[63,64] As such, the use of steroids for ARDS remains a controversial therapy at this time.

As previously described, fluid overload has a significant detrimental role on the physiology and outcome of adults and children with ALI,[1,40,65–67] specifically when greater than 10% to 15%.[1,66] No rigorous clinical trial has attempted to replicate the 2006 ARDSNet fluid management trial[65] in children. Nonetheless, conservative fluid management while ensuring adequate cardiac output is a common strategy in patients with ALI.[52]

The use of paralytic agents in patients with ARDS has recently shown promise. The judicious use of neuromuscular blockade has been used to improve patient-ventilator synchrony, although concerns about prolonged muscle weakness have persisted. In an adult study, the use of cisatricurium within 48 hours of ARDS onset was demonstrated to improve adjusted 90-day mortality and time off the ventilator, without an increased incidence of muscle weakness.[68] No pediatric data currently exist to guide the use of neuromuscular blocking agents in respiratory failure.

Asthma

The mechanics of respiratory failure due to asthma and other obstructive pulmonary processes are different than those related to ARDS and pneumonia, and require different management strategies. As previously described, obstructive lung disease results in air trapping and an increase in end expiratory lung volume over FRC, resulting in increased intrinsic pulmonary pressure at end expiration, termed auto-PEEP. This places the respiratory system at a mechanical disadvantage, in the face of increased work of breathing required to initiate inspiration (to overcome the auto-PEEP) as well as to overcome the resistance to airflow.

The act of intubation and initiation of positive pressure ventilation in a patient with high levels of auto-PEEP bears additional risks, such as barotrauma and resultant air leak syndrome. Adding positive pressure can further impair venous return to the heart, which can result in compromised cardiac output and cardiac arrest. Significant efforts are therefore made to prevent intubation of asthmatic patients. These include anti-inflammatory therapy with steroids, and bronchodilation with inhaled or intravenous β-agonists. Other acute asthma adjuncts include magnesium, anticholinergics, and methylxanthines. In-depth discussion on these therapies is beyond the scope of this article.

The use of BiPAP has been advocated as a safe and effective way to realize some of the benefits of positive pressure ventilation on the sick asthmatic patient without some of the risks inherent in endotracheal intubation.[49,69,70] By providing assistance to inspiratory flow, BiPAP can help unload the respiratory muscles and decrease work of breathing. Perhaps more importantly, the PEEP maintained at end exhalation stents the small airways open, reducing airway collapse due to elevated intrathoracic pressures and dynamic compression, and relieves hyperinflation. Further, PEEP decreases the amount of negative intrathoracic pressure required to initiate a breath, reducing the work of breathing.[71]

Helium-oxygen (heliox) gas mixture may be considered for severe asthma. Helium is less dense than air, reducing the Reynolds number, improves laminar flow to and from obstructed airways, and may help in delivery of aerosolized particles to the distal airways.[71,72] Heliox is available in concentrations ranging from 80%: 20% to 60%: 40% helium: oxygen, with the highest benefit derived from the highest helium concentration. Heliox has been used to drive albuterol nebulization, and can be blended into BiPAP and ventilator circuits. Limited studies have failed to show consistent benefit with the use of heliox, with the suggestion of benefit in the most severe patients.[71–73] More rigorous study is indicated before heliox can be routinely recommended for asthmatic individuals with respiratory failure.

Intubation and mechanical ventilation may be required in patients who fail noninvasive therapy. The general approach most frequently advocated is a prolonged exhalatory phase, targeted to allow complete exhalation and reversal of the dynamic hyperinflation. Monitoring should ensure that a complete exhalation has taken place before the next ventilator breath is delivered, preventing worsening dynamic hyperinflation, compromising gas exchange and cardiac function further. This requires low respiratory rates with limitation of minute ventilation and accepting a concomitant respiratory acidosis. A pH above 7.20 and $PaCO_2$ below 90 are generally accepted goals.[74,75] Volume control modes of ventilation offer a fixed tidal volume in patients with dynamic changes in airway resistance, whose delivered volumes in pressure control modes may vary significantly from breath to breath.

The role of PEEP for mechanically ventilated asthmatic individuals is controversial. The use of PEEP may help overcome increased respiratory effort needed to overcome auto-PEEP in the spontaneously breathing patient. In addition, PEEP may assist in stenting open distal airways during exhalation, preventing dynamic collapse during exhalation; however, PEEP itself provides an obstruction to exhalatory flow, with the potential to worsen intrinsic air trapping.[74–76]

Another approach to the intubated asthmatic individual is the use of pressure support ventilation. Pressure support assistance during inspiration helps overcome the resistance to airflow and decreases work of breathing. The patient determines the rate, inspiratory and expiratory times, and flow pattern. High levels of PEEP are applied to match the intrinsic PEEP created by the air trapping, titrated to the clinical assessment of the patient's work of breathing. By remaining unparalyzed, the patient contributes to the reversal of hyperinflation with active exhalation. Although only case reports on this approach are published to date, the possibility of minimizing the use of paralytics in patients already at risk of muscle weakness caused by corticosteroid use is attractive and bears further investigation.[77]

Bronchiolitis

Bronchiolitis is the result of airway inflammation, with subsequent secretions and cellular debris, resulting in obstructive pulmonary disease. As a viral process, there is no specific therapy and treatment is supportive. Multiple pharmacologic interventions, including β-2 agonists, racemic epinephrine, and corticosteroids, have been studied without convincing evidence of their efficacy.[78] Nasal CPAP is frequently used for respiratory support in the sick individual with bronchiolitis. High-flow nasal cannula appears to be a potential alternative, although further study is warranted.[79] If unresponsive to noninvasive therapy, intubation and pulmonary support while allowing for lung recovery is indicated.

It is important to differentiate RSV bronchiolitis from RSV pneumonia, which tends have a more prolonged course with greater lung injury.[80] Those with RSV pneumonia frequently meet ALI and ARDS criteria, and therapy is directed in that manner.

Extracorporeal Membrane Oxygenation

Extracorporeal membrane oxygenation (ECMO) has been used for cases of refractory respiratory and cardiorespiratory failure since its widespread deployment in the late 1970s and early 1980s. Overall survival is 57% in pediatric patients (30 days to 18 years old), with wide variation based on diagnosis, ranging from 39% (pertussis) to 83% (asthma).[81] As ECMO circuits have become more compact and easier to manage, and greater expertise has been developed, ECMO has been offered to more complex patients. Patients can be considered eligible candidates even after prolonged mechanical ventilation for longer than 14 days.[82] Nevertheless, ECMO remains a highly invasive, costly, labor-intensive therapy that can be used only in centers experienced in its use.

PROGNOSIS AND OUTCOME

Overall, the mortality from ALI is relatively high (22%–27%) compared with the general PICU population, although lower than in adults (35%–45%).[37,83] Fortunately, mortality for ALI continues to improve in children, recently reported as low as 8%,[56] although higher for recipients of stem cell transplantation.[84] Interestingly, children with ARDS secondary to RSV have a significantly lower mortality rate of approximately 5% compared with ARDS from other causes.[80] The degree of hypoxemia, as described by PaO_2/Fio_2 ratio, SaO_2/Fio_2 ratio, OI, or OSI, and alveolar dead space fraction ($PaCO_2$-$PETCO_2/PaCO_2$), is associated with increased risk of death.[11,42,43,83] The presence of central nervous system (CNS) dysfunction and non-CNS organ dysfunction are also associated with an increased risk of mortality.[37]

Although the prevalence of asthma in the pediatric population has increased in recent years, the outcome in even those with respiratory failure is generally good. The rate of invasive mechanical ventilation ranges from 3% to 47%, with an overall mortality rate of 7% to 8%.[85,86] Most are intubated outside the PICU (56%), with those intubated in the PICU requiring longer durations of mechanical ventilation.

Survivors of acute hypoxemia respiratory failure have risk for both restrictive and obstructive lung disease,[12,87–91] similar to adult survivors. Although most children will have physiologic evidence of obstructive or restrictive disease after discharge from the hospital, pulmonary function continues to recover over the first year after the acute illness.[89] Little improvement is seen subsequently, and evidence of altered pulmonary function persists.[88] Subjectively, though, many will have complete functional recovery,[88,91] although bronchodilators may be needed during exercise or an intercurrent viral illness.

Outcome reports vary, likely related to the timing of the follow-up. It has been suggested that patient evaluations should occur 6 to 12 months after the acute illness, after which any significant recovery of pulmonary function is unlikely.[89,92–94]

REFERENCES

1. Arikan AA, Zappitelli M, Goldstein SL, et al. Fluid overload is associated with impaired oxygenation and morbidity in critically ill children. Pediatr Crit Care Med 2012;13(3):253.
2. WHO. World Health Statistics 2012: part III global health indicators. WHO; 2012. Available at: http://www.who.int/gho/publications/world_health_statistics/2012.
3. West JB. Respiratory physiology the essentials. Baltimore, MD: Lippincott Williams & Wilkins; 2008.
4. Turi JL, Cheifetz IM. Acute respiratory failure. Resuscitation and stabilization of the critically ill child. London: Springer; 2009. p. 1–9.
5. McFadden E Jr, Lyons HA. Arterial-blood gas tension in asthma. N Engl J Med 1968;278(19):1027.
6. Powell F, Heldt G, Haddad G. Respiratory physiology. In: David N, editor. Anonymous. Philadelphia: Lippincott Williams &Wilkins; 2008. p. 631.
7. Braun N, Arora NS, Rochester DF. Respiratory muscle and pulmonary function in polymyositis and other proximal myopathies. Thorax 1983;38(8):616–23.
8. Roussos C, Macklem PT. The respiratory muscles. N Engl J Med 1982;307(13): 786–97.
9. Randolph AG, Meert KL, O'Neil ME, et al. The feasibility of conducting clinical trials in infants and children with acute respiratory failure. Am J Respir Crit Care Med 2003;167(10):1334–40.
10. Zimmerman JJ, Akhtar SR, Caldwell E, et al. Incidence and outcomes of pediatric acute lung injury. Pediatrics 2009;124(1):87–95.
11. Flori HR, Glidden DV, Rutherford GW, et al. Pediatric acute lung injury. Am J Respir Crit Care Med 2005;171(9):995–1001.
12. Dahlem P, Van Aalderen W, Hamaker M, et al. Incidence and short-term outcome of acute lung injury in mechanically ventilated children. Eur Respir J 2003;22(6): 980–5.
13. Shay DK, Holman RC, Newman RD, et al. Bronchiolitis-associated hospitalizations among US children, 1980-1996. JAMA 1999;282(15):1440–6.
14. Hall CB, Weinberg GA, Iwane MK, et al. The burden of respiratory syncytial virus infection in young children. N Engl J Med 2009;360(6):588–98.
15. Stockman LJ, Curns AT, Anderson LJ, et al. Respiratory syncytial virus-associated hospitalizations among infants and young children in the United States, 1997–2006. Pediatr Infect Dis J 2012;31(1):5.
16. Carroll CL, Smith SR, Collins MS, et al. Endotracheal intubation and pediatric status asthmaticus: site of original care affects treatment. Pediatr Crit Care Med 2007;8(2):91.
17. Weil M. Patient evaluation, "vital signs," and initial care. Critical Care: state of the art, Fullerton. In: Shoemaker WC, Thompson WL, editors. Soc Crit Care Med 1980;1(1).
18. Gravelyn TR, Weg JG. Respiratory rate as an indicator of acute respiratory dysfunction. JAMA 1980;244(10):1123–5.
19. Cretikos MA, Bellomo R, Hillman K, et al. Respiratory rate: the neglected vital sign. Med J Aust 2008;188(11):657.
20. Tobin MJ, Perez W, Guenther SM, et al. Does rib cage-abdominal paradox signify respiratory muscle fatigue? J Appl Physiol 1987;63(2):851–60.

21. Harrison V, Heese HV, Klein M. The significance of grunting in hyaline membrane disease. Pediatrics 1968;41(3):549–59.
22. Kirubakaran C, Gnananayagam JE, Sundaravalli EK. Comparison of blood gas values in arterial and venous blood. Indian J Pediatr 2003;70(10):781–5.
23. Khemani RG, Bart RD, Newth CJ. Respiratory monitoring during mechanical ventilation. Paediatr Child Health 2007;17(5):193–201.
24. Yıldızdaş D, Yapıcıoğlu H, Yılmaz H, et al. Correlation of simultaneously obtained capillary, venous, and arterial blood gases of patients in a paediatric intensive care unit. Arch Dis Child 2004;89(2):176–80.
25. Harrison AM, Lynch JM, Dean JM, et al. Comparison of simultaneously obtained arterial and capillary blood gases in pediatric intensive care unit patients. Crit Care Med 1997;25(11):1904–8.
26. Courtney SE, Weber KR, Breakie LA, et al. Capillary blood gases in the neonate: a reassessment and review of the literature. Arch Pediatr Adolesc Med 1990; 144(2):168.
27. Bilan N, Behbahan AG, Khosroshahi A. Validity of venous blood gas analysis for diagnosis of acid-base imbalance in children admitted to pediatric intensive care unit. World J Pediatr 2008;4(2):114–7.
28. Lima AP, Beelen P, Bakker J. Use of a peripheral perfusion index derived from the pulse oximetry signal as a noninvasive indicator of perfusion. Crit Care Med 2002; 30(6):1210–3.
29. Felice C, Latini G, Vacca P, et al. The pulse oximeter perfusion index as a predictor for high illness severity in neonates. Eur J Pediatr 2002;161(10):561–2.
30. Knowles G, Clark T. Pulsus paradoxus as a valuable sign indicating severity of asthma. Lancet 1973;302(7842):1356–9.
31. Hartert TV, Wheeler AP, Sheller JR. Use of pulse oximetry to recognize severity of airflow obstruction in obstructive airway disease: correlation with pulsus paradoxus. Chest 1999;115(2):475–81.
32. Khemani RG, Markovitz BP, Curley MA. Characteristics of children intubated and mechanically ventilated in 16 PICUs. Chest 2009;136(3):765–71.
33. Tobias JD, Flanagan JFK, Wheeler TJ, et al. Noninvasive monitoring of end-tidal CO_2 via nasal cannulas in spontaneously breathing children during the perioperative period. Crit Care Med 1994;22(11):1805.
34. Hart LS, Berns SD, Houck CS, et al. The value of end-tidal CO_2 monitoring when comparing three methods of conscious sedation for children undergoing painful procedures in the emergency department. Pediatr Emerg Care 1997; 13(3):189–93.
35. Miner JR, Heegaard W, Plummer D. End-tidal carbon dioxide monitoring during procedural sedation. Acad Emerg Med 2002;9(4):275–80.
36. Bernard GR, Artigas A, Brigham KL, et al. Report of the American-European Consensus conference on acute respiratory distress syndrome: definitions, mechanisms, relevant outcomes, and clinical trial coordination. J Crit Care 1994;9(1):72–81.
37. Seeley E, McAuley DF, Eisner M, et al. Predictors of mortality in acute lung injury during the era of lung protective ventilation. Thorax 2008;63(11):994–8.
38. Trachsel D, McCrindle BW, Nakagawa S, et al. Oxygenation index predicts outcome in children with acute hypoxemic respiratory failure. Am J Respir Crit Care Med 2005;172(2):206–11.
39. Erickson S, Schibler A, Numa A, et al. Acute lung injury in pediatric intensive care in Australia and New Zealand-A prospective, multicenter, observational study. Pediatr Crit Care Med 2007;8(4):317–23.

40. Flori HR, Church G, Liu KD, et al. Positive fluid balance is associated with higher mortality and prolonged mechanical ventilation in pediatric patients with acute lung injury. Crit Care Res Pract 2011;2011:854142.
41. Bayrakci B, Josephson C, Fackler J. Oxygenation index for extracorporeal membrane oxygenation: is there predictive significance? J Artif Organs 2007; 10(1):6–9.
42. Thomas NJ, Shaffer ML, Willson DF, et al. Defining acute lung disease in children with the oxygenation saturation index. Pediatr Crit Care Med 2010;11(1):12.
43. Khemani RG, Thomas NJ, Venkatachalam V, et al. Comparison of SpO2 to PaO2 based markers of lung disease severity for children with acute lung injury. Crit Care Med 2012;40(4):1309.
44. Rice TW, Wheeler AP, Bernard GR, et al. Comparison of the SpO2/FIO2 ratio and the PaO2/FIO2 ratio in patients with acute lung injury or ARDS. Chest 2007; 132(2):410–7.
45. Bernet V, Hug MI, Frey B. Predictive factors for the success of noninvasive mask ventilation in infants and children with acute respiratory failure. Pediatr Crit Care Med 2005;6(6):660.
46. Kramer N, Meyer TJ, Meharg J, et al. Randomized, prospective trial of noninvasive positive pressure ventilation in acute respiratory failure. Am J Respir Crit Care Med 1995;151(6):1799–806.
47. Teague WG. Noninvasive ventilation in the pediatric intensive care unit for children with acute respiratory failure. Pediatr Pulmonol 2003;35(6):418–26.
48. Fortenberry JD, Del Toro J, Jefferson LS, et al. Management of pediatric acute hypoxemic respiratory insufficiency with bilevel positive pressure (BiPAP) Nasal Mask Ventilation. Chest 1995;108(4):1059–64.
49. Carroll CL, Schramm CM. Noninvasive positive pressure ventilation for the treatment of status asthmaticus in children. Ann Allergy Asthma Immunol 2006;96(3): 454–9.
50. Birnkrant DJ, Pope JF, Eiben RM. Topical review: management of the respiratory complications of neuromuscular diseases in the pediatric intensive care unit. J Child Neurol 1999;14(3):139–43.
51. Ventilation with lower tidal volumes as compared with traditional tidal volumes for acute lung injury and the acute respiratory distress syndrome. N Engl J Med 2000;342(18):1301–8.
52. Randolph AG. Management of acute lung injury and acute respiratory distress syndrome in children. Crit Care Med 2009;37(8):2448–54.
53. Albuali WH, Singh RN, Fraser DD, et al. Have changes in ventilation practice improved outcome in children with acute lung injury? Pediatr Crit Care Med 2007;8(4):324–30.
54. Ventre KM, Arnold JH. High frequency oscillatory ventilation in acute respiratory failure. Paediatr Respir Rev 2004;5(4):323–32.
55. Relvas MS, Silver PC, Sagy M. Prone positioning of pediatric patients with ARDS results in improvement in oxygenation if maintained >12 h daily. Chest 2003; 124(1):269–74.
56. Curley MA, Hibberd PL, Fineman LD, et al. Effect of prone positioning on clinical outcomes in children with acute lung injury. JAMA 2005;294(2):229–37.
57. Gattinoni L, Tognoni G, Pesenti A, et al. Effect of prone positioning on the survival of patients with acute respiratory failure. N Engl J Med 2001;345(8):568–73.
58. Sud S, Friedrich JO, Taccone P, et al. Prone ventilation reduces mortality in patients with acute respiratory failure and severe hypoxemia: systematic review and meta-analysis. Intensive Care Med 2010;36(4):585–99.

59. Sokol J, Jacobs SE, Bohn D. Inhaled nitric oxide for acute hypoxic respiratory failure in children and adults: a meta-analysis. Anesth Analg 2003;97(4):989–98.
60. Willson DF, Thomas NJ, Markovitz BP, et al. Effect of exogenous surfactant (calfactant) in pediatric acute lung injury. JAMA 2005;293(4):470–6.
61. Seger N, Soll R. Animal derived surfactant extract for treatment of respiratory distress syndrome. Cochrane Database Syst Rev 2009;(2):CD007836.
62. Duffett M, Choong K, Ng V, et al. Surfactant therapy for acute respiratory failure in children: a systematic review and meta-analysis. Crit Care 2007;11(3):R66.
63. Meduri GU, Headley AS, Golden E, et al. Effect of prolonged methylprednisolone therapy in unresolving acute respiratory distress syndrome. JAMA 1998;280(2): 159–65.
64. Meduri GU, Marik PE, Chrousos GP, et al. Steroid treatment in ARDS: a critical appraisal of the ARDS network trial and the recent literature. Intensive Care Med 2008;34(1):61–9.
65. National Heart, Lung, and Blood Institute Acute Respiratory Distress Syndrome (ARDS) Clinical Trials Network, Wiedemann HP, Wheeler AP, Bernard GR, et al. Comparison of two fluid-management strategies in acute lung injury. N Engl J Med 2006;354(24):2564–75.
66. Foland JA, Fortenberry JD, Warshaw BL, et al. Fluid overload before continuous hemofiltration and survival in critically ill children: a retrospective analysis. Crit Care Med 2004;32(8):1771.
67. Upadya A, Tilluckdharry L, Muralidharan V, et al. Fluid balance and weaning outcomes. Intensive Care Med 2005;31(12):1643–7.
68. Papazian L, Forel J, Gacouin A, et al. Neuromuscular blockers in early acute respiratory distress syndrome. N Engl J Med 2010;363(12):1107–16.
69. Thill PJ, McGuire JK, Baden HP, et al. Noninvasive positive-pressure ventilation in children with lower airway obstruction. Pediatr Crit Care Med 2004;5(4):337.
70. Beers SL, Abramo TJ, Bracken A, et al. Bilevel positive airway pressure in the treatment of status asthmaticus in pediatrics. Am J Emerg Med 2007;25(1):6–9.
71. Levine DA. Novel therapies for children with severe asthma. Curr Opin Pediatr 2008;20(3):261–5.
72. Piva JP, Menna Barreto SS, Zelmanovitz F, et al. Heliox versus oxygen for nebulized aerosol therapy in children with lower airway obstruction. Pediatr Crit Care Med 2002;3(1):6.
73. Rodrigo G, Pollack C, Rodrigo C, et al. Heliox for nonintubated acute asthma patients. Cochrane Database Syst Rev 2006;(4):CD002884.
74. Leatherman JW, McArthur C, Shapiro RS. Effect of prolongation of expiratory time on dynamic hyperinflation in mechanically ventilated patients with severe asthma. Crit Care Med 2004;32(7):1542–5.
75. Stather DR, Stewart TE. Clinical review: mechanical ventilation in severe asthma. Crit Care 2005;9(6):581.
76. Oddo M, Feihl F, Schaller MD, et al. Management of mechanical ventilation in acute severe asthma: practical aspects. Intensive Care Med 2006;32(4):501–10.
77. Wetzel RC. Pressure-support ventilation in children with severe asthma. Crit Care Med 1996;24(9):1603.
78. Nagakumar P, Doull I. Current therapy for bronchiolitis. Arch Dis Child 2012;97(9): 827–30.
79. McKiernan C, Chua LC, Visintainer PF, et al. High flow nasal cannulae therapy in infants with bronchiolitis. J Pediatr 2010;156(4):634–8.
80. Hammer J, Numa A, Newth C. Acute respiratory distress syndrome caused by respiratory syncytial virus. Pediatr Pulmonol 1997;23(3):176–83.

81. Zabrocki LA, Brogan TV, Statler KD, et al. Extracorporeal membrane oxygenation for pediatric respiratory failure: survival and predictors of mortality. Crit Care Med 2011;39(2):364.

82. Domico MB, Ridout DA, Bronicki R, et al. The impact of mechanical ventilation time before initiation of extracorporeal life support on survival in pediatric respiratory failure: a review of the extracorporeal life support registry. Pediatr Crit Care Med 2012;13(1):16.

83. Ghuman AK, Newth CJL, Khemani RG. The association between the end tidal alveolar dead space fraction and mortality in pediatric acute hypoxemic respiratory failure. Pediatr Crit Care Med 2012;13(1):11.

84. DiCarlo JV, Alexander SR, Agarwal R, et al. Continuous veno-venous hemofiltration may improve survival from acute respiratory distress syndrome after bone marrow transplantation or chemotherapy. J Pediatr Hematol Oncol 2003;25(10):801.

85. Roberts JS, Bratton SL, Brogan TV. Acute severe asthma: differences in therapies and outcomes among pediatric intensive care units. Crit Care Med 2002;30(3):581.

86. Bratton SL, Newth CJL, Zuppa AF, et al. Critical care for pediatric asthma: wide care variability and challenges for study. Pediatr Crit Care Med 2012;13(4):407–14.

87. Knoester H, Grootenhuis MA, Bos AP. Outcome of paediatric intensive care survivors. Eur J Pediatr 2007;166(11):1119–28.

88. Weiss I, Ushay HM, DeBruin W, et al. Respiratory and cardiac function in children after acute hypoxemic respiratory failure. Crit Care Med 1996;24(1):148.

89. Golder N, Lane R, Tasker R. Timing of recovery of lung function after severe hypoxemic respiratory failure in children. Intensive Care Med 1998;24(5):530–3.

90. Fanconi S, Kraemer R, Weber J, et al. Long-term sequelae in children surviving adult respiratory distress syndrome. J Pediatr 1985;106(2):218–22.

91. Ben-Abraham R, Weinbroum AA, Roizin H, et al. Long-term assessment of pulmonary function tests in pediatric survivors of acute respiratory distress syndrome. Med Sci Monit 2002;8(3):CR153–7.

92. Ghio AJ, Elliott CG, Crapo RO, et al. Impairment after adult respiratory distress syndrome: an evaluation based on American Thoracic Society recommendations. Am J Respir Crit Care Med 1989;139(5):1158–62.

93. Hudson LD. What happens to survivors of the adult respiratory distress syndrome? Chest 1994;105(Suppl 3):123S–6S.

94. Dahlem P, Van Aalderen W, Bos A. Pediatric acute lung injury. Paediatr Respir Rev 2007;8(4):348–62.

Pediatric Postoperative Cardiac Care

George Ofori-Amanfo, MBChB*, Ira M. Cheifetz, MD, FCCM

KEYWORDS

- Congenital heart disease • Cardiac surgery • Cardiac output • Right ventricle
- Left ventricle • Pediatric • Neonatal • Cardiopulmonary bypass

KEY POINTS

- Postoperative care of cardiac patients requires a comprehensive and multidisciplinary approach to critically ill patients with cardiac disease whose care requires a clear understanding of cardiovascular physiology.
- Finely balanced multiorgan interaction maintained during health can be profoundly deranged in disease states.
- When a patient fails to progress along the projected course or decompensates acutely, prompt evaluation with bedside assessment, laboratory evaluation, and echocardiography is essential.
- When things do not add up, cardiac catheterization must be seriously considered. With continued advancements in the field of neonatal and pediatric postoperative cardiac care, continued improvements in overall outcomes for this specialized population are anticipated.

INTRODUCTION

Postoperative care of pediatric cardiac patients has evolved dramatically over the past 2 decades, with significant improvement in survival. These improvements are attributable, at least in part, to improvements in diagnostic modalities, surgical techniques, cardiopulmonary bypass (CPB) support, anesthetic management, postoperative care, and the use of extracorporeal life support to manage postoperative refractory shock.[1,2]

Despite an overall increase in complexity, mortality has decreased in both short-term and long-term follow-up.[3] Several factors have contributed to this improvement in outcome, including advances in prenatal and preoperative evaluation and diagnosis,[4,5] anesthetic and intraoperative management,[6] and standardized approaches to postoperative care.[7–9] For example, recent advances in the surgical and perioperative

Division of Pediatric Critical Care Medicine, Duke Children's Hospital, Duke University Medical Center, DUMC 3046, 2300 Erwin Road, Durham, NC 27710, USA
* Corresponding author.
E-mail address: george.ofori@duke.edu

Crit Care Clin 29 (2013) 185–202
http://dx.doi.org/10.1016/j.ccc.2013.01.003
0749-0704/13/$ – see front matter Published by Elsevier Inc.
criticalcare.theclinics.com

management of congenital heart disease in neonates have allowed early primary repair of cardiac lesions, such as tetralogy of Fallot, with results comparable to delayed repair.[10]

The growing implementation of multidisciplinary clinical care teams with expertise in cardiac surgery, critical care, cardiology, cardiac anesthesia, neonatology, electrophysiology, nursing, respiratory care, pharmacology, and nutritional support have had a positive impact on the care delivered to these complex patients. The development of these dedicated teams along with improved outcomes in premature and low-birth-weight infants have changed the demographics of patients managed in pediatric cardiac ICUs.[11]

Optimal postoperative care in the ICU requires an accurate preoperative assessment, use of intraoperative findings and data, careful patient risk stratification, and meticulous anticipatory management. When patients fail to progress along their predicted clinical course, prompt hands-on reassessment at the bedside is essential. In some cases, deviations from the predicted clinical course necessitate urgent cardiac catheterization and angiography for diagnostic and therapeutic purposes.

PREOPERATIVE ASSESSMENT

Preoperative assessment of pediatric patients with congenital heart disease is essential to optimal intraoperative and postoperative management. The goal of preoperative evaluation is to compile data in a systematic fashion to aid in the establishment of an accurate diagnosis, a determination of patient risk level, and a preliminary formulation of postoperative expectations.

Congenital heart defects can be complex. The preoperative data should be carefully collected, appropriately organized, and synthesized based on the underlying physiologic problems. Clinical assessment should focus on identifying factors that can be modified to optimize a patient's preoperative clinical status as well as those that could potentially affect the intraoperative and postoperative courses. The optimal approach to assessing patients with congenital heart disease is influenced by age category (ie, neonate or non-neonate) and underlying physiology (ie, pulmonary overcirculation, impaired systemic output, impaired pulmonary blood flow, or parallel circulations).

For neonatal severe congenital heart disease, infants may present from the delivery room with a prenatal diagnosis, may be transferred from another institution, or may present via an emergency department with cyanosis, respiratory distress, and/or circulatory collapse. In most cases, an intensivist has the opportunity to assess patients and develop an overall plan for postoperative management before surgery. The preoperative evaluation of these infants must focus on the clinical effects of the current physiology and the anticipated impact on intraoperative and postoperative courses.

The situation with non-neonates varies in that these children are often admitted from the operating room (OR) after an elective primary repair or staged palliation, and, thus, an intensivist may not have had the opportunity to meet and assess the patient preoperatively. The intensivist must gather and synthesize preexisting data from the cardiologist and cardiothoracic surgeon for risk stratification and guidance of the postoperative course. A comprehensive and systematic handoff from the OR team is essential to optimal postoperative care.

Pulmonary Overcirculation

Cardiac lesions associated with pulmonary overcirculation are marked by intracardiac (eg, atrial septal defect, ventricular septal defect [VSD], and atrioventricular [AV] septal defect) or extracardiac (eg, patent ductus arteriosus) left-to-right shunting. Infants with such lesions are generally acyanotic and their clinical presentation is one of excessive pulmonary blood flow and congestive heart failure. In this category of lesions, the pulmonary and systemic circulations are not ductus dependent, and these infants generally do not present an acute surgical emergency. Over time, however, they may develop frequent respiratory infections (especially viral) and failure to thrive.

Impaired Systemic Output

This group includes patients with obstructive left-sided heart lesions, such as critical aortic valve stenosis, critical coactation of the aorta, and hypoplastic left heart syndrome (HLHS). Systemic output depends on right-to-left shunting through a patent ductus arteriosus; hence, these neonates are prostaglandin (PGE) dependent. In the event of closure of the ductus arteriosus, these infants appear dusky and can rapidly develop acute circulatory shock due to lack of systemic output.

Aortic stenosis is one of the few congenital heart lesions that present as an acute surgical/interventional catheterization emergency. Critical aortic valve stenosis is only treatable by urgent relief of the obstruction, which, in most cases, can be accomplished by cardiac catheterization. In the situation of critical aortic valve stenosis, PGE infusion provides systemic blood flow; however, profound left ventricular (LV) hypertrophy and elevated LV end-diastolic pressure impede coronary perfusion, potentially resulting in poor LV function.

Impaired Pulmonary Blood Flow

Lesions in this category include pulmonary atresia or severe pulmonary stenosis. A PGE infusion is required to provide pulmonary blood flow. For infants with pulmonary atresia and an intact ventricular septum, cardiac catherization is usually required to define the coronary anatomy before determining a surgical plan.

Parallel Circulation

The prototype congenital heart lesion in this category is transposition of the great arteries. In this situation, the pulmonary circulation runs parallel to the systemic circulation. As such, the only means of delivering oxygenated blood to the systemic circulation is by intracardiac mixing. Inadequate mixing presents as profound cyanosis that may require an urgent balloon atrial septostomy.

HISTORY, PHYSICAL EXAMINATION, AND LABORATORY TESTING

Regardless of physiology and patient age, preoperative assessment requires a complete review of the cardiac and noncardiac history, a thorough physical examination, laboratory tests, ECGs, echocardiograms, and/or other cardiac imaging as available and clinically indicated, including cardiac catheterization, angiograms, and MRI. The critical care team must have an accurate understanding of the anatomic diagnoses and cardiac physiology as well as a clear outline of issues that are likely to have an impact on the postoperative course.

The history and physical examination should ascertain and assess each patient's cardiopulmonary status, including any comorbid conditions. A detailed review of systems, past medical history, and surgical history is necessary for appropriate risk stratification and planning for the postoperative period. A recent intercurrent illness, especially respiratory infection, can be a manifestation of chronic pulmonary overcirculation and can prolong postoperative mechanical ventilation and ICU length of stay. A history of clinically significant arrhythmias can be an additional risk factor for patients in the postoperative period. Although there are no data indicating that postoperative events repeat themselves, knowledge of events of prior surgeries, such as postoperative arrhythmia, chylous effusions, and unexplained pulmonary hypertensive crises, is important.

Genetic defects and syndromes/dysmorphisms may have important clinical implications for the perioperative course. For example, Down syndrome is associated with a significant risk of upper and lower airway anomalies, endocrinopathies, hematologic derangements, and immune deficiencies.[12–14] Patients with conotruncal anomalies may also have chromosome 22q11 deletion and its associated T-cell dysfunction and derangements in calcium metabolism.[15]

As a minimum, laboratory evaluation should include routine complete blood cell count and serum electrolytes. A high white blood cell count may indicate infection. The hemoglobin level may provide valuable information as to how well a patient is responding to chronic cyanosis, and an adequate platelet count is important for patients undergoing CPB. Electrolyte derangements and acid-base disturbances may be a reflection of the effects of preoperative medications, such as diuretics. Although these pieces of information are necessary for preparing patients for surgery, they may also have implications for the cardiac anesthesiologist. Additional laboratory tests, such as coagulation profile and liver function panels, may be dictated by a patient's clinical status and institutional practice.

Chest radiography is necessary to assess the cardiac silhouette and lung fields at baseline. An ECG is an important part of the preoperative evaluation to demonstrate a patient's cardiac rhythm as well as to assess conduction intervals, QRS duration, and T-wave morphology. ECGs may be helpful to identify the presence of subtle arrhythmias, such as first-degree or second-degree heart block.

Echocardiography and MRI

Echocardiography is an essential imaging tool in diagnosing congenital heart disease. Recent advances in technology, including Doppler measurements, 3-D echocardiography, and strain rate imaging, have enhanced the diagnostic accuracy and allowed prenatal diagnosis of cardiac disease as early as the first trimester of gestation.[16,17] In addition to the anatomic diagnoses, physiologic information can be inferred from an echocardiogram, but intensivists must be aware of the limitations of these data. For instance, right ventricular (RV) volume overload should be carefully assessed if the RV is compared with an underfilled LV. The RV pressure estimate from the jet of tricuspid regurgitation requires an optimal Doppler envelope and a fair estimate of right atrial (RA) pressure, because the number obtained is a pressure gradient between the RV and the RA. When assessing a pressure gradient across an obstruction via echocardiography, it must be remembered that the gradient is flow dependent. For example, the pressure gradient across the aortic valve is dependent on the stroke volume and myocardial contractility. Pressure gradients measured on the venous side of the cardiovascular system and at the interatrial level may be low yet have significant clinical implications.

Furthermore, echocardiography also has some limitations in assessing myocardial function. Although the assessment of ventricular systolic function using volumetric measurements of the LV is accurate, the complex geometry of the RV makes assessment of function challenging.[18]

In spite of the limitations, echocardiography indicates cardiac situs, intracardiac anatomy, myocardial function, AV and semilunar valve function, and anatomy of the great vessels. It also assesses the pulmonary and systemic venous systems and in the prenatal stage can be used in the diagnosis of arrhythmias. Echocardiography, transthoracic and/or transesophageal, is an essential tool throughout the perioperative period.

In recent years, MRI and magnetic resonance angiography have played an increasingly important role in the noninvasive evaluation of cardiac patients. Because most patients undergoing cardiac MRI have had prior echocardiograms, the cardiac MRI can be targeted and able to characterize the precise location and anatomic severity of primary cardiac lesions. Also identifiable are associated defects and the functional consequences of the primary lesions. For example, cardiac MRI can assess ejection fractions as an indicator of biventricular function. Thus, regurgitant fraction across valves and Qp:Qs in shunt lesions can be calculated.[19] CT scan with angiography can also be used in the preoperative evaluation, but its use has been limited by the high doses of radiation required and the increasing availability of MRI.

Cardiac Catheterization and Angiography

Due to advances in noninvasive imaging modalities, diagnostic cardiac catheterization is no longer indicated in the routine preoperative evaluation of most congenital heart defects. It is used in circumstances, however, in which the anatomy of the congenital heart disease is inadequately defined by noninvasive means or in cases where specific anatomic details or hemodynamic data, such as pulmonary vascular resistance (PVR), are necessary to optimize surgical management.[20] When cardiac catheterization has been performed, intensivists must know the hemodynamic data, in particular any information that may have an impact on a patient's physiology and postoperative course. For example, pulmonary venous desaturation may suggest the presence of lung disease. Qp:Qs may provide an objective measure of pulmonary overcirculation. Pulmonary hypertension can be more accurately measured and diastolic function can be better assessed using ventricular end-diastolic pressures.

POSTOPERATIVE PERIOD

The intensivist and other members of the critical care team assume the postoperative management after a patient has been successfully transitioned to the ICU environment. This transition includes full monitoring on the ICU (not transport) devices, appropriate support of the respiratory system without manual ventilation, and medication infusions administered via the appropriate ICU equipment. A systematic and comprehensive surgical and anesthesia handoff is essential to optimal patient management.

A comprehensive OR to ICU handoff should include patient history; airway and anesthetic management (including the most recent doses of anesthetic, paralytic, and antimicrobial agents); and detailed description of operative findings, the repair procedure, intraoperative complications, CPB time, cross-clamp time, deep hypothermic circulatory arrest time, presence of intraoperative arrhythmias, and current infusions (eg, vasoactive agents, inotropes, and sedatives/analgesics). Difficulties with airway management, such as a difficult intubation, and problems with myocardial protection must be clearly communicated to the ICU team. Specific cardiac data to be communicated from the conclusion of surgery include systemic arterial pressure, central venous pressure required to maintain a targeted systemic blood pressure, pulmonary arterial pressure, if measured, and systemic oxygen saturation. Vasoactive medication usage, arrhythmias, and atrial or ventricular pacing are also critical components of the handoff. The results of an intraoperative echocardiogram (generally transesophageal) should be reported, including the results of the repair, any known residual defects, and ventricular function. An example of a scripted postoperative handoff sheet is provided in **Fig. 1.**

Postoperative assessment requires a complete initial physical examination followed by regular, focused examinations dictated by a patient's clinical condition. Laboratory

Surgery/Procedure:

Induction...........................Intubation: Easy/difficult, Blade............... ETT........@.......

Lines: PIV........................ RA............... IJ.......... Art............ PICC............ Other CVL............

Times- CPB............... X-Clamp................ DHCA........... Regional cerebral perfusion............

Intra-operative Events and Interventions..

....

TEE:..

Medications

	Pre Transp Vitals
Epi...........Mil..........NiCardipine.............. Vasop.......... NitroGLYCErine............ Other............	HR..............
Fent.....................Morphine......................Midazolam.....................Precedex......................	RR.............. BP..............
Time of last: Neuromuscular blockade.................... Antibiotics................ Tylenol	CVP............
Intr-op Vol: Plasmanate........... Crystalloid........ PRBC................ Plt.................. FFP............	O₂Sat..........
Cryo................ aVII.................. Cell Saver/MUF ....Urine Output..................	Cereb O₂Sat ......
Last ACT...... Last ABG: pH...... PCO₂..... PO₂...... K...... Ca...... Lactate...... Hct....... BE.........	

Post-op Rhythm.............   Paced Y/N   Mode........................@........../min

Pacing Wires: Atrial................   Ventricular.................   Skin................

Vent Settings: PIP.............PEEP...............TV..............FiO₂..............

Chest Tubes: Mediastinal.............. Pleural CT (R)............. (L)............. PD Cath...........

Other...

Fig. 1. Example of a scripted postoperative handoff sheet from the OR to ICU for pediatric patients status postsurgery for congenital heart disease.

data include blood gas analyses, serum electrolytes and glucose, complete blood count, coagulation profile, serum lactate, chest radiograph, and a 12-lead or 15-lead ECG. Preoperative, intraoperative, and postoperative data should be used to determine a patient's risk level and to help direct the postoperative management plan.

The Risk Adjustment in Congenital Heart Surgery and the Aristotle basic complexity scoring systems have been used to evaluate risk of mortality, morbidity, and quality of care in patients undergoing congenital heart surgery.[19,21–23] Although these tools are relevant in the care of cardiac ICU patients, they are designed to describe populations of patients and not individual patients. The intensivist's stratification should aim to group each patient based on the following categories: potential for early extubation, risk of major postoperative complications, and risk of prolonged ICU and/or hospital admission. These risk strata not only create a sense of awareness of patient acuity but also help direct clinical efforts toward mitigating risk factors and improving outcomes.[24]

Early extubation after CPB has been shown to be safe,[25,26] but the practice requires strong collaboration among the ICU, cardiac surgery, and cardiac anesthesia teams. Patients must be carefully selected to minimize the risk of reintubation, which may lead to increased morbidity and an increased total length of mechanical ventilation. Younger age, longer CPB time, and increased inotrope requirement are risk factors for failed early extubation.[25]

The risk for postoperative complications may be anticipated based on a patient's complexity of diagnoses and surgical repair, presence of intraoperative complications or pulmonary hypertension, excessive bleeding, refractory arrhythmias, and the presence of low cardiac output syndrome (LCOS). Those with complications have a higher risk of cardiac arrest and may have a tendency to drift into the prolonged hospitalization risk category. ICU management should focus on preventing this adverse drift.

Patients at risk for chronic hospitalization tend to be those who develop complications, such as persistent chylous effusions, thrombosis of major vessels, airway problems (eg, vocal cord and diaphragmatic compromise), and difficulty feeding.

Postoperative Monitoring

The goals of postoperative monitoring are to establish an objective assessment of each patient's overall clinical status, predict potential adverse events, and guide proactive management. The level of monitoring is dictated by complexity of diagnoses, surgical repair, and hemodynamic and respiratory data. All patients should have continuous ECG monitoring, invasive or noninvasive blood pressure monitoring, and respiratory monitoring, including pulse oximetry. Assessment of urine output (with or without a Foley catheter) is essential in the immediate postoperative period. In mechanically ventilated patients, other noninvasive respiratory data can be obtained, including end-tidal carbon dioxide, carbon dioxide elimination, dead space ventilation (V_D/V_T ratio of physiologic dead space over tidal volume), respiratory compliance, and airway resistance. The use of capnography is steadily increasing.

Cerebral near-infrared spectroscopy is gaining popularity in postoperative management. Trends in cerebral oximetry for individual patients may be a helpful marker of alterations in cardiac output, and the use of this approach has been suggested as a predictor of outcome after cardiac surgery.[27–29]

Central venous pressure monitoring is standard for most patients who have undergone CPB. This can be monitored continuously through a percutaneously placed central venous line or a surgically placed transthoracic line. RA pressure monitoring provides a continuous assessment of filling pressures so that low RA pressures in hypotensive patients may suggest the need for fluid resuscitation. Elevated RA pressures may be an indicator of cardiac tamponade resulting from a pericardial effusion, poor RV function/compliance, or acute pulmonary processes, such as pneumothorax.

Indirect assessment of cardiac output can be determined by measuring mixed venous saturation (SVo_2) on a specimen drawn from the RA. The arteriovenous oxygen difference ($AVDo_2$) may reflect cardiac output. A difference of approximately 25% suggests a normal output, and this is applicable for patients with mixing lesions with systemic oxygen desaturation as well. Patients with left to RA level shunts have elevated SVo_2, and the $AVDo_2$ may not necessarily reflect cardiac output. LA and pulmonary artery lines are seldom used in the current era of cardiac critical care, but LA lines can provide useful objective data in the management of patients with LV dysfunction, mitral valve disease, and/or abnormalities in coronary artery perfusion.

Low Cardiac Output Syndrome

LCOS is a common postoperative complication after CPB and occurs within the first 6 to 12 hours after surgery. It is reported in approximately 25% of patients undergoing CPB for congenital heart surgery and has been defined by a constellation of signs and symptoms of low cardiac output state: tachycardia, poor peripheral perfusion, and oliguria. LCOS requires increased inotropic support and may result in cardiac arrest.[30]

The factors believed to account for LCOS are hemodynamically significant residual lesions, myocardial dysfunction probably resulting from prolonged periods of cardioplegia, myocardial ischemia, and reperfusion injury. Other factors include inflammatory response to CPB, with a resulting increase in systemic vascular resistance, PVR, capillary leak, and pulmonary dysfunction.[31,32] The risk of LCOS is greatest among neonates undergoing complex surgeries. Additional risk factors are prolonged CPB time, prolonged cross-clamp time, preoperative circulatory collapse, and preoperative ventricular dysfunction.[33] The hallmarks of management beyond prevention are careful anticipation and aggressive cardiorespiratory treatment.

Patients should be critically evaluated, and the evaluation should start with a focused physical examination to identify a cause. For instance, physical examination may reveal murmurs consistent with a residual VSD or AV valve regurgitation. This is followed by laboratory evaluation to help make the diagnosis and to discern the clinical repercussions of the LCOS, such as worsening acidosis and resultant end-organ dysfunction. Additional tests, such as an echocardiogram, may be necessary. Diagnosis of residual lesions is often accurately made in the ICU, but their absolute contribution to a patient's clinical deterioration may be difficult to ascertain. Therefore, the intensivist may need to err on the side of being more aggressive, which may include cardiac catheterization with angiography.

After the evaluation, the cause of LCOS must be stratified into 2 main categories: those requiring surgical intervention and those amenable to medical therapy. For instance, neonates who undergo *tetralogy of Fallot* repair generally do not tolerate a significant residual VSD, and infants who have undergone AV canal defect repair generally do not tolerate a persistent patent ductus arteriosus. These clinical scenarios present significant hemodynamic problems with refractory LCOS and often require urgent reoperation.

Therapy for LCOS should be individualized and a patient's response to interventions closely monitored. Medical therapy is geared toward the perceived cause but all patients must receive adequate fluid resuscitation to maintain preload and systemic blood pressure followed by appropriate use of inotropic agents to support myocardial contractility and afterload, reducing agents to decrease ventricular work load, enhance cardiac output, and improve perfusion.[34] Although the PRIMACORP study has proposed the use of milrinone prophylactically against postoperative LCOS,[30] there are institutional variations in agents used to prevent or treat LCOS, including low-dose epinephrine alone or in combination with milrinone. Several studies have shown drugs, such as milrinone, dopamine, and epinephrine, to have significant arryhythmogenicity in the postoperative period.[35,36]

In the absence of a surgical cause, when LCOS remains refractory to medical therapy, mechanical support should be considered. Extracorporeal membrane oxygenation (ECMO) has been used with good results in postoperative cardiac patients, including those placed on ECMO for an inability to wean from CPB and those with severe hemodynamic instability with refractory LCOS, and as rescue from cardiac arrest.[37–39] Because of the associated morbidity, timing of ECMO poses a major decision challenge. Therefore, early engagement of the multidisciplinary team, involving critical care, surgery, anesthesiology, and cardiology, is crucial. Any delay in initiation of extracorporeal life support may have grave repercussions for patients.

Pulmonary Hypertension

Elevated PVR and resultant pulmonary arterial hypertension (PAH) is a common postoperative complication after congenital heart surgery. PAH can acutely elevate RV afterload with resultant RV dysfunction and is a common cause of cardiac arrest in the postoperative period. Several factors contribute to its development, including CPB, which is associated with a systemic inflammatory response syndrome, involving mediators, such as interleukin 6, interleukin 10, tumor necrosis factor α, P-selectin and E-selectin, leptin, soluble intercellular adhesion molecule and vascular cell adhesion molecule, and fractalkine.[40] Patient factors that contribute to pulmonary hypertension include cardiac physiology, comorbid conditions, and some genetic syndromes.

The cardiac physiologies most at risk for development of PAH are

1. Those associated with an increased pressure load to the pulmonary arterial system, such as truncus arteriosus communis, VSD, AV canal defect, aortopulmonary window, and patent ductus arteriosus
2. Those associated with impaired egress of blood from the pulmonary arterial tree (eg, obstructed total anomalous pulmonary venous connections), mitral valve stenosis, or restrictive atrial communication in cases of HLHS
3. Heart transplant patients with preexisting pulmonary hypertension (eg, restrictive cardiomyopathy)

Comorbid conditions, such as congenital diaphragmatic hernia, may also pose an independent risk to the development of PAH, and some genetic syndromes, in particular Down syndrome, can also be a risk factor.

The postoperative implication of PAH is pulmonary vascular reactivity. In this setting, a vasospastic stimulus can trigger a potentially lethal episodic pulmonary hypertensive crisis that can result in acute RV failure, tricuspid regurgitation, decreased cardiac output, and myocardial ischemia.[41] The initial approach to postoperative pulmonary hypertension is prevention. Noxious stimuli must be minimized. For example, in a mechanically ventilated patient, endotracheal suctioning should be performed carefully. This might mean limiting suctioning to the tip of the *endotracheal tube* and administering additional sedation/analgesia/neuromuscular blockade in labile patients. Hypercarbia should be avoided, and supplemental oxygen should be used judiciously for its pulmonary vasodilatory benefit.

Inhaled nitric oxide decreases vascular tone and is an effective agent in the treatment of pulmonary hypertension in the postoperative period. Although its prophylactic use remains controversial,[42–44] preemptive use should be considered in those critically ill patients who are less likely to tolerate an acute decompensation. Other agents used to treat postoperative pulmonary hypertension include inhaled illoprost[42] and intravenous sildenafil.[45]

Postoperative Arrhythmia

Postoperative arrhythmias, with a reported incidence of 15% to 50%, can cause significant hemodynamic compromise. Although most arrhythmias are clinically unimportant, junctional ectopic tachycardia (JET), reentrant supraventricular tachycardia, ectopic atrial tachycardia (EAT), and ventricular tachycardia , when they occur, can result in prolonged mechanical ventilation, increased inotrope use, prolonged ICU length of stay, increased risk of cardiac arrest, and decreased survival.[36,46,47] Risk factors for the development of tachyarrhythmias include younger age at surgery, long CPB and cross-clamp times, and use of deep hypothermic circulatory arrest.[46,48] Ventricular tachycardia, although not common in the postoperative period, can lead to rapid hemodynamic compromise. It presents as a wide complex tachycardia that must be rapidly differentiated from an aberrantly conducted supraventricular tachycardia.

Accurate diagnosis of the arrhythmia is paramount to optimal management. Narrow complex tachycardias are classified into automatic or reentrant rhythm. Reentrant arrhythmias have sudden onset and respond to pharmacologic agents (eg, adenosine) or electrical cardioversion. They also respond to overdrive pacing and have the characteristic of abrupt termination. The automatic arrhythmias (JET and EAT) demonstrate warm-up and cool-down phenomena (ie, slow increase and slow decline in heart rate); they are catecholamine responsive and do not respond to overdrive pacing or cardioversion. A 12-lead or 15-lead ECG with rhythm strip may be necessary to make the diagnosis, and in some cases an atrial electrogram is necessary to identify the location of P waves.

Although there is some suggestion of prophylactic amiodarone for prevention of postoperative JET,[49] the hallmark of prevention of JET and other postoperative tachy-arrhythmia is aggressive repletion of electrolytes and treatment of significant acid-base disturbances. In cases of the automatic arrhythmias, minimizing a patient's catechol-amine state (eg, avoidance of fever, instituting appropriate sedation, when indicated, and adequate neuromuscular blockade) may decrease risk of arrhythmia. Once arrhythmia occurs, the treatment algorithm largely depends on whether a patient is hemodynamically stable or unstable.

Fig. 2 provides a suggested diagnostic algorithm and a guide to the approach to therapy. Ventricular tachycardia is managed per the Pediatric Advanced Life Support algorithm. supraventricular tachycardia with aberrant conduction may appear, electrographically, similar to ventricular tachycardia. The type of supraventricular tachycardia needs to be established and treated appropriately. The recommended treatment of stable reentrant tachycardia is vagal maneuvers, adenosine, or β-blockers. Unstable patients should be treated with adenosine (if it can be administered promptly) or synchronized cardioversion. For EAT, β-blockers (eg, esmolol) are effec-tive initial therapy.[50] For JET, the traditional therapeutic modalities should be imple-mented: cooling to approximately 36°C, decreasing catechol infusions as tolerated, adequate sedation, and appropriate neuromuscular blockade. Cooling must be cautiously performed because shivering can cause a catecholamine surge and coun-teract the therapy. Amiodarone is a suggested first-line pharmacologic therapy for JET.[51] It can be effective, but its dose-related adverse effects (ie, α-blockade) should be considered.[52]

Bradyarrhythmias encountered in the postoperative period include sinus brady-cardia, as seen in sick sinus syndrome, and varying degrees of AV node block. These

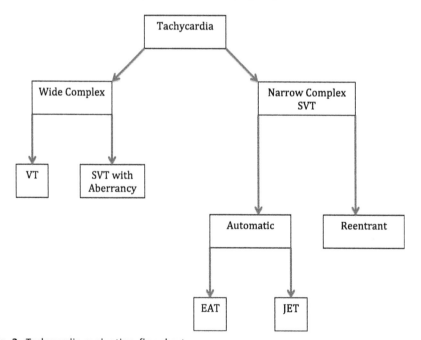

Fig. 2. Tachycardia evaluation flowchart.

respond well to pacing using temporary pacing wires placed at the time of surgery. In isolated sick sinus syndrome, atrial pacing alone is adequate. AV node block often requires AV sequential pacing.

Respiratory Management

Positive pressure ventilation may have major influences on hemodynamics after congenital heart surgery. Patients most affected are those with significantly impaired myocardial function, pulmonary vascular disease, and passive pulmonary blood flow (eg, bidirectional Glenn or Fontan circulation). The key to optimal mechanical ventilation is to adopt strategies to achieve adequate gas exchange while minimizing the adverse effects on hemodynamics.

In terms of postoperative respiratory management, the increasingly common approach is early extubation.[25,26,53] Advantages of early extubation include minimizing the need for postoperative sedation, reducing the length of ICU admission, reducing the incidence of nosocomial infection, and improving family and patient satisfaction.[25] A discussion regarding the candidacy for early extubation should be made in consultation among the intensivist, cardiothoracic surgeon, and anesthesiologist.

Once extubated, most patients require supplemental oxygen via a standard nasal cannula. Others, however, require increased support including high-flow nasal cannula (HFNC) and noninvasive ventilation (NIV), whereas a small subset requires reintubation. Although a comprehensive discussion of high-flow oxygen therapy and NIV is beyond the scope of this article, a few key points are provided.

High-flow nasal cannula is an increasingly common approach to the management of patients who require mild-to-moderate respiratory support.[54] Although definitive data are lacking in the pediatric population, there is growing evidence that such an approach is well tolerated with minimal adverse effects. The concept underlying this approach is to provide patients with an elevated flow of oxygen-enriched, warmed, and humidified gas.[55] Flow rates of up to 8 L per minute and 40 L per minute are used for infants and children, respectively.

Multiple mechanisms of action have been proposed for the beneficial effects of high-flow nasal cannula therapy.[56] The increased flow of gas provides pressure to the airways, similar to a continuous positive airway pressure approach. Data show, however, that the pressure generated by HFNC is lower than with continuous positive airway pressure. Thus, this mechanism alone is unlikely to be the sole benefit. Other proposed mechanisms of action include the beneficial secretion clearing and positive mucosal effects of heated and humidified gas, the washout of deadspace by the continuous flow of gas to the upper airways, and the providence of inspiratory gas flow that more closely approaches that of spontaneous respiration, thus minimizing the entrainment of room air.[57,58] Further investigation on the mechanisms of action for HFNC therapy is under way.

As an intermediate step between HFNC and invasive mechanical ventilation, NIV can be considered. NIV involves the administration of airway pressure at either single-level (continuous positive airway pressure) or bilevel positive airway pressure without the need for intubation. The advantage of NIV focuses on the lack of an endotracheal tube, which is associated with a reduced need for pharmacologic sedation and a reduction in the incidence of ventilator associated pneumonia. The downside of NIV in the pediatric population is a lack of Food and Drug Administration–approved devices and interfaces to efficiently provide this respiratory support for all infants and children.

Cardiorespiratory Interactions

When management of postoperative patients requires the use of positive airway pressure (regardless of modality), the cardiorespiratory effects of such an approach must be considered. Positive airway pressure by definition increases the mean intrathoracic pressure. If the increase in mean intrathoracic pressure is significant, systemic venous return can be reduced due to a decreased pressure gradient between the superior and inferior vena cava and the RA. The result is decreased RV output, and such a situation can be corrected by volume augmentation. The volume required is approximately 5 mL/kg, which can be repeated as clinically indicated.

This physiologic effect is most prominent in those patients with passive pulmonary blood flow (eg, bidirectional Glenn shunt or Fontan shunt), who rely on a low pulmonary artery pressure to establish a flow gradient between the systemic and pulmonary venous systems. In these patients, either high mean airway pressure or atelectasis can adversely affect venous return and cardiac output by compromising the flow gradient.[59] Although there is often hesitation to use positive end-expiratory pressure in such patients, avoidance of positive end-expiratory pressure could cause atelectasis with untoward hemodynamic consequences.

The effects of mechanical ventilation on PVR and RV afterload are variable and dependent on lung volume. PVR and RV afterload are optimized at an optimal lung volume, approximating functional residual capacity. Hyperinflation increases PVR by alveolar overdistension and subsequent compression of perialveolar capillaries.[60,61] Pulmonary hypoinflation, alternatively, causes lung collapse and elevated PVR from hypoxia-induced pulmonary vasoconstriction[62] and increased impedance of the large pulmonary vessels. Therefore, in patients with RV dysfunction, in whom elevated PVR adds further stress to the RV, it is crucial to ventilate with settings that prevent overdistension and avoid atelectasis.

In terms of the LV, the preload effects are variable and principally dependent on the effects of mechanical ventilation on the RV. This exemplifies the concept of ventricular interdependence. The effects of mechanical ventilation on LV afterload are clearer. The mean intrathoracic pressure generated by positive pressure ventilation reduces LV afterload by reducing the LV transmural pressure.[63] Thus, mechanical ventilation can be an effective approach to patients with LV dysfunction. As an example, patient status postimplantation of anomalous left coronary artery from the pulmonary artery will likely benefit from mechanical ventilation. Similarly, in patients with poor LV function, clinicians should anticipate a possible deterioration in hemodynamics after extubation. Furthermore, mechanical ventilation may benefit patients with ventricular dysfunction/failure by reducing the respiratory work of breathing (ie, reducing oxygen consumption).

Cardiac support

Cardiac support for postoperative patients with congenital heart disease must be directed by patient pathophysiology, including an assessment of changes in loading conditions (described previously). Clinicians must consider the effects of the various inotropes/vasoactive agents available in relation to patient physiology. The physiologic balance most commonly involves reducing the afterload to the ventricles, optimizing ventricular contractility, and providing an appropriate perfusion pressure for both ventricles.[64] Additionally, it should be acknowledged that with the lack of definitive data showing that any one approach is more beneficial than another, institutional preference often plays a large role in clinical decision making. A common approach for postoperative management includes the use of milrinone as an inodilator with supplemental low-dose epinephrine as clinically indicated.

Inhaled nitric oxide

For those patients with significant RV dysfunction and/or pulmonary hypertension, inhaled nitric oxide may represent a beneficial approach.[65] As a selective pulmonary vasodilator, inhaled nitric oxide reduces PVR and may benefit those patients with pulmonary hypertension.[66] More controversial is the use of inhaled nitric oxide for patients with normal PVR and RV dysfunction/failure. Some data suggest that the administration of inhaled nitric oxide despite a normal pulmonary vasculature may improve RV performance.[67]

Special Considerations in the Postoperative Period

Although it is impossible to comprehensively describe all clinical considerations in a review article, a few special considerations should be discussed. One example is patients with significant chest tube or surgical site bleeding refractory to blood product administration, including platelets, cryoprecipitate, and fresh frozen plasma. Once the platelet count and clotting parameters have been corrected (ie, medical bleeding) and active bleeding continues, a surgical reason must be considered. Close communication with the surgeon throughout such a process is important.

A second group requiring reoperation is shunt-dependent patients with an acute shunt occlusion (eg, thrombosis). With shunt-dependent pulmonary blood flow, an acute desaturation without clear explanation and resolution requires prompt evaluation of the shunt by echocardiography. Once shunt malfunction or occlusion is suspected, evaluation and therapy must be initiated promptly and concurrently. Appropriate therapy includes aggressive fluid administration and heparin bolus followed by continuous infusion. Unless shunt occlusion/malfunction is conclusively ruled out with the initial evaluation, urgent cardiac catheterization with intervention or surgical exploration is the appropriate next step. The effects of profound cyanosis, acidosis, aggressive fluid resuscitation, and/or high doses of pharmacologic cardiovascular agents may have a negative impact on clinical status and elevate the surgical risk for the reoperation.

Special consideration should also be provided for cardiac patients undergoing noncardiac surgery. This population presents unique preoperative and postoperative issues that require careful consideration and assessment. A key example is a single ventricle patient who has undergone stage I palliation with a Blalock-Taussig shunt who may be at risk for acute shunt thrombosis from dehydration. The preoperative and intraoperative management must include careful consideration of this complex physiology. Preoperative intravenous hydration while patients are withheld food and fluids is essential. Also, close consideration should be given to obtaining a preoperative echocardiogram. Careful attention to hydration status and perfusing pressures is essential throughout the perioperative period. Also, during the intraoperative course, abdominal insufflation during laparoscopic gastric tube placement can increase systemic vascular resistance and compromise cardiac output. Support of the function of the single ventricle as clinically indicated is essential.

EXTRACORPOREAL MEMBRANE OXYGENATION

ECMO can be life saving for patients with refractory cardiac and/or respiratory failure, including during the postoperative period. The decision to proceed with ECMO support is subjective and must be made in conjunction with a patient's clinical course and trajectory. It should be stressed that ECMO does not correct cardiac and/or respiratory failure but is rather a bridge to recovery, transplantation, or decision making. In cases of planned cardiac transplantation due to a failure of ventricular recovery, ECMO can be transitioned to a ventricular assist device as a bridge to transplantation.

Although ECMO in the postoperative period can be life saving, overall mortality rates for the neonatal and pediatric populations remain suboptimal at 40% and 49%, respectively (Extracoporeal Life Support Organization Database, July 2012). The optimal timing for ECMO cannulation and the best candidates for ECMO remain controversial.

One of the growing uses of ECMO in the postoperative congenital heart population is in the situation of cardiac arrest (extracorporeal cardiopulmonary resuscitation). Extracorporealcardiopulmonary resuscitation is the extension of cardiopulmonary resuscitation to ECMO when standard resuscitative efforts are failing. Reported survival with good neurologic outcomes has been reported as 30% to 40%.[68–71] As ECMO systems become simpler and can be set up more quickly, it is reasonable to expect the use of extracorporeal cardiopulmonary resuscitation to continue to grow. Additional outcomes-based research is needed.

SUMMARY

Postoperative care of cardiac patients requires a comprehensive and multidisciplinary approach to critically ill patients with cardiac disease whose care requires a clear understanding of cardiovascular physiology, multiorgan system function, and organ interactions in health and in disease. When patients fail to progress along the projected course or decompensate acutely, prompt evaluation with bedside assessment, laboratory evaluation, and echocardiography is essential. When things do not add up, cardiac catheterization must be seriously considered. With continued advancements in the field of neonatal and pediatric postoperative cardiac care, continued improvements in overall outcomes for this specialized population are anticipated.

REFERENCES

1. Knowles RL, Bull C, Wren C, et al. Mortality with congenital heart defects in England and Wales, 1959-2009: exploring technological change through period and birth cohort analysis. Arch Dis Child 2012;97(10):861–5.
2. Thiagarajan RR, Laussen PC. Mortality as an outcome measure following cardiac surgery for congenital heart disease in the current era. Paediatr Anaesth 2011; 21(5):604–8.
3. Larsen SH, Emmertsen K, Johnsen SP, et al. Survival and morbidity following congenital heart surgery in a population-based cohort of children—up to 12 years of follow-up. Congenit Heart Dis 2011;6(4):322–9.
4. Browne LP, Krishnamurthy R, Chung T. Preoperative and postoperative MR evaluation of congenital heart disease in children. Radiol Clin North Am 2011;49(5): 1011–24.
5. Levey A, Glickstein JS, Kleinman CS, et al. The impact of prenatal diagnosis of complex congenital heart disease on neonatal outcomes. Pediatr Cardiol 2010; 31(5):587–97.
6. Kin N, Weismann C, Srivastava S, et al. Factors affecting the decision to defer endotracheal extubation after surgery for congenital heart disease: a prospective observational study. Anesth Analg 2011;113(2):329–35.
7. Fernandes AM, Mansur AJ, Caneo LF, et al. The reduction in hospital stay and costs in the care of patients with congenital heart diseases undergoing fast-track cardiac surgery. Arq Bras Cardiol 2004;83(1):27–34, 18–26, [in English, Portuguese].
8. Srinivasan C, Sachdeva R, Morrow WR, et al. Standardized management improves outcomes after the Norwood procedure. Congenit Heart Dis 2009;4(5):329–37.
9. Brown DW, Connor JA, Pigula FA, et al. Variation in preoperative and intraoperative care for first-stage palliation of single-ventricle heart disease: a report from

the Joint Council on Congenital Heart Disease National Quality Improvement Collaborative. Congenit Heart Dis 2011;6(2):108–15.

10. Vohra HA, Adamson L, Haw MP. Is early primary repair for correction of tetralogy of Fallot comparable to surgery after 6 months of age? Interact Cardiovasc Thorac Surg 2008;7(4):698–701.

11. Padley JR, Cole AD, Pye VE, et al. Five-year analysis of operative mortality and neonatal outcomes in congenital heart disease. Heart Lung Circ 2011;20(7): 460–7.

12. Khan I, Malinge S, Crispino J. Myeloid leukemia in down syndrome. Crit Rev Oncog 2011;16(1–2):25–36.

13. Anah MU, Ansa VO, Etiuma AU, et al. Recurrent pericardial effusion associated with hypothyroidism in down syndrome: a case report. West Afr J Med 2011; 30(3):210–3.

14. Bruwier A, Chantrain CF. Hematological disorders and leukemia in children with Down syndrome. Eur J Pediatr 2012;171(9):1301–7.

15. McLean-Tooke A, Spickett GP, Gennery AR. Immunodeficiency and autoimmunity in 22q11.2 deletion syndrome. Scand J Immunol 2007;66(1):1–7.

16. Koestenberger M. Transthoracic echocardiography in children and young adults with congenital heart disease. ISRN Pediatr 2012;2012:753481.

17. Hartge DR, Weichert J, Krapp M, et al. Results of early foetal echocardiography and cumulative detection rate of congenital heart disease. Cardiol Young 2011; 21(5):505–17.

18. Crean A, Maredia N, Ballard G, et al. 3D Echo systematically underestimates right ventricular volumes compared to cardiovascular magnetic resonance in adult congenital heart disease patients with moderate or severe RV dilatation. J Cardiovasc Magn Reson 2011;13(1):78.

19. Woodard PK, Bhalla S, Javidan-Nejad C, et al. Cardiac MRI in the management of congenital heart disease in children, adolescents, and young adults. Curr Treat Options Cardiovasc Med 2008;10(5):419–24.

20. Feltes TF, Bacha E, Beekman RH 3rd, et al. Indications for cardiac catheterization and intervention in pediatric cardiac disease: a scientific statement from the American Heart Association. Circulation 2011;123(22):2607–52.

21. O'Brien SM, Clarke DR, Jacobs JP, et al. An empirically based tool for analyzing mortality associated with congenital heart surgery. J Thorac Cardiovasc Surg 2009;138(5):1139–53.

22. Jacobs JP, Wernovsky G, Elliott MJ. Analysis of outcomes for congenital cardiac disease: can we do better? Cardiol Young 2007;17(Suppl 4):145–58.

23. Lacour-Gayet F, Jacobs ML, Jacobs JP, et al. The need for an objective evaluation of morbidity in congenital heart surgery. Ann Thorac Surg 2007;84(1):1–2.

24. Pagowska-Klimek I, Pychynska-Pokorska M, Krajewski W, et al. Predictors of long intensive care unit stay following cardiac surgery in children. Eur J Cardiothorac Surg 2011;40(1):179–84.

25. Meißner U, Scharf J, Dötsch J, et al. Very early extubation after open-heart surgery in children does not influence cardiac function. Pediatr Cardiol 2008; 29(2):317–20.

26. Mittnacht AJ, Thanjan M, Srivastava S, et al. Extubation in the operating room after congenital heart surgery in children. J Thorac Cardiovasc Surg 2008; 136(1):88–93.

27. Kussman BD, Wypij D, DiNardo JA, et al. Cerebral oximetry during infant cardiac surgery: evaluation and relationship to early postoperative outcome. Anesth Analg 2009;108(4):1122–31.

28. Tweddell JS, Ghanayem NS, Hoffman GM. Pro: NIRS is "standard of care" for postoperative management. Semin Thorac Cardiovasc Surg Pediatr Card Surg Annu 2010;13(1):44–50.
29. Phelps HM, Mahle WT, Kim D, et al. Postoperative cerebral oxygenation in hypoplastic left heart syndrome after the Norwood procedure. Ann Thorac Surg 2009; 87(5):1490–4.
30. Hoffman TM, Wernovsky G, Atz AM, et al. Prophylactic intravenous use of milrinone after cardiac operation in pediatrics (PRIMACORP) study. Prophylactic Intravenous Use of Milrinone After Cardiac Operation in Pediatrics. Am Heart J 2002;143(1):15–21.
31. Nagashima M, Imai Y, Seo K, et al. Effect of hemofiltrated whole blood pump priming on hemodynamics and respiratory function after the arterial switch operation in neonates. Ann Thorac Surg 2000;70(6):1901–6.
32. Burrows FA, Williams WG, Teoh KH, et al. Myocardial performance after repair of congenital cardiac defects in infants and children. Response to volume loading. J Thorac Cardiovasc Surg 1988;96(4):548–56.
33. Brown KL, Ridout DA, Hoskote A, et al. Delayed diagnosis of congenital heart disease worsens preoperative condition and outcome of surgery in neonates. Heart 2006;92(9):1298–302.
34. Butts RJ, Scheurer MA, Atz AM, et al. Comparison of maximum vasoactive inotropic score and low cardiac output syndrome as markers of early postoperative outcomes after neonatal cardiac surgery. Pediatr Cardiol 2012;33(4):633–8.
35. Hoffman TM, Bush DM, Wernovsky G, et al. Postoperative junctional ectopic tachycardia in children: incidence, risk factors, and treatment. Ann Thorac Surg 2002;74(5):1607–11.
36. Smith AH, Owen J, Borgman KY, et al. Relation of milrinone after surgery for congenital heart disease to significant postoperative tachyarrhythmias. Am J Cardiol 2011;108(11):1620–4.
37. Beiras-Fernandez A, Deutsch MA, Kainzinger S, et al. Extracorporeal membrane oxygenation in 108 patients with low cardiac output - a single-center experience. Int J Artif Organs 2011;34(4):365–73.
38. Ravishankar C, Dominguez TE, Kreutzer J, et al. Extracorporeal membrane oxygenation after stage I reconstruction for hypoplastic left heart syndrome. Pediatr Crit Care Med 2006;7(4):319–23.
39. Wernovsky G, Kuijpers M, Van Rossem MC, et al. Postoperative course in the cardiac intensive care unit following the first stage of Norwood reconstruction. Cardiol Young 2007;17(6):652–65.
40. Avni T, Paret G, Thaler A, et al. Delta chemokine (fractalkine)—a novel mediator of pulmonary arterial hypertension in children undergoing cardiac surgery. Cytokines 2010;52(3):143–5.
41. Adatia I, Beghetti M. Immediate postoperative care. Cardiol Young 2009; 19(Suppl 1):23–7.
42. Loukanov T, Bucsenez D, Springer W, et al. Comparison of inhaled nitric oxide with aerosolized iloprost for treatment of pulmonary hypertension in children after cardiopulmonary bypass surgery. Clin Res Cardiol 2011;100(7):595–602.
43. Gorenflo M, Gu H, Xu Z. Peri-operative pulmonary hypertension in paediatric patients: current strategies in children with congenital heart disease. Cardiology 2010;116(1):10–7.
44. Ofori-Amanfo G, Hsu D, Lamour JM, et al. Heart transplantation in children with markedly elevated pulmonary vascular resistance: impact of right ventricular failure on outcome. J Heart Lung Transplant 2011;30(6):659–66.

45. Fraisse A, Butrous G, Taylor MB, et al. Intravenous sildenafil for postoperative pulmonary hypertension in children with congenital heart disease. Intensive Care Med 2011;37(3):502–9.

46. Rekawek J, Kansy A, Miszczak-Knecht M, et al. Risk factors for cardiac arrhythmias in children with congenital heart disease after surgical intervention in the early postoperative period. J Thorac Cardiovasc Surg 2007;133(4):900–4.

47. Shamszad P, Cabrera AG, Kim JJ, et al. Perioperative atrial tachycardia is associated with increased mortality in infants undergoing cardiac surgery. J Thorac Cardiovasc Surg 2012;144(2):396–401.

48. Delaney JW, Moltedo JM, Dziura JD, et al. Early postoperative arrhythmias after pediatric cardiac surgery. J Thorac Cardiovasc Surg 2006;131(6):1296–300.

49. Imamura M, Dossey AM, Garcia X, et al. Prophylactic amiodarone reduces junctional ectopic tachycardia after tetralogy of Fallot repair. J Thorac Cardiovasc Surg 2012;143(1):152–6.

50. Garnock-Jones KP. Esmolol: a review of its use in the short-term treatment of tachyarrhythmias and the short-term control of tachycardia and hypertension. Drugs 2012;72(1):109–32.

51. Kovacikova L, Hakacova N, Dobos D, et al. Amiodarone as a first-line therapy for postoperative junctional ectopic tachycardia. Ann Thorac Surg 2009;88(2): 616–23.

52. Saul JP, Scott WA, Brown S, et al. Intravenous amiodarone for incessant tachyarrhythmias in children: a randomized, double-blind, antiarrhythmic drug trial. Circulation 2005;112(22):3470–7.

53. Manrique AM, Feingold B, Di Filippo S, et al. Extubation after cardiothoracic surgery in neonates, children, and young adults: one year of institutional experience. Pediatr Crit Care Med 2007;8(6):552–5.

54. Spentzas T, Minarik M, Patters AB, et al. Children with respiratory distress treated with high-flow nasal cannula. J Intensive Care Med 2009;24(5):323–8.

55. Lee JH, Rehder KJ, Williford L, et al. Use of high flow nasal cannula in critically ill infants, children, and adults: a critical review of the literature. Intensive Care Med 2012. [Epub ahead of print].

56. Urbano J, del Castillo J, Lopez-Herce J, et al. High-flow oxygen therapy: pressure analysis in a pediatric airway model. Respir Care 2012;57(5):721–6.

57. Dysart K, Miller TL, Wolfson MR, et al. Research in high flow therapy: mechanisms of action. Respir Med 2009;103(10):1400–5.

58. Frizzola M, Miller TL, Rodriguez ME, et al. High-flow nasal cannula: impact on oxygenation and ventilation in an acute lung injury model. Pediatr Pulmonol 2011;46(1):67–74.

59. Duke GJ. Cardiovascular effects of mechanical ventilation. Crit Care Resusc 1999;1(4):388–99.

60. Cheifetz IM, Meliones JN. Hemodynamic effects of high-frequency oscillatory ventilation: a little volume goes a long way. Crit Care Med 2000;28(1):282–4.

61. Polglase GR, Morley CJ, Crossley KJ, et al. Positive end-expiratory pressure differentially alters pulmonary hemodynamics and oxygenation in ventilated, very premature lambs. J Appl Phys 2005;99(4):1453–61.

62. Michelakis ED, Thebaud B, Weir EK, et al. Hypoxic pulmonary vasoconstriction: redox regulation of O_2-sensitive $K+$ channels by a mitochondrial O_2-sensor in resistance artery smooth muscle cells. J Mol Cell Cardiol 2004;37(6):1119–36.

63. Kocis KC, Meliones JN. Cardiopulmonary interactions in children with congenital heart disease: physiology and clinical correlates. Prog Pediatr Cardiol 2000; 11(3):203–10.

64. Bronicki RA, Anas NG. Cardiopulmonary interaction. Pediatr Crit Care Med 2009; 10(3):313–22.
65. Lindberg L, Olsson AK, Jogi P, et al. How common is severe pulmonary hypertension after pediatric cardiac surgery? J Thorac Cardiovasc Surg 2002;123(6): 1155–63.
66. Buzzarro M, Gross I. Inhaled nitric oxide for the postoperative management of pulmonary hypertension in infants and children with congenital heart disease. Anesth Analg 2006;102(3):964.
67. Haddad F, Doyle R, Murphy DJ, et al. Right ventricular function in cardiovascular disease, part II: pathophysiology, clinical importance, and management of right ventricular failure. Circulation 2008;117(13):1717–31.
68. Joffe AR, Lequier L, Robertson CM. Pediatric outcomes after extracorporeal membrane oxygenation for cardiac disease and for cardiac arrest: a review. ASAIO J 2012;58(4):297–310.
69. Huang SC, Wu ET, Chen YS, et al. Extracorporeal membrane oxygenation rescue for cardiopulmonary resuscitation in pediatric patients. Crit Care Med 2008;36(5): 1607–13.
70. Huang SC, Wu ET, Wang CC, et al. Eleven years of experience with extracorporeal cardiopulmonary resuscitation for paediatric patients with in-hospital cardiac arrest. Resuscitation 2012;83(6):710–4.
71. Morris MC, Wernovsky G, Nadkarni VM. Survival outcomes after extracorporeal cardiopulmonary resuscitation instituted during active chest compressions following refractory in-hospital pediatric cardiac arrest. Pediatr Crit Care Med 2004;5(5):440–6.

Pediatric Sepsis
Challenges and Adjunctive Therapies

William Hanna, MD[a,b], Hector R. Wong, MD[a,b,*]

KEYWORDS

- Epidemiology • Outcomes • Antibiotics • Quality improvement • Corticosteroids
- Hemofiltration • Hemoadsorption • Plasmapheresis

KEY POINTS

- Sepsis continues to be a major challenge in pediatric critical care medicine.
- Studies of sepsis outcomes should include both short-term and long-term outcomes, and should also focus on functional outcomes.
- The issue of timeliness and appropriateness of antibiotics is an appropriate and important area for quality improvement in pediatric sepsis.
- The issue of corticosteroids as an adjunctive therapy in pediatric septic shock remains largely unresolved and requires formal testing by way of clinical trials.
- Hemofiltration, hemoperfusion, and plasmapheresis are potential adjunctive therapies for pediatric sepsis, but require formal testing by way of clinical trials.
- A new multi-biomarker–based model has been developed to reliably stratify the outcome risk in children with septic shock.

INTRODUCTION

Sepsis remains a major challenge in pediatric critical care medicine. Several recent publications cover the general principles of sepsis management, as well as pathophysiology in a developmental context.[1–5] This review intends to provide an appraisal of adjunctive therapies for sepsis and to highlight opportunities for meeting selected challenges in the field.

EPIDEMIOLOGIC AND QUALITY-IMPROVEMENT CHALLENGES

Sepsis is estimated to be the leading cause of death in infants and children worldwide, with an annual mortality of approximately 1.6 million per year. In the United States,

Funded by: NIH (RO1 GM096994; RO1 GM099773).

[a] Division of Critical Care Medicine, Cincinnati Children's Hospital Research Foundation, Cincinnati Children's Hospital Medical Center, University of Cincinnati College of Medicine, 3333 Burnet Avenue, Cincinnati, OH 45229, USA; [b] Department of Pediatrics, University of Cincinnati College of Medicine, 3333 Burnet Avenue, Cincinnati, OH 45229, USA
* Corresponding author. Division of Critical Care Medicine, Cincinnati Children's Hospital Medical Center, MLC2005, 3333 Burnet Avenue, Cincinnati, OH 45229.
E-mail address: hector.wong@cchmc.org

approximately 42,000 cases of severe sepsis occur annually and in-hospital mortality is estimated at 10.3%.[6,7] The mean length of stay and cost for a child with severe sepsis in the United States are estimated to be 31 days and more than $40,000, respectively. Clearly sepsis remains an important public health issue in both underdeveloped and developed countries, and consequently brings many opportunities for translational research and efforts at quality improvement.

The ability to benchmark outcomes, based on a reliable outcome metric (ie, reliable outcome prediction), is fundamental to quality-improvement efforts and improvement science.[8] Unfortunately, there is no quality metric or outcome benchmark specific to pediatric sepsis. Scoring systems based on physiologic and clinical variables, such as the Pediatric Risk of Mortality (PRISM) score and the Pediatric Index of Mortality (PIM), are very robust for predicting outcomes of general pediatric intensive care unit (ICU) populations, but begin to perform less well when applied to specific diseases, such as sepsis.[9] Recently a multi-biomarker–based outcome risk model that reliably predicts outcome in children with severe sepsis and septic shock was developed and validated.[10,11] Although the model requires further prospective testing, it is hoped it will enhance currently available scoring systems and therefore provide a sepsis-specific quality metric to better assess short-term outcomes of pediatric sepsis.

While short-term outcomes (ie, acute mortality or survival) will continue to be important considerations in translational research efforts and clinical trials, increasingly greater attention is now focused on sepsis-related morbidity and mortality beyond the acute phase. Quartin and colleagues[12] reported that adults who initially recover from the acute stage of sepsis have an increased risk of death for up 5 years after discharge, even after accounting for the effects of comorbidities. Karlsson and colleagues[13] documented a 2-year mortality rate of 45% for adults after severe sepsis and decreased quality of life in sepsis survivors at a median of 17 months after the acute episode of severe sepsis.

Similar data are now being reported in pediatric survivors of severe sepsis. Czaja and colleagues[14] retrospectively studied more than 7000 pediatric cases of severe sepsis. Almost one-half of the patients who were discharged after the initial admission were readmitted at least once, at a median of 3 months after discharge. Respiratory infection was the most common indication for readmission, and greater than 30% of these readmissions were in children without comorbidities. An additional 6.5% of patients died during these readmissions. Thus sepsis has important long-term consequences and there is a need to more robustly assess long-term outcomes, as well as functional outcomes beyond the acute dichotomy of alive or dead.

The Functional Status Scale (FSS) was recently developed to specifically meet the need of assessing functional outcomes of critically ill children.[15] The FSS incorporates several relevant functional assessments including mental status, sensory functioning, communication, motor functioning, feeding, and respiratory status, and is designed to be applied in diverse and time-limited environments. The FSS appears to have very good interrater reliability, and its performance compares favorably with more complex and labor-intensive functional outcome tools. A major challenge moving forward, as stated by the FSS investigators, is the development of subgroup-specific versions of FSS (eg, sepsis specific).[15]

APPROPRIATENESS AND TIMING OF ANTIBIOTICS

Along with aggressive fluid resuscitation, prompt and appropriate administration of antibiotics continues to be a cornerstone of therapy for patients with severe sepsis and septic shock. The 2008 Surviving Sepsis Campaign guidelines, using a grading scheme involving both strength of recommendation and quality of evidence, assigned a level 1B recommendation for the use of broad-spectrum intravenous antibiotics within the first hour of septic shock.[16] There are 2 major components to this recommendation: appropriateness and timing of antibiotics.

Although it seems intuitive that inappropriate antibiotic usage in septic shock is likely to be associated with poorer outcome, corroboration with existing proof-of-concept literature provides further support. Notable studies include a prospective cohort study involving 492 critically ill adults with documented bloodstream infections, 147 (29.9%) of whom received inadequate antimicrobial treatment, defined as infection with an organism that was not susceptible to the antimicrobials being used at the time of positive culture results.[17] Patients not adequately treated had a mortality rate of 61.9%, whereas patients who were adequately treated had a mortality rate of 28.4%. Similarly, a retrospective review of 5175 adult patients with septic shock, in 3 countries, reported 5-fold increase in hospital mortality for those receiving inappropriate antibiotics. In this study, inappropriate antibiotics were defined based on sensitivity testing or, in the case of culture negative septic shock, expert clinical opinion and existing guidelines. These and other related studies strongly support the importance of appropriate antimicrobial therapy in severe sepsis and septic shock.

Kumar and colleagues[18] have provided compelling experimental evidence supporting the importance of early antibiotic treatment of sepsis (ie, timing of antibiotics) in animal models. In mice undergoing intraperitoneal implantation of an *Escherichia coli*–laced, gelatin capsule–encased fibrinogen clot, treatment with antibiotics at 12 hours or less after implantation resulted in 20% or less mortality. By comparison, antibiotic administration at least 15 hours after implantation resulted in greater than 85% mortality. Of note, significant hypotension was noted by 12 hours after implantation in untreated mice, leading the investigators to propose the existence of a "critical inflection point" for the impact of antibiotics on survival.

A large, retrospective, multicenter study of adults with septic shock followed this laboratory-based study.[19] The overall in-hospital mortality for this cohort was 56.2%; however, for patients who received appropriate antibiotics within the first hour of hypotension the in-hospital mortality was 20.1%. Of interest, following onset of hypotension mortality was found to increase by an average of 7.6% for every hour untreated over the subsequent 6 hours. Similarly, a study involving 291 adults with sepsis in the emergency department reported that whereas longer times between initial triage and antibiotic administration were not independently associated with increased mortality, delay in treatment following recognition of shock was independently associated with increased mortality.[20]

Studies on a similar scale do not exist in the pediatric sepsis literature. One small retrospective study involving children with community-acquired pneumonia and the need for mechanical ventilation (N = 45) assessed the impact of antibiotic timeliness and appropriateness on surrogate outcomes.[21] Delays in antibiotic administration as short as 2 to 4 hours were independently associated with longer duration of mechanical ventilation, and longer lengths of stay in the ICU and hospital.

Collectively these data provide substantial support that the readily tangible concept of timeliness of appropriate antibiotics is an important area of focus for quality-improvement efforts in clinical sepsis. In this regard, Cruz and colleagues[22] recently reported the implementation of a protocol to optimize antibiotic administration in children with signs of sepsis and presenting to the emergency department of a large, tertiary-care children's hospital. Before protocol implementation, the median time from initial triage to antibiotic administration was 130 minutes. The median time from initial triage to antibiotic administration decreased to 38 minutes after protocol implementation.

FLUID RESUSCITATION

More than 20 years ago, Carcillo and colleagues[23] reported that in children with septic shock, fluid resuscitation in excess of 40 mL/kg within the first hour of presentation was associated with improved survival, without an increase in the risk of cardiogenic pulmonary edema or acute respiratory distress syndrome. Since that time, aggressive fluid resuscitation has been a mainstay of both adult and pediatric guidelines for the management of septic shock.[5,16] In addition, subsequent observational and interventional studies further support and corroborate the importance of aggressive fluid resuscitation early in septic shock.[24–27]

Although seemingly one of the most fundamental principles in critical care medicine, aggressive fluid resuscitation in septic shock has been recently questioned and critiqued as being weakly supported.[28] Indeed, cohort studies have reported an association between positive fluid balance and mortality.[29–32] Most recently, The Fluid Expansion as Supportive Therapy (FEAST) study compared fluid boluses of 20 to 40 mL/kg with no bolus in more than 3000 acutely ill African children.[33] FEAST reported a significantly increased mortality risk in the group randomized to the fluid-bolus arm.

These data should not lead one directly to the premature and erroneous conclusion that fluid resuscitation is intrinsically deleterious for patients with septic shock. The concepts of fluid overload and aggressive volume resuscitation are certainly related, but are also distinct temporally and mechanistically. None of the observational studies linking fluid overload and mortality have clearly proved a cause-and-effect relationship. Positive fluid balance could simply be a marker of increased severity of illness leading to increased vascular leak and increased third spacing of fluid, rather than a direct cause of increased mortality. Moreover, the results of the FEAST study need to be carefully considered contextually.[34] For example, the definition of shock in the FEAST study has been called into question, and 57% of the patients in this study had a positive blood smear for malaria. In addition, 32% of the participants had a hemoglobin concentration of less than 5 g/dL. Thus the results of the FEAST study could reflect the inclusion of a large number of participants for whom fluid administration may indeed be intrinsically deleterious, particularly in a low-resource setting, rather than leading to the conclusion that fluid administration is intrinsically deleterious in septic shock.[34]

Fundamental aspects of sepsis biology and physiology, including vascular leak, increased fluid loss, and increased vascular capacitance, well support the need for aggressive volume resuscitation, particularly at an early stage in the course of septic shock.[1] Since the 1991 study by Carcillo and colleagues,[23] the concept of aggressive fluid resuscitation in septic shock has remained well supported.[24–27] The important clinical question that needs to be addressed is not should patients with septic shock receive fluid resuscitation, but rather how much fluid resuscitation is most optimal.[35]

CORTICOSTEROIDS AND SEPSIS

The hypothalamic-pituitary-adrenal (HPA) axis is a neurohormonal feedback mechanism well described in human physiology (**Fig. 1**). In addition to the sympathoadrenal axis, the HPA axis serves a vital role in homeostatic adaptation to physiologic and biologic stress. Under normal circumstances, pituitary adrenocorticotropic hormone (ie, corticotropin) release is stimulated by hypothalamic corticotropin-releasing hormone

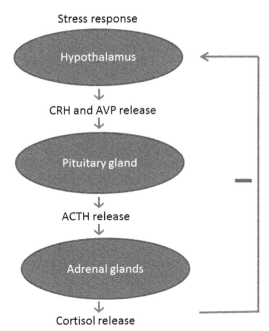

Fig. 1. The hypothalamic-pituitary-adrenal axis. ACTH, corticotropin; AVP, arginine vaso-pressin production; CRH, corticotropin-releasing hormone.

(CRH) and arginine vasopressin production (AVP), and in turn stimulates cortisol production from the adrenal cortex. Cortisol acts through a myriad of mechanisms to maintain homeostasis, including modulating inflammation, glucose availability, and vascular reactivity.[36]

Both adult and pediatric studies suggest a form of HPA-axis impairment in critical illness and sepsis.[37–43] Critical illness–related corticosteroid insufficiency (CIRCI) is a recently coined term intended to describe a group of critically ill patients who seemingly have an inadequate cortisol response relative to their degree of illness. The mechanisms of this relative adrenal insufficiency are thought to include both deficiency of cortisol production and tissue resistance to cortisol.[44]

Corticosteroids have been considered as potential adjunctive therapy in sepsis for decades. Initial efforts, centered around the concept of sepsis as an excessive and dysregulated proinflammatory condition, primarily studied short courses of high-dose corticosteroids intended for inflammatory suppression, often using single bolus doses of up to 30 mg/kg of methylprednisolone or equivalent steroid dosing. However, results were inconsistent; with meta-analyses arising in the 1980s to 1990s suggesting either no survival benefit or a trend toward increased mortality, the use of steroids in sepsis and septic shock began to fall out of favor.[45–47]

The pediatric literature during the same time largely consisted of case studies and several trials investigating high-dose steroid therapy in dengue shock syndrome. The first of these involved a randomized, double-blind, placebo-controlled trial of 98 children with dengue shock syndrome, and showed a significant mortality improvement (19% vs 44% case fatality rate) with corticosteroid administration.[48] However, subsequent trials failed to replicate this benefit.[49,50] In addition, a randomized trial of dexamethasone therapy, before antibiotic administration, failed to improve the outcome in a cohort of African children with sepsis from causes other than dengue.[51]

More recently, the CIRCI and relative adrenal insufficiency concepts have renewed interest in adjunctive corticosteroid therapy in sepsis. Annane and colleagues[52] conducted the initial study supporting the concept of relative adrenal insufficiency. These investigators described 3 classes of adults with septic shock based on random cortisol levels and cortisol levels resulting from a corticotropin-stimulation test. In a cohort of 189 adult patients with septic shock, a class of patients with "high" baseline cortisol levels ($\geq$34 μg/dL) and a "poor" response to a high-dose corticotropin-stimulation test (change in serum cortisol concentration of $\leq$9 μg/dL) had the highest mortality rate (82%) among the 3 classes. This study thus initiated the concept that a class of identifiable patients with septic shock and relative adrenal insufficiency may exist, which has the potential to benefit from corticosteroid replacement. The pediatric literature suggests a similar phenomenon in children with septic shock, but it is challenging to interpret the data because of the small cohort sizes and the high degree of heterogeneity in study design, definitions of relative adrenal insufficiency, and approaches to corticotropin stimulation.[37,39–42]

Menon and colleagues[38] conducted the most comprehensive study to date of relative adrenal insufficiency in critically ill children. This prospective study included 381 critically ill children across 7 tertiary-care pediatric ICUs in Canada. The primary goal of the study was to determine the prevalence of relative adrenal insufficiency in a general population of critically ill children (ie, not just in children with septic shock). The study examined various definitions of adrenal insufficiency, but the primary analysis for prevalence was based on a low-dose corticotropin-stimulation test (1 μg) and the resulting increment of serum cortisol concentration; a cortisol increment of 9 μg/dL or less after corticotropin stimulation was considered diagnostic of relative adrenal insufficiency.

Menon and colleagues reported a 30.2% overall prevalence of relative adrenal insufficiency in this cohort. Subgroup analyses revealed that patients suffering from trauma had the highest prevalence (62.5%), whereas the prevalence in patients with sepsis was 32.8%. Increasing age was associated with a higher prevalence of relative adrenal insufficiency, with each additional year of age increasing the odds of relative adrenal insufficiency by 11%. The study also demonstrated that relative adrenal insufficiency was associated with a greater need for the number of catecholamines, a greater duration of catecholamine requirement, and a greater need for volume resuscitation. This study well supports the concept of relative adrenal insufficiency, including functional consequences, in pediatric critical illness.

Given the potential functional implications of relative adrenal insufficiency, the more recent interventional trials have focused on lower doses of corticosteroids, with a primary intention of replacing a putative defective cortisol response rather than globally inhibiting the inflammatory response of sepsis. Annane and colleagues[43] conducted a randomized, placebo-controlled trial of simultaneous hydrocortisone (50 mg every 6 hours) and fludrocortisone (50 μg once per day) administration for 7 days, in 300 adults with septic shock. Relative adrenal insufficiency (ie, nonresponders) was defined as a serum cortisol concentration increment of 9 μg/dL or less after corticotropin stimulation, and the outcome analysis was stratified based on the response to corticotropin stimulation. There was a significant mortality benefit in nonresponders treated with hydrocortisone and fludrocortisone (hazard ratio, 0.67; 95% confidence interval [CI], 0.47–0.95; P = .02), whereas there was no benefit in the responders. In addition, the duration of vasopressor therapy was shorter in the nonresponders treated with hydrocortisone and fludrocortisone. Finally, there was no difference in adverse events between the treatment and placebo groups, irrespective of the response to corticotropin stimulation.

This study by Annane and colleagues[43] led to much enthusiasm for the use of cortisol measurements, corticotropin stimulation, and hydrocortisone replacement therapy in both adults and children with septic shock. However, the study by Annane and colleagues[43] was followed by the Corticosteroid Therapy for Septic Shock (CORTICUS) study by Sprung and colleagues,[53] which also evaluated the efficacy of hydrocortisone replacement in patients with septic shock, based on responder and nonresponder classifications after corticotropin stimulation. The study involved 499 patients across multiple European ICUs. This study showed no mortality difference between hydrocortisone-treated patients and placebo-treated patients, irrespective of the responder/nonresponder status. The duration of time until reversal of shock was shorter across all patients treated with hydrocortisone, but there was also a higher rate of shock relapse in the patients treated with hydrocortisone, possibly related to new infections.

There are some important differences worth mentioning between the initial study by Annane and colleagues and the subsequent CORTICUS study. The patients in the study by Annane and colleagues had an overall higher level of illness severity and possibly more profound shock compared with the patients in the CORTICUS study. In addition, enrollment in the Annane study was restricted to a relatively narrow window of within 8 hours of meeting study-entry criteria, whereas the CORTICUS study had a 72-hour window for enrollment. Although these differences may account for the divergence in the results between the two studies, the aftermath of CORTICUS study has nonetheless profoundly influenced the enthusiasm for hydrocortisone replacement as an adjunctive therapy in septic shock.

In the context of the aforementioned studies, the 2008 Surviving Sepsis Campaign guidelines recommend against corticotropin-stimulation testing to identify subsets of patients who may benefit from hydrocortisone, and that the decision to initiate hydrocortisone therapy should be predicated on confirmation that blood pressure is poorly responsive to fluid resuscitation and vasopressor therapy (**Fig. 2**).[16] In direct contrast to this recommendation, a recently published, single-author, evidence-based guide for physicians provides a decision tree for the use of hydrocortisone in adults with septic shock, which is based on both specific vasopressor requirements and results from corticotropin-stimulation testing.[54]

The most recent specific pediatric guidelines differ somewhat from the adult guidelines, reflecting the relative lack of pediatric data.[5] The pediatric guidelines recommend the use of corticosteroids for patients with fluid-resistant and catecholamine-resistant septic shock, and evidence of adrenal insufficiency (see **Fig. 2**). The definition of catecholamine resistance is somewhat subjective, and the recommendation implies the need to conduct corticotropin-stimulation testing, in contrast to the adult-specific recommendations.

There are retrospective, pediatric-specific data that should raise some doubts in the mind of the practitioner concerning the efficacy of corticosteroids in pediatric septic shock. Markovitz and colleagues[55] analyzed more than 6000 cases of pediatric severe sepsis in the Pediatric Health Information System (PHIS) administrative database, with the goal of determining correlates of outcome, including the use of corticosteroids. The use of corticosteroids was an independent predictor of mortality (relative risk, 1.7; 95% CI, 1.7–2.2). Although the lack of illness-severity data leaves open the possibility that more severely ill children received steroids, at the very least this retrospective study could not find evidence for a benefit of corticosteroids in pediatric severe sepsis. In agreement with this observation, Zimmerman and Williams[56] conducted a post hoc analysis of the RESOLVE database (n = 477), which is derived from the largest interventional clinical trial in

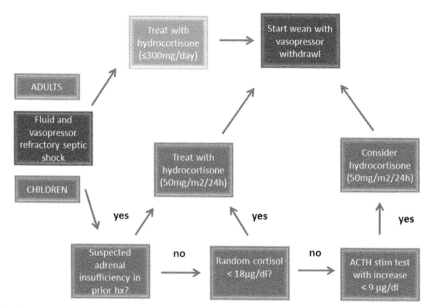

Fig. 2. Recommendations for adjunctive corticosteroid administration in septic shock. The adult recommendations do not include the use of serum cortisol concentrations or corticotropin-stimulation (ACTH stim) testing.[16] The pediatric recommendations, however, recommend measurement of serum cortisol concentrations and corticotropin-stimulation testing.[5]

pediatric severe sepsis conducted to date.[57] Their analysis of the RESOLVE data could not find any evidence to support the efficacy of adjunctive corticosteroids in pediatric severe sepsis.

For children with septic shock who are at risk for classic adrenal insufficiency (eg, patients receiving chronic steroids, or patients with hypothalamic, pituitary, or adrenal disease), adjunctive corticosteroids are clearly indicated. For the general pediatric patient with septic shock, however, the current evidence does not definitively support the use of adjunctive corticosteroids, and it should be kept in mind that the risk profile of adjunctive corticosteroids may not be benign.[58] Thus it is imperative that we unite as a critical care community and organize a robust, multicenter, prospective, randomized trial to objectively test the efficacy of adjunctive corticosteroids in pediatric septic shock.[58]

Several fundamental issues must be resolved in the design of such a trial. Such concerns include standardized, consensus definitions of refractory shock and relative adrenal insufficiency, a standardized approach to corticotropin-stimulation testing, and strong consideration for pre-enrollment outcome risk stratification. An important issue that has emerged surrounds the measurement of free cortisol, as opposed to the more commonly used laboratory test that measures total cortisol.[59] Finally, consideration must be given to the issue of tissue resistance to corticosteroid stimulation, which has not been directly addressed in any clinical trial to date.

Genome-wide expression studies in children with septic shock recently highlighted the issue of tissue resistance to corticosteroid stimulation.[60–62] These studies revealed and validated the existence of at least 3 pediatric septic shock classes based on differential patterns of gene expression. Of importance, 1 of the 3 subclasses has a higher level of illness severity and mortality rate, compared with the other 2 gene-expression–based subclasses. The gene signature that defines the subclasses includes a large number of genes corresponding to the glucocorticoid receptor signaling pathway, and these genes are repressed in the subclass of patients with the highest illness severity and mortality. These observations support the concept that there may be a subset of patients with septic shock who are relatively unresponsive to conventional doses of corticosteroids, and if this were true it would represent an enormous confounding factor for any trial seeking to establish the efficacy of adjunctive corticosteroids in pediatric septic shock.

BLOOD-PURIFICATION STRATEGIES

Whitehouse one of them much heated and fortiegued on his arrivall drank a very hearty draft of water and was taken almost instantly extreemly ill. His pulse were full and I therefore bled him plentifully from which he felt great relief. I had no other instrument with which to perform this operation but my penknife, however it answered very well.
    –Captain Meriwether Lewis, during the portage of the Great Falls of the Missouri River, June 26, 1805.

The concept of blood purification can be traced at least to medieval times, when barbers would "bleed" patients for a variety of ailments with the goal of removing "evil humors." Ample evidence for this concept can also be found in the journals of the Lewis and Clark expedition, which contain multiple entries documenting the deliberate "bleeding" of expedition members for a variety of ailments. Though not a randomized trial, it is noteworthy that 59 individuals took part in the Lewis and Clark expedition, all but 1 of whom survived the over the 2-year long journey across the North American continent (98.3% survival; 95% CI, 91–100).

The concept of blood purification persists today in the modern ICU.[63] The "evil humors" are now a plethora of soluble mediators and toxins thought to be involved in the pathobiology of sepsis. Bloodletting is now replaced by a variety of extracorporeal techniques that remove blood, purify the blood in some manner, and return the blood to the patient (**Box 1**).

Hemofiltration

Given the size (5–60 kDa) and water-soluble nature of putative sepsis mediators (eg, cytokines), hemofiltration through continuous renal replacement therapy (CRRT) has been studied with increasing interest as a nonspecific approach to mediator removal. Randomized controlled trials to date focusing on standard filtration rates in adults, however, have largely failed to support the use of CRRT for the purpose of blood purification in sepsis.[64–66] For example, Payen and colleagues[64] studied 76 ICU patients with severe sepsis/septic shock in the absence of renal dysfunction, with the primary study end point being the degree of organ failure. A hemofiltration rate of 25 mL/kg/h, initiated within the first 24 hours of the first organ failure, failed to reduce plasma concentrations of inflammatory mediators, and did not reduce the degree of organ failure. In fact, the patients assigned to the hemofiltration arm had a significantly higher degree of organ failure.

A common criticism of these trials is that the hemofiltration rate is not sufficient to clear inflammatory mediators from the blood compartment. Accordingly, the use of high-volume hemofiltration (HVHF; often defined as >35 mL/kg/h) has been increasingly studied as a plausible solution, and this approach showed some initial promise in terms of reduction of inflammatory mediators and improvements in clinical outcomes.[67–69] One very large trial involved 1505 critically ill adults with acute kidney injury that were randomized to standard CRRT or HVHF, with the primary measure

---

Box 1
Major differences between hemofiltration, hemoadsorption, and plasmapheresis as blood-purification strategies for sepsis

Blood-Purification Modalities

Hemofiltration

1. Uses property of convection to filter solutes through semipermeable membrane
2. Largely nonspecific removal of solutes, including potentially harmful inflammatory mediators
3. Standard hemofiltration rates have shown no benefit in sepsis from existing randomized controlled trials
4. Use of high-volume hemofiltration is still being investigated for efficacy in septic shock (IVOIRE)

Hemoadsorption

1. Uses property of adsorption, with solutes binding to sorbent via molecular interactions
2. Posited as contributing to nonspecific inflammatory mediator removal in standard continuous renal replacement therapy
3. Specific forms include polymyxin B hemoperfusion, largely targeting gram-negative endotoxin
4. Existing trials with polymyxin B show promise, with a large randomized controlled trial pending (EUPHRATES)

Plasmapheresis

1. Uses cell separator to remove and replace plasma component of blood (plasma exchange)
2. Also may lead to nonspecific removal of mediators, with added benefit of plasma replacement
3. May be beneficial in sepsis-related thrombocytopenia-related multisystem organ failure (TAMOF)
4. Existing study links TAMOF with ADAMTS-13 deficiency, similar to thrombotic thrombocytopenic purpura pathophysiology

---

being death within 90 days after randomization.[70] There was no difference in mortality for the overall study population or for the predefined subgroup of patients with sepsis. Thus, the efficacy of HVHF as a blood-purification approach in general critical illness and in sepsis remains to be demonstrated.[71]

In the pediatric population, estimates suggest that roughly 40% of those with multi-organ dysfunction syndrome and receiving CRRT concomitantly have sepsis. The advent of the Prospective Pediatric Continuous Replacement Therapy Registry Group (ppCRRT) in 2000 has led to a comprehensive characterization of critically ill children receiving CRRT.[32,72–77] However, despite provocative findings such as associations between increased volume status at initiation of therapy and mortality, few data exist with sufficient granularity to evaluate specifically the efficacy of CRRT as a blood-purification strategy in pediatric sepsis. One recent retrospective study analyzed 22 pediatric patients undergoing CRRT and having concomitant systemic inflammatory response syndrome and multiple organ dysfunction syndrome.[78] The study reported no improvement in hemodynamic and respiratory parameters while accounting for lack of weight change during 48 hours of therapy. In addition to the lack of a control group, the study allowed for large heterogeneity among patients, and no analyses of ultrafiltration rates were performed.

An international consensus statement published in 2010 recommends against the use of HVHF in patients with sepsis in the absence of acute kidney injury, citing a lack of both "strong, scientific rationale" and "reproducible, proof-of-principle efficacy" in existing clinical trials.[79] Although this strong consensus statement is based primarily on adult data, at this time there is no reason to think that the recommendation should be any different for the pediatric population. The highly anticipated IVOIRE (High Volume in Intensive Care) trial (clinicaltrials.gov identifier: NCT00241228), a large, randomized multicenter trial comparing ultrafiltration rates of 35 versus 70 mL/kg/h in adult patients with septic shock and acute kidney injury, with 28-day mortality as the primary outcome measure, may help clarify the current value of CRRT in sepsis and concomitant acute kidney injury.

Hemoadsorption

The concepts reviewed in the previous section are centered on the convective filtration properties of CRRT. There has also been interest in the adsorptive properties of various hemofilters as a potential mechanism for mediator removal. Studies have shown decreases in mediator concentrations approximately 1 hour after CRRT initiation and with frequent filter changes, suggesting initial efficacy through adsorption, with subsequent membrane saturation.[67] A similar principle has led to the use of polymyxin B–coated filters as a means to remove endotoxin in patients with sepsis.[80] It is estimated that more than 80,000 patients have been treated with extracorporeal removal of endotoxin via polymyxin B–coated filters in Japan since 1994, and the procedure is covered by the Japanese national health insurance system.[81]

The EUPHAS (Early Use of Polymyxin B Hemoperfusion in Abdominal Sepsis) trial randomized 64 adults, with septic shock and requiring emergency surgery for intra-abdominal infection, to conventional therapy or conventional therapy plus 2 sessions of polymyxin B hemoperfusion.[82] The group undergoing polymyxin B hemoperfusion showed significant improvements in hemodynamics, improvements in organ dysfunction, and decreased mortality. Although this trial is thought to be underpowered, a systematic review of 28 publications, including 9 randomized trials, lends further support for the potential efficacy of this approach.[83]

Similar to the EUPHAS trial in design and outcome measures, the ongoing EUPHRATES trial (clinicaltrials.gov identifier: NCT01046669) anticipates enrollment of 360 adult patients in 15 centers, with an estimated completion date of January 2015. The primary end point for the EUPHRATES trial is all-cause 28-day mortality. Of importance, the entry criteria include a requirement for an increased blood concentration of endotoxin, as measured by a rapid assay platform. Thus, this trial is using the concept of pre-enrollment stratification based on a biological mechanism, a refreshing approach in human septic shock trials.

There is one report in the literature describing the successful application of polymyxin B hemoperfusion in a child with sepsis.[84] One could surmise that the quintessential pediatric critical illness, meningococcemia, which is characterized by a profound systemic load of endotoxin, would be potentially amenable to this approach. However, experimental data indicate that polymyxin B does not bind endotoxin from *Neisseria meningitidis* as effectively as endotoxin from *E coli*.[85]

Plasmapheresis

Plasmapheresis is another extracorporeal approach to blood purification, but is based on separation, removal, and replacement of the plasma component of blood.[86]

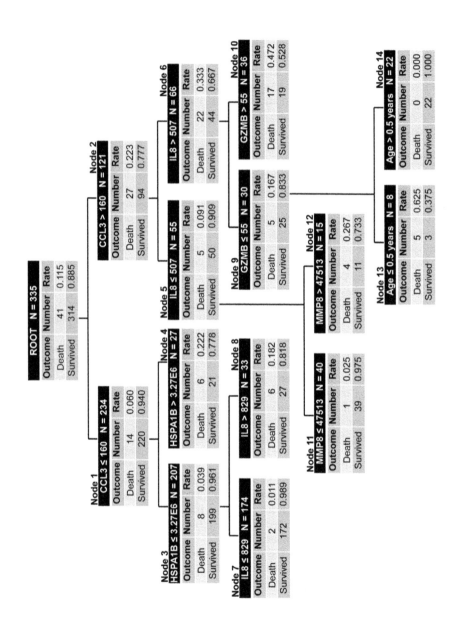

Plasmapheresis is thought to derive its efficacy from 2 basic principles: (1) removal of pathologic molecules contributing to the disease process, and (2) replacement of molecules vital to homeostasis and found to be endogenously deficient because of the disease. Much like the use of hemofiltration, the removal of such molecules is often of a nonspecific nature, and may not have a clear therapeutic objective in mind. An added component, however, is the replacement of plasma for that removed, more accurately termed plasma exchange, which may account for potential differences in clinical results.

Stegmayr and colleagues[87] reported a large case series of 76 adult patients with disseminated intravascular coagulation (DIC) and multiple organ dysfunction syndrome, including acute renal failure. These patients underwent rescue therapy with plasmapheresis until DIC was reversed (median of 2 treatments, with a range of 1–14 treatments). Eighty-two percent of these patients survived, compared with a historical rate of 20% with similar clinical characteristics. Busund and colleagues[88] randomized 106 adults with severe sepsis to conventional therapy versus conventional therapy plus plasmapheresis. This study reported an absolute 28-day mortality risk reduction of 20% and relative risk of death in the plasmapheresis group of 0.6. Other reports focused on meningococcemia and plasmapheresis in children and young adults, and reported improved survival rates of 70% to 80% when compared with historical controls and projected mortality based on clinical scores.[89,90]

The most recent iteration of the use of plasmapheresis in sepsis is centered on the concept of thrombocytopenia-associated multiorgan failure (TAMOF) as a complication of sepsis.[86] TAMOF has been compared with thrombotic thrombocytopenic purpura (TTP). TTP is an acute thrombotic microangiopathy thought to be primarily caused by deficiency or inhibition of the enzyme ADAMTS13, which is responsible for cleaving procoagulant multimers of von Willebrand factor into small, less procoagulant units. Plasmapheresis has become the standard of care for TTP in that it can eliminate the inhibitory ADAMTS13 factor and replace ADAMTS13.[91,92]

Nguyen and colleagues[93] described 37 children with a least 2 organ failures and suspected sepsis, of whom 76% had thrombocytopenia, defined as platelet counts of less than 100,000/mm^3. The subset of patients with thrombocytopenia (ie, TAMOF, n = 28) had decreased ADAMTS13 activity compared with patients with organ failure, but no thrombocytopenia (n = 9). All of the nonsurvivors in this cohort (n = 7) met clinical criteria for TAMOF and demonstrated von Willebrand factor–rich microvascular thrombosis at autopsy. The same investigators then randomized 10 children with TAMOF to plasmapheresis or conventional therapy, and showed improvements in 28-day organ dysfunction scores and mortality in the patients treated with plasmapheresis.

Fig. 3. Classification tree for PERSEVERE based on 355 subjects.[10] The classification tree consists of 6 biomarker-based decision rules, 1 age-based decision rule, and 14 daughter nodes. The classification tree includes 5 stratification biomarkers: C-C chemokine ligand 3 (CCL3), heat-shock protein 70 kDa 1B (HSPA1B), interleukin-8 (IL8), granzyme B (GZMB), and matrix metalloproteinase-8 (MMP8). Each node provides the total number of subjects in the node, the biomarker serum concentration–based or age-based decision rule, and the number of survivors and nonsurvivors with the respective rates. The serum concentrations of all stratification biomarkers are provided in pg/mL. Terminal nodes 7, 11, and 14 are low-risk nodes, with mortality probabilities ranging from 0.0% to 2.5%. Terminal nodes 4, 8, 10, 12, and 13 are high-risk terminal nodes, with mortality probabilities ranging from 18.2% to 62.5%.

Current guidelines of the American Society of Apheresis list the use of plasmaphe-resis in "sepsis with multiorgan failure" as a category III recommendation (optimum role of plasmapheresis is not established and decision making should be individual-ized) with a 2B grade (weak recommendation, moderate-quality evidence).[94] In summary, the use of plasmapheresis in both adult and pediatric sepsis may have value, but remains to be demonstrated. Similarly, it could be argued that TAMOF is a construct, rather than a genuine clinical entity. These issues can only be resolved through equipoise and the conduct of rigorous, prospective clinical trials, which are currently being planned.[95]

RISK STRATIFICATION

The adjunctive therapies for sepsis already discussed, as well as therapies not dis-cussed (eg, extracorporeal life support), all have biological and physiologic plausibility in terms of efficacy, but require more rigorous testing. Moving forward with testing, consideration should be given to objective and effective outcome risk stratification as means of optimizing clinical trial design. The therapeutic successes of our oncology colleagues are, in large part, predicated on effective outcome risk stratifica-tion. In an analogous manner, we must develop tools that allow early assessment of outcome risk, and thus provide a means for excluding patients with low mortality risk while simultaneously selecting patients with higher mortality risk for trial inclusion. Experts in critical care medicine have strongly stated that currently available, physiology-based scoring systems should not be used for risk stratification in clinical trials.[9]

Recently a multi-biomarker–based risk model, which robustly predicts outcome (ie, 28 day mortality) in children with septic shock, was derived and successfully tested.[10,11] The biomarkers for the risk model are readily measured serum proteins, and were selected objectively based on a series of extensive, exploratory, genome-wide–expres-sion studies in children with septic shock.[96,97] Of importance, the biomarker measure-ments are conducted within the first 24 hours of meeting criteria for septic shock, an optimal time point for clinically relevant outcome risk stratification. The risk model is based on a classification and regression tree (CART) approach, which has the potential to discover predictor-variable interactions that may not be apparent by more traditional modeling approaches.[98]

The model is called PERSEVERE (PEdiatRic SEpsis biomarkEr Risk modEl) and has the following test characteristics for predicting death in a cohort of 355 children with septic shock from 17 different institutions in the United States: sensitivity of 93%, specificity of 74%, positive predictive value of 32%, negative predictive value of 99%, and an area under the receiver-operating curve of 0.883.[10] Of importance is that the model outperforms a physiology-based scoring system, and the false posi-tives generated by the model (ie, patients predicted to die, but actually survive) have a higher degree of illness severity than the true negatives generated by the model (ie, patients predicted to survive and actually survive), as measured by persistence of organ failure and length of stay in the ICU. The PERSEVERE classification tree is shown in **Fig. 3**.

It has been proposed that PERSEVERE can enhance current tools for the selection of patients for interventional trials by providing a means to exclude and include patients with low and high mortality risks, respectively. This type of approach would have the potential to optimize the risk-to-benefit ratio of an experimental therapy that carries more than minimal risk, such as the experimental therapies described in the previous sections.

REFERENCES

1. Wong HR, Nowak JE, Standage S, et al. Sepsis and septic shock. In: Fuhrman BP, Zimmerman JJ, editors. Pediatric critical care medicine. 4th edition. St Louis (MO): Mosby; 2011. p. 1413–29.
2. Cornell TT, Wynn J, Shanley TP, et al. Mechanisms and regulation of the gene-expression response to sepsis. Pediatrics 2010;125:1248–58.
3. Wynn JL, Wong HR. Pathophysiology and treatment of septic shock in neonates. Clin Perinatol 2010;37:439–79.
4. Wynn J, Cornell TT, Wong HR, et al. The host response to sepsis and developmental impact. Pediatrics 2010;125:1031–41.
5. Brierley J, Carcillo JA, Choong K, et al. Clinical practice parameters for hemodynamic support of pediatric and neonatal septic shock: 2007 update from the American College of Critical Care Medicine. Crit Care Med 2009;37:666–88.
6. Watson RS, Carcillo JA, Linde-Zwirble WT, et al. The epidemiology of severe sepsis in children in the United States. Am J Respir Crit Care Med 2003;167: 695–701.
7. Watson RS, Carcillo JA. Scope and epidemiology of pediatric sepsis. Pediatr Crit Care Med 2005;6:S3–5.
8. Marcin JP, Pollack MM. Review of the acuity scoring systems for the pediatric intensive care unit and their use in quality improvement. J Intensive Care Med 2007;22:131–40.
9. Vincent JL, Opal SM, Marshall JC. Ten reasons why we should NOT use severity scores as entry criteria for clinical trials or in our treatment decisions. Crit Care Med 2010;38:283–7.
10. Wong HR, Salisbury S, Xiao Q, et al. The pediatric sepsis biomarker risk model. Crit Care 2012;16:R174.
11. Kaplan JM, Wong HR. Biomarker discovery and development in pediatric critical care medicine. Pediatr Crit Care Med 2011;12:165–73.
12. Quartin AA, Schein RM, Kett DH, et al. Magnitude and duration of the effect of sepsis on survival. Department of Veterans Affairs Systemic Sepsis Cooperative Studies Group. JAMA 1997;277:1058–63.
13. Karlsson S, Ruokonen E, Varpula T, et al. Long-term outcome and quality-adjusted life years after severe sepsis. Crit Care Med 2009;37:1268–74.
14. Czaja AS, Zimmerman JJ, Nathens AB. Readmission and late mortality after pediatric severe sepsis. Pediatrics 2009;123:849–57.
15. Pollack MM, Holubkov R, Glass P, et al. Functional Status Scale: new pediatric outcome measure. Pediatrics 2009;124:e18–28.
16. Levy MM, Dellinger RP, Townsend SR, et al. The Surviving Sepsis Campaign: results of an international guideline-based performance improvement program targeting severe sepsis. Crit Care Med 2010;38:367–74.
17. Ibrahim EH, Sherman G, Ward S, et al. The influence of inadequate antimicrobial treatment of bloodstream infections on patient outcomes in the ICU setting. Chest 2000;118:146–55.
18. Kumar A, Haery C, Paladugu B, et al. The duration of hypotension before the initiation of antibiotic treatment is a critical determinant of survival in a murine model of Escherichia coli septic shock: association with serum lactate and inflammatory cytokine levels. J Infect Dis 2006;193:251–8.
19. Kumar A, Roberts D, Wood KE, et al. Duration of hypotension before initiation of effective antimicrobial therapy is the critical determinant of survival in human septic shock. Crit Care Med 2006;34:1589–96.

20. Puskarich MA, Trzeciak S, Shapiro NI, et al. Association between timing of antibiotic administration and mortality from septic shock in patients treated with a quantitative resuscitation protocol. Crit Care Med 2011;39:2066–71.

21. Muszynski JA, Knatz NL, Sargel CL, et al. Timing of correct parenteral antibiotic initiation and outcomes from severe bacterial community-acquired pneumonia in children. Pediatr Infect Dis J 2011;30:295–301.

22. Cruz AT, Perry AM, Williams EA, et al. Implementation of goal-directed therapy for children with suspected sepsis in the emergency department. Pediatrics 2011; 127:e758–66.

23. Carcillo JA, Davis AL, Zaritsky A. Role of early fluid resuscitation in pediatric septic shock. JAMA 1991;266:1242–5.

24. Han YY, Carcillo JA, Dragotta MA, et al. Early reversal of pediatric-neonatal septic shock by community physicians is associated with improved outcome. Pediatrics 2003;112:793–9.

25. de Oliveira CF, de Oliveira DS, Gottschald AF, et al. ACCM/PALS haemodynamic support guidelines for paediatric septic shock: an outcomes comparison with and without monitoring central venous oxygen saturation. Intensive Care Med 2008;34:1065–75.

26. Rivers E, Nguyen B, Havstad S, et al. Early goal-directed therapy in the treatment of severe sepsis and septic shock. N Engl J Med 2001;345:1368–77.

27. Smith SH, Perner A. Higher vs. lower fluid volume for septic shock: clinical characteristics and outcome in unselected patients in a prospective, multicenter cohort. Crit Care 2012;16:R76.

28. Hilton AK, Bellomo R. A critique of fluid bolus resuscitation in severe sepsis. Crit Care 2012;16:302.

29. Vincent JL, Sakr Y, Sprung CL, et al. Sepsis in European intensive care units: results of the SOAP study. Crit Care Med 2006;34:344–53.

30. Boyd JH, Forbes J, Nakada TA, et al. Fluid resuscitation in septic shock: a positive fluid balance and elevated central venous pressure are associated with increased mortality. Crit Care Med 2011;39:259–65.

31. Murphy CV, Schramm GE, Doherty JA, et al. The importance of fluid management in acute lung injury secondary to septic shock. Chest 2009;136:102–9.

32. Goldstein SL, Somers MJ, Baum MA, et al. Pediatric patients with multi-organ dysfunction syndrome receiving continuous renal replacement therapy. Kidney Int 2005;67:653–8.

33. Maitland K, Kiguli S, Opoka RO, et al. Mortality after fluid bolus in African children with severe infection. N Engl J Med 2011;364:2483–95.

34. Duke T. What the African fluid-bolus trial means. Lancet 2011;378:1685–7.

35. Russell JA. How much fluid resuscitation is optimal in septic shock? Crit Care 2012;16:146.

36. Prigent H, Maxime V, Annane D. Science review: mechanisms of impaired adrenal function in sepsis and molecular actions of glucocorticoids. Crit Care 2004;8:243–52.

37. Hebbar K, Rigby MR, Felner EI, et al. Neuroendocrine dysfunction in pediatric critical illness. Pediatr Crit Care Med 2009;10:35–40.

38. Menon K, Ward RE, Lawson ML, et al. A prospective multicenter study of adrenal function in critically ill children. Am J Respir Crit Care Med 2010;182:246–51.

39. Casartelli CH, Garcia PC, Branco RG, et al. Adrenal response in children with septic shock. Intensive Care Med 2007;33:1609–13.

40. Hebbar KB, Stockwell JA, Leong T, et al. Incidence of adrenal insufficiency and impact of corticosteroid supplementation in critically ill children with systemic

inflammatory syndrome and vasopressor-dependent shock. Crit Care Med 2011; 39:1145–50.

41. Pizarro CF, Troster EJ, Damiani D, et al. Absolute and relative adrenal insufficiency in children with septic shock. Crit Care Med 2005;33:855–9.

42. Sarthi M, Lodha R, Vivekanandhan S, et al. Adrenal status in children with septic shock using low-dose stimulation test. Pediatr Crit Care Med 2007;8:23–8.

43. Annane D, Sebille V, Charpentier C, et al. Effect of treatment with low doses of hydrocortisone and fludrocortisone on mortality in patients with septic shock. JAMA 2002;288:862–71.

44. Marik PE, Pastores SM, Annane D, et al. Recommendations for the diagnosis and management of corticosteroid insufficiency in critically ill adult patients: consensus statements from an international task force by the American College of Critical Care Medicine. Crit Care Med 2008;36:1937–49.

45. Lefering R, Neugebauer EA. Steroid controversy in sepsis and septic shock: a meta-analysis. Crit Care Med 1995;23:1294–303.

46. Cronin L, Cook DJ, Carlet J, et al. Corticosteroid treatment for sepsis: a critical appraisal and meta-analysis of the literature. Crit Care Med 1995;23:1430–9.

47. The Veterans Administration Systemic Sepsis Cooperative Study Group. Effect of high-dose glucocorticoid therapy on mortality in patients with clinical signs of systemic sepsis. N Engl J Med 1987;317:659–65.

48. Min M, U T, Aye M, et al. Hydrocortisone in the management of dengue shock syndrome. Southeast Asian J Trop Med Public Health 1975;6:573–9.

49. Tassniyom S, Vasanawathana S, Chirawatkul A, et al. Failure of high-dose methylprednisolone in established dengue shock syndrome: a placebo-controlled, double-blind study. Pediatrics 1993;92:111–5.

50. Sumarmo, Talogo W, Asrin A, et al. Failure of hydrocortisone to affect outcome in dengue shock syndrome. Pediatrics 1982;69:45–9.

51. Slusher T, Gbadero D, Howard C, et al. Randomized, placebo-controlled, double blinded trial of dexamethasone in African children with sepsis. Pediatr Infect Dis J 1996;15:579–83.

52. Annane D, Sebille V, Troche G, et al. A 3-level prognostic classification in septic shock based on cortisol levels and cortisol response to corticotropin. JAMA 2000; 283:1038–45.

53. Sprung CL, Annane D, Keh D, et al. Hydrocortisone therapy for patients with septic shock. N Engl J Med 2008;358:111–24.

54. Annane D. Corticosteroids for severe sepsis: an evidence-based guide for physicians. Ann Intensive Care 2011;1:7.

55. Markovitz BP, Goodman DM, Watson RS, et al. A retrospective cohort study of prognostic factors associated with outcome in pediatric severe sepsis: what is the role of steroids? Pediatr Crit Care Med 2005;6:270–4.

56. Zimmerman JJ, Williams MD. Adjunctive corticosteroid therapy in pediatric severe sepsis: observations from the RESOLVE study. Pediatr Crit Care Med 2011;12:2–8.

57. Nadel S, Goldstein B, Williams MD, et al. Drotrecogin alfa (activated) in children with severe sepsis: a multicentre phase III randomised controlled trial. Lancet 2007;369:836–43.

58. Zimmerman JJ. A history of adjunctive glucocorticoid treatment for pediatric sepsis: moving beyond steroid pulp fiction toward evidence-based medicine. Pediatr Crit Care Med 2007;8:530–9.

59. Zimmerman JJ, Donaldson A, Barker RM, et al. Real-time free cortisol quantification among critically ill children. Pediatr Crit Care Med 2011;12:525–31.

60. Wong HR, Cvijanovich NZ, Allen GL, et al. Validation of a gene expression-based subclassification strategy for pediatric septic shock. Crit Care Med 2011;39: 2511–7.
61. Wong HR, Wheeler DS, Tegtmeyer K, et al. Toward a clinically feasible gene expression-based subclassification strategy for septic shock: proof of concept. Crit Care Med 2010;38:1955–61.
62. Wong HR, Cvijanovich N, Lin R, et al. Identification of pediatric septic shock subclasses based on genome-wide expression profiling. BMC Med 2009;7:34.
63. Rimmele T, Kellum JA. Clinical review: blood purification for sepsis. Crit Care 2011;15:205.
64. Payen D, Mateo J, Cavaillon JM, et al. Impact of continuous venovenous hemofiltration on organ failure during the early phase of severe sepsis: a randomized controlled trial. Crit Care Med 2009;37:803–10.
65. Sander A, Armbruster W, Sander B, et al. Hemofiltration increases IL-6 clearance in early systemic inflammatory response syndrome but does not alter IL-6 and TNF alpha plasma concentrations. Intensive Care Med 1997;23:878–84.
66. Cole L, Bellomo R, Hart G, et al. A phase II randomized, controlled trial of continuous hemofiltration in sepsis. Crit Care Med 2002;30:100–6.
67. De Vriese AS, Colardyn FA, Philippe JJ, et al. Cytokine removal during continuous hemofiltration in septic patients. J Am Soc Nephrol 1999;10:846–53.
68. Cole L, Bellomo R, Journois D, et al. High-volume haemofiltration in human septic shock. Intensive Care Med 2001;27:978–86.
69. Honore PM, Jacobs R, Boer W, et al. New insights regarding rationale, therapeutic target and dose of hemofiltration and hybrid therapies in septic acute kidney injury. Blood Purif 2012;33:44–51.
70. Bellomo R, Cass A, Cole L, et al. Intensity of continuous renal-replacement therapy in critically ill patients. N Engl J Med 2009;361:1627–38.
71. Rimmele T, Kellum JA. High-volume hemofiltration in the intensive care unit: a blood purification therapy. Anesthesiology 2012;116:1377–87.
72. Fleming GM, Walters S, Goldstein SL, et al. Nonrenal indications for continuous renal replacement therapy: a report from the Prospective Pediatric Continuous Renal Replacement Therapy Registry Group. Pediatr Crit Care Med 2012;13: e299–304.
73. Goldstein SL. Advances in pediatric renal replacement therapy for acute kidney injury. Semin Dial 2011;24:187–91.
74. Sutherland SM, Zappitelli M, Alexander SR, et al. Fluid overload and mortality in children receiving continuous renal replacement therapy: the prospective pediatric continuous renal replacement therapy registry. Am J Kidney Dis 2010;55: 316–25.
75. Zappitelli M, Goldstein SL, Symons JM, et al. Protein and calorie prescription for children and young adults receiving continuous renal replacement therapy: a report from the Prospective Pediatric Continuous Renal Replacement Therapy Registry Group. Crit Care Med 2008;36:3239–45.
76. Flores FX, Brophy PD, Symons JM, et al. Continuous renal replacement therapy (CRRT) after stem cell transplantation. A report from the prospective pediatric CRRT Registry Group. Pediatr Nephrol 2008;23:625–30.
77. Hackbarth R, Bunchman TE, Chua AN, et al. The effect of vascular access location and size on circuit survival in pediatric continuous renal replacement therapy: a report from the PPCRRT registry. Int J Artif Organs 2007;30:1116–21.
78. Naran N, Sagy M, Bock KR. Continuous renal replacement therapy results in respiratory and hemodynamic beneficial effects in pediatric patients with severe

systemic inflammatory response syndrome and multiorgan system dysfunction. Pediatr Crit Care Med 2010;11:737–40.

79. Brochard L, Abroug F, Brenner M, et al. An Official ATS/ERS/ESICM/SCCM/SRLF Statement: prevention and Management of Acute Renal Failure in the ICU Patient: an international consensus conference in intensive care medicine. Am J Respir Crit Care Med 2010;181:1128–55.

80. Shoji H, Tani T, Hanasawa K, et al. Extracorporeal endotoxin removal by poly-myxin B immobilized fiber cartridge: designing and antiendotoxin efficacy in the clinical application. Ther Apher 1998;2:3–12.

81. Tani T, Shoji H, Guadagni G, et al. Extracorporeal removal of endotoxin: the poly-myxin B-immobilized fiber cartridge. Contrib Nephrol 2010;167:35–44.

82. Cruz DN, Antonelli M, Fumagalli R, et al. Early use of polymyxin B hemoperfusion in abdominal septic shock: the EUPHAS randomized controlled trial. JAMA 2009; 301:2445–52.

83. Cruz DN, Perazella MA, Bellomo R, et al. Effectiveness of polymyxin B-immobi-lized fiber column in sepsis: a systematic review. Crit Care 2007;11:R47.

84. Morishita Y, Kita Y, Ohtake K, et al. Successful treatment of sepsis with polymyxin B-immobilized fiber hemoperfusion in a child after living donor liver transplanta-tion. Dig Dis Sci 2005;50:757.

85. Baldwin G, Alpert G, Caputo GL, et al. Effect of polymyxin B on experimental shock from meningococcal and *Escherichia coli* endotoxins. J Infect Dis 1991; 164:542–9.

86. Nguyen TC, Kiss JE, Goldman JR, et al. The role of plasmapheresis in critical illness. Crit Care Clin 2012;28:453–68.

87. Stegmayr BG, Banga R, Berggren L, et al. Plasma exchange as rescue therapy in multiple organ failure including acute renal failure. Crit Care Med 2003;31: 1730–6.

88. Busund R, Koukline V, Utrobin U, et al. Plasmapheresis in severe sepsis and septic shock: a prospective, randomised, controlled trial. Intensive Care Med 2002;28:1434–9.

89. van Deuren M, Santman FW, van Dalen R, et al. Plasma and whole blood exchange in meningococcal sepsis. Clin Infect Dis 1992;15:424–30.

90. Gardlund B, Sjolin J, Nilsson A, et al. Plasmapheresis in the treatment of primary septic shock in humans. Scand J Infect Dis 1993;25:757–61.

91. Rock GA, Shumak KH, Buskard NA, et al. Comparison of plasma exchange with plasma infusion in the treatment of thrombotic thrombocytopenic purpura. Cana-dian Apheresis Study Group. N Engl J Med 1991;325:393–7.

92. Zheng XL, Kaufman RM, Goodnough LT, et al. Effect of plasma exchange on plasma ADAMTS13 metalloprotease activity, inhibitor level, and clinical outcome in patients with idiopathic and nonidiopathic thrombotic thrombocytopenic purpura. Blood 2004;103:4043–9.

93. Nguyen TC, Han YY, Kiss JE, et al. Intensive plasma exchange increases a disin-tegrin and metalloprotease with thrombospondin motifs-13 activity and reverses organ dysfunction in children with thrombocytopenia-associated multiple organ failure. Crit Care Med 2008;36:2878–87.

94. Szczepiorkowski ZM, Winters JL, Bandarenko N, et al. Guidelines on the use of therapeutic apheresis in clinical practice–evidence-based approach from the Apheresis Applications Committee of the American Society for Apheresis. J Clin Apheresis 2010;25:83–177.

95. Fortenberry JD, Paden ML. Extracorporeal therapies in the treatment of sepsis: experience and promise. Semin Pediatr Infect Dis 2006;17:72–9.

96. Wong HR. Genetics and genomics in pediatric septic shock. Crit Care Med 2012; 40:1618–26.
97. Wong HR. Clinical review: sepsis and septic shock—the potential of gene arrays. Crit Care 2012;16:204.
98. Che D, Liu Q, Rasheed K, et al. Decision tree and ensemble learning algorithms with their applications in bioinformatics. Adv Exp Med Biol 2011;696:191–9.

Pediatric Traumatic Brain Injury in 2012

The Year with New Guidelines and Common Data Elements

Michael J. Bell, MD[a,b,c,*], Patrick M. Kochanek, MD[a]

KEYWORDS

- Pediatric TBI guidelines • Pediatric TBI common data elements
- Evidenced-based medicine • Children • Severe traumatic brain injury

KEY POINTS

- By any measure, there has been an enormous effort within the pediatric neurotrauma community to identify the optimal practices that can lead to improved outcomes for traumatic brain injury (TBI), a disorder that is the leading killer of children.
- It is equally obvious that the current state of TBI literature is such that a wide variety of clinical approaches can fall "within" the guidelines because of the lack of data regarding the superiority of clinical decisions that are made every day for children with severe injuries.
- With the development of common data elements, it is possible that some of these questions may be answered by combining clinical trials in the future for secondary analyses.
- Alternatively, the time may be right for an observational study of pediatric TBI that uses novel statistical methods for comparing the effectiveness of these commonly used TBI therapies as they are currently used in clinical practice.

Disclosures: Both Drs Bell and Kochanek were selected by the Brain Trauma Foundation to develop the *Guidelines for the Medical Management of Severe Traumatic Brain Injury for Infants, Children and Adolescents* but were not compensated for their work. In addition, Dr Bell was selected by the National Institute of Neurological Disorders and Stroke to participate in development of the Common Data Elements for Pediatric TBI, but he was not compensated for his work. Dr Kochanek is supported by several Federal grants (U44 NS070324, T32HD040686 from the NIH and W81XWH-09-2-0187 and W81XWH-10-0623 from the US Army), as is Dr Bell (U01 HD049981, R01 NS069247, R01 NS072308 from the NIH).

[a] Department of Critical Care Medicine, Safar Center for Resuscitation Research, University of Pittsburgh, 3434 Fifth Avenue, Pittsburgh, PA 15260, USA; [b] Department of Neurological Surgery, Safar Center for Resuscitation Research, University of Pittsburgh, 3434 Fifth Avenue, Pittsburgh, PA 15260, USA; [c] Department of Pediatrics, Safar Center for Resuscitation Research, University of Pittsburgh, 3434 Fifth Avenue, Pittsburgh, PA 15260, USA
* Corresponding author. Critical Care Medicine, Pediatric Neurocritical Care, Neurological Surgery and Pediatrics, Pediatric Neurotrauma Center, Safar Center for Resuscitation Research, 3434 Fifth Avenue, Pittsburgh, PA 15260.
E-mail address: bellmj4@upmc.edu

Crit Care Clin 29 (2013) 223–238
http://dx.doi.org/10.1016/j.ccc.2012.11.004
0749-0704/13/$ – see front matter © 2013 Elsevier Inc. All rights reserved.

PEDIATRIC TBI GUIDELINES: HISTORY AND METHODOLOGY

In March 2000, the process ultimately culminating in the first edition of the *Guidelines for Medical Management of Severe Traumatic Brain Injury for Infants, Children, and Adolescents* (referred to as the Guidelines from this point forward) was initiated during the fifth Annual Aspen Neurobehavioral Conference. Participants in the conference from the Evidence-Based Practice Center (EPC) of Oregon Health and Science University agreed to form a panel of experts to develop guidelines for the medical management of children with severe traumatic brain injury (TBI).[1–19] Using the previously completed guidelines developed for adult victims of TBI as a guide,[20] the panel identified topics that are relevant to pediatric TBI needs; specifically, topics that are widely believed to be related to outcomes and TBI systems for children with severe injuries. A reference librarian searched Medline (1966–2001) for articles related to the various topics using an inclusive search strategy. Abstracts were reviewed by primary and secondary authors identified for each topic and then articles were reviewed for possible inclusion. The basic requirement for inclusion was the ability (1) to identify children with severe TBI and (2) to discern outcomes within the article. Data were classified into 3 categories of evidence: class I from randomized controlled trials; class II from clinical studies with prospective data collection; class III from retrospective data, case reports, and expert opinion. Altogether the information available for these first guidelines included data from virtually all sources, including all forms of pediatric studies, expert opinions, and even suggestions from adult studies. Ultimately, recommendations were made regarding the strength of the evidence: standards for accepted principles that "reflect a high degree of clinical certainty," guidelines that "reflect a moderate clinical certainty," and options that reflect an "unclear clinical certainty."

The resulting articles were watershed works for pediatric neurotrauma and pediatric critical care as a whole, serving as a virtual template on issues that were related to the severely brain-injured child. As the first evidenced-based guideline for a pediatric critical care illness or syndrome, it was divided into sections regarding systems of care, thresholds for therapies, and specific treatments. The first 3 chapters focused on the system of caring for children with severe TBI, including the trauma systems, prehospital airway management, and resuscitation. The next 4 chapters focused on intracranial hypertension, including indications for implementing monitoring modalities, thresholds for treatments, technology related to the devices themselves, and management of cerebral perfusion pressure (CPP; a measure derived from the arithmetical difference between the mean arterial blood pressure and intracranial pressure [ICP]). The remaining chapters focused on therapies for children with severe TBI, including those for intracranial hypertension (cerebrospinal fluid drainage, hyperosmolar therapies, hyperventilation, barbiturates, decompressive surgery, temperature control, corticosteroids) and supportive care (sedatives/neuromuscular antagonists and nutrition). Finally, a suggested algorithm for management of acute intracranial hypertension was developed based on the expert opinions of the Committee. The overall tenor of this revolutionary document is a combination of a comprehensive review of the literature combined with expert opinions to act as a user's guide for pediatric TBI. Within the various chapters, a wide variety of quality of evidence was shown (**Table 1**). Of note, there were no topics with sufficient evidence for the expert panel to define a standard, thus showing that the state of the literature is insufficient to compel clinicians toward various specific aspects of TBI care. Nevertheless, valuable information can be gleaned from the Guidelines and options that are outlined.

A total of 5 guidelines were identified concerning trauma systems, hypoxia/airway management, hypotension, CPP thresholds, and corticosteroid usage. Based on

Table 1
Summary of standards, guidelines, and options generated from the 2003 pediatric TBI guidelines

Topic	Level of Evidence	Recommendation
Trauma systems, pediatric trauma centers, and the neurosurgeon	Guideline	"In a metropolitan area, pediatric patients with severe TBI should be transported directly to a pediatric trauma center, if available"
	Option	"…should be treated in a pediatric trauma center or in an adult trauma center with added qualifications to treat children in preference to a level I or II adult trauma center without added qualifications…"
Prehospital airway management	Guideline	"Hypoxia must be avoided … and attempts made to correct it immediately. Supplemental oxygen should be administered … no evidence to support an advantage of endotracheal intubation over bag-valve-mask ventilation…"
	Option	"If prehospital endotracheal intubation is instituted…, then specialized training and use of end-tidal CO_2 detectors is necessary"
Resuscitation of blood pressure and oxygenation	Guideline	"Hypotension should be identified and corrected … defined as systolic blood pressure below fifth percentile for age or by clinical signs of shock…"
	Option	"Airway control should be obtained in children with a GCS ≤ 8 to avoid hypoxemia, hypercarbia and aspiration … hypoxia should be identified and corrected … blood pressure should be monitored frequently and accurately…"
Indications for intracranial pressure monitoring	Option	"ICP monitoring is appropriate … (GCS ≤ 8). The presence of an open fontanelle and/or sutures does not preclude the development of intracranial hypertension or negate the utility of ICP monitoring"
Threshold for treatment of intracranial hypertension	Option	"Treatment for intracranial hypertension … should begin at an ICP ≥ 20 mm Hg"
Intracranial pressure monitoring technology	Option	"…a ventricular catheter or an external strain gauge transducer or catheter tip pressure transducer device is an accurate and reliable method of monitoring ICP"
Cerebral perfusion pressure	Guideline	"A CPP >40 mm Hg … should be maintained"

(continued on next page)

Table 1 (continued)		
Topic	**Level of Evidence**	**Recommendation**
	Option	"A CPP between 40 and 65 mm Hg probably represents an age-related continuum for optimal treatment threshold ... Hypotension should be avoided"
Sedation and neuromuscular blockade	Option	"...the choice and dosing of sedatives, analgesics and neuromuscular blocking agents ... should be left to the treating physician..."
Hyperosmolar therapies	Option	"Hypertonic saline is effective at control of increased ICP ... Mannitol is effective for control of increased ICP..."
Hyperventilation	Option	"...Prophylactic hyperventilation ... should be avoided. Mild hyperventilation ($Paco_2$ 30–35 mm Hg) may be considered for longer periods of intracranial hypertension ... Aggressive hyperventilation ($Paco_2$ <30 mm Hg) may be considered as a second tier option in the setting of refractory intracranial hypertension..."
Barbiturates	Option	"High-dose barbiturate therapy may be considered in hemodynamically stable patients with refractory intracranial hypertension ... appropriate hemodynamic monitoring and cardiovascular support are essential..."
Temperature control	Option	"...Hyperthermia should be avoided..."
Surgical treatment of intracranial hypertension	Option	"Decompressive craniectomy should be considered...."
Corticosteroids	Guideline	"The use of steroids significantly reduces endogenous cortisol production ... may have an associated increased risk of complications of infection"
	Option	"The use of steroids is not recommended for improving outcome or reducing ICP..."
Nutritional support	Option	"Replace 130%–160% of resting metabolism expenditure ... nutritional support should begin by 72 h with full replacement by 7 d"

Abbreviations: CPP, cerebral perfusion pressure (mean arterial blood pressure minus intracranial pressure); GCS, Glasgow Coma Scale; ICP, intracranial pressure.
   Data from Refs.[1–19]

a study by Johnson and Krishnamurthy,[21] the benefits of a pediatric trauma center were demonstrated. In their prospective study of 225 children, children who were directly transferred to a Level 1 Pediatric Trauma Center had improved mortality compared with those who had been "indirectly" transferred (1.9% vs 4.7% mortality). This study, in concert with other supporting data from retrospective studies of patients from Pennsylvania, Oregon, and Washington,[22,23] led to the guideline that children within urban centers should be transferred directly to specialized pediatric trauma centers. Two guidelines generated from this document involved prehospitalization management of hypoxia and hypotension. In a series of 4 studies regarding airway management, it was determined that although hypoxia was to be avoided, a firm recommendation regarding the superiority of tracheal intubation or bag-valve-mask ventilation could not be discerned.[24–27] In 4 other studies from the 1980s and 1990s, the effect of hypoxia and hypotension was measured. Based on data from the Traumatic Coma Databank project and including more than 1900 children, Luerssen and colleagues[28] demonstrated that hypotension was independently associated with an increased mortality rate in children with TBI, although hypoxia was not measured in this cohort. In single-center experiences within the United States, Michaud and colleagues[29] found an increased mortality rate in hypotensive children with severe TBI in a study of 75 children, and Pigula and colleagues[30] reported improved survival without hypotension and hypoxia in 58 children. In a study from Kuala Lumpur,[31] hypotension and hypoxia were associated with increased poor outcome, with hypoxia increasing the risk of poor outcome by 2- to 4-fold. The fourth guideline regarding a CPP threshold was generated from a study by Downard and colleagues,[32] who reported no survivors in a total of 118 patients, with a mean CPP of less than 40 mm Hg. Finally, the guideline recommending against corticosteroid use to either decrease ICP or improve outcome was generated from 2 small randomized studies from several decades ago.[33,34]

In addition to these guidelines, a large number of optional therapies were outlined. Of particular significance are: (1) 14 studies providing evidence that ICP monitoring is helpful for children with Glasgow Coma Scale (GCS) score of 8 or less; (2) 5 studies that provided support for the ICP threshold of 20 mm Hg; (3) 4 studies that demonstrated some efficacy of hypertonic saline solutions in lowering ICP; and (4) 3 small studies demonstrating that decompressive surgery can lead to decreased ICP and some improvement in outcomes. However, in this document a significant proportion of these optional recommendations were from expert opinion. For instance, the recommendation that high-dose barbiturate therapy be used in conjunction with hemodynamic monitoring is valuable information for practitioners, yet there are obviously no studies randomizing children receiving barbiturates to varying levels in invasive hemodynamic monitoring. Obviously this represents prudent advice from the experts who have decades of experience in caring for such children. Similarly, the recommendations regarding hyperventilation were based on a very limited data set of approximately 36 patients.[35,36] However, the advice generated—avoid prophylactic hyperventilation when ICP is not a problem, judicious use of hyperventilation as an adjuvant therapy for ICP when first-tier measures are operational, and aggressive use of it during times of crisis—is a thoroughly reasonable approach for this maneuver. Nonetheless, these optional recommendations rest on the vast experience of the expert panel and not on the experience of large clinical trials. The culmination of the guidelines and options within the guideline, along with the expertise of the panel, is a treatment algorithm for intracranial hypertension (**Fig. 1**), which has served as a template for clinical protocols for patient care and research.

NEW GUIDELINES: A DIFFERENT APPROACH LEADS TO NEW RESULTS

Almost a decade after the generation of the first edition of the Guidelines, the Brain Trauma Foundation convened another panel of experts to begin the process of reexamining the literature to generate new recommendations in 2009. In the interval

A

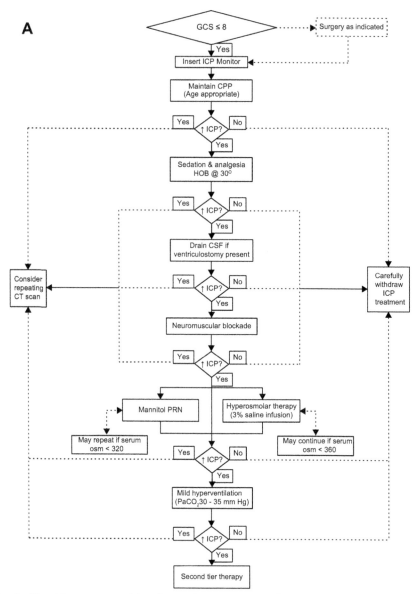

Fig. 1. Algorithm generated by the Brain Trauma Foundation Committee for the first edition of the *Guidelines for the Medical Management of Severe Traumatic Brain Injury in Infants, Children, and Adolescents* for first-tier therapies (*A*) and second-tier therapies (*B*). AFDO₂, arteriovenous difference in oxygen; CBF, cerebral blood flow; CPP, cerebral perfusion pressure; CSF, cerebrospinal fluid; CT, computed tomography; EEG, electroenceph-alogram; GCS, Glasgow Coma Scale; HOB, head of bed; ICP, intracranial pressure; PaCO₂, partial pressure of carbon dioxide; PRN, as needed; SjO₂, jugular bulb venous oxygen satu-ration. (*From* Adelson, PD, Bratton SL, Carney NA, et al. Guidelines for the acute medical management of severe traumatic brain injury in infants, children, and adolescents. Chapter 17. Critical pathway for the treatment of established intracranial hypertension in pediatric traumatic brain injury. Pediatr Crit Care Med 2003;4(Suppl 3):S65–7; with permission.)

B

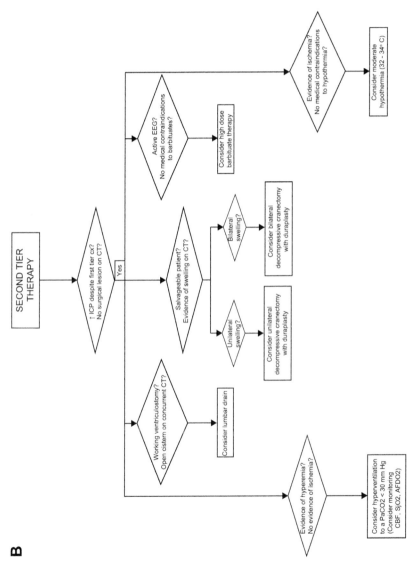

Fig. 1. (*continued*)

between the reviews of the literature, a large body of work had been performed including the largest randomized controlled trial of therapeutic hypothermia in children, the implementation of monitoring for brain-tissue oxygen pressure, a randomized controlled trial of immune-enhanced nutrition, and many reports regarding fundamental aspects of pediatric TBI care. Therefore, several topics were added (advanced neuro-monitoring, neuroimaging, cerebrospinal fluid drainage, antiseizure prophylaxis) and others were eliminated (trauma systems, prehospital airway management, resuscitation of blood pressure and oxygenation, intracranial pressure monitoring technology, and the critical pathway). The result is that the new guidelines are considerably more focused on therapies for improvements in outcomes (either overall outcomes or surrogate outcomes) and hospital-based procedures rather than on issues related to prehospital or system-based approaches. In addition, the standards for evidenced-based medicine guidelines had evolved in the intervening time, decreasing the emphasis on expert opinion and relying on rigorous definitions of inclusion/exclusion criteria for articles that are included within these types of guidelines. These advances led to a quite different guideline document, which was published in early 2012.[37]

Methodologically there were several significant changes within the procedure that generated the new Guidelines. Although the methods of gathering articles for consideration were largely similar (scanning of search engines using keywords specific for the topic by a librarian as well as from the knowledge of the committee members), a priori inclusion criteria for articles within the new guidelines were agreed to include: severe TBI (GCS <9), human subjects only, English-language articles only, pediatric patients (age $\leq$18 years), randomized controlled trials (N$\geq$25), cohort studies (prospective or retrospective, N$\geq$25), case-control studies (N$\geq$25), and case series (N$\geq$5). Articles were excluded for exclusively including penetrating brain injuries, animal studies, cadaver studies, and those including adult subjects (>15% of adult subjects) or those with brain injuries other than TBI (>15% of subjects with conditions other than TBI). Case studies, editorials, letters to the editors, and commentary works were also excluded. The intervention needed to be specific to the topic and the outcome must be a relevant health outcome (normally mortality, favorable outcome, or a surrogate outcome specific for the intervention).

There were also significant changes in the assessments of the quality of the evidence. For this version of the Guidelines, epidemiologists and staff from the Evidence-Based Practice Center of Oregon Health and Science University developed criteria and procedures for the quality assessments of individual studies and assigned a level of evidence for each topic. Specifically, criteria for classification of evidence were derived from several international sources of other evidence-based methodologies, and assignment of evidence to levels I, II, and III was adjudicated by members of the staff. Overall, Class I evidence was defined as having been derived from high-quality randomized controlled trials, with adequate randomization, allocation concealment, blinded assessments, adequate statistical power, and follow-up rates greater than 85%. Class II evidence was defined as having been derived from clinical studies in which data were either prospectively collected or retrospectively collected with clearly reliable data, representing observational, cohort, prevalence, and case-control studies, along with randomized controlled trials of lower quality. These studies required unbiased selection of subjects, statistical analysis for confounders, clear differentiation of treatment groups, and blinded assessments of outcomes. Lastly, Class III evidence was defined as data derived from purely observational studies including registries, case series, or databases. These articles lacked some of the more rigorous controls outlined for the other classifications. The strength of the overall evidence within a given topic was assessed as high, moderate, or low, based on a grading system adopted by the Agency for Healthcare Research and Quality,[38] including the risk of bias from individual studies, consistency of findings across studies, directness of the evidence, and precision of the findings.

As a result of these changes and of the new review of the literature, 27 new articles were added to the Guidelines. However, following the procedures outlined here, 25 articles that were included in the first version of the Guidelines were excluded from this revised version. The reasons for exclusion of articles varied, but centered around lack of clarity regarding admission GCS score (thereby leaving the diagnosis of the severity of TBI in doubt), inclusion of subjects with diagnoses other than TBI, inclusion of adult subjects (without the ability to discern the effect of the therapy on children only), and lack of a relevant outcome as defined here. In contrast to the previous guideline, the classification of standards, guidelines, and options were replaced with evidence Class I, II, and III, respectively. These criteria were generally regarded as therapies that "must be done," "should be considered," and "may be considered," respectively.

Overall, again, there were no topics that generated data of sufficient quality to generate Class I evidence. There were 4 Class II recommendations generated; disappointingly, only one of these recommendations was supportive of a therapeutic approach (**Table 2** summarizes the recommendations). For hyperosmolar therapies, 2 studies were judged to be of Class II quality.[39,40] Fisher and colleagues[39] performed a randomized controlled trial including 18 children of 3% saline compared with 0.9% saline during a 2-hour trial period. The group receiving the hypertonic saline had lower ICP and decreased need for other ICP-related therapies. Simma and colleagues[40] performed a small randomized controlled trial comparing the utility of hypertonic saline solution (1.7% saline) with that of isotonic solutions (lactated Ringer solution) over a 3-day period after TBI. Although there was no difference in overall outcomes, the hypertonic saline group required fewer ICP-related interventions during the study period. Both studies were judged to be of moderate quality.

The other 3 Class II recommendations involved avoiding therapies. In perhaps the most important clinical trial in pediatric neurotrauma and neurocritical care to date, Hutchison and colleagues[41] completed the Hyp-HIT study, a randomized controlled trial of early, moderate hypothermia for pediatric TBI. In this landmark study, 225 children were randomized (205 were available for follow-up) to an experimental group who were cooled to 32° to 33°C for 24 hours (initiation of cooling within 8 hours, rewarming at 0.5°C per hour). The study was confounded in a few ways (the normothermia group had greater exposure to hypertonic saline therapies, both groups received aggressive hyperventilation [$Paco_2$ <30 mm Hg] at frequencies >40%, decreases in CPP were noted in the hypothermia group), but the experimental group failed to demonstrate a benefit from the treatment and even trended toward a worse outcome at 6 months after injury ($P = .08$). These findings led to a Class II recommendation to avoid the use of therapeutic hypothermia to improve outcome, and along with the stopping of the Pediatric Traumatic Brain Injury Consortium: Hypothermia (the "Cool Kids" trial) for reasons of futility, this leaves the future of the use of therapeutic hypothermia to improve overall outcome after TBI in doubt. Despite these findings, there are also data of Class II quality demonstrating that therapeutic hypothermia is associated with decreased ICP in some cases.[42] The second Class II recommendation is also generated from a new randomized controlled trial, studying the use of an immune-modulating diet to improve outcomes. Briassoulis and colleagues[43] randomized 40 children to receive an immune-modulated diet (with increased glutamine, arginine, antioxidants, and ω-3 fatty acids) using a protocol that standardized the amount of support within both groups. Unfortunately, there were no significant differences in mortality or other outcomes measures tested, thereby generating the Class II evidence

Table 2
Summary of evidence generated from the 2012 pediatric TBI guidelines

Topic	Level of Evidence	Recommendation
Indications for ICP monitoring	Level III	"Use of ICP monitoring may be considered…"
Threshold for treatment of intracranial hypertension	Level III	"Treatment of ICP may be considered at a threshold of 20 mm Hg"
Cerebral perfusion pressure thresholds	Level III	"A minimum CPP of 40 mm Hg may be considered … A CPP threshold of 40–50 mm Hg may be considered…"
Advanced neuromonitoring	Level III	"If brain oxygenation monitoring is used, maintenance of a partial pressure of brain-tissue oxygen ($Pbto_2$) $\geq$10 mm Hg may be considered"
Neuroimaging	Level III	"In the absence of neurologic deterioration … routine repeat CT scan … may not be indicated…"
Hyperosmolar therapy	Level II	"Hypertonic saline should be considered … for intracranial hypertension … effective doses … range between 6.5 and 10 mL/kg"
	Level III	"Hypertonic saline should be considered … effective doses as a continuous infusion of 3% saline range between 0.1 and 1.0 mL/kg/h administered on a sliding scale…"
Temperature control	Level II	"Moderate hypothermia … for only 24 h duration should be avoided … moderate hypothermia starting within 8 h after injury and lasting for 48 h duration should be considered to reduce ICP … rewarming at a rate of 0.5°C/h should be avoided"
	Level III	"Moderate hypothermia … for 48 h duration may be considered"
Cerebrospinal fluid drainage	Level III	"CSF drainage through an externalized ventricular drain … may be considered … The addition of a lumbar drain may be considered…"
Barbiturates	Level III	"High-dose barbiturate therapy may be considered in hemodynamically stable patients with refractory intracranial hypertension … continuous arterial blood pressure monitoring and cardiovascular support to maintain adequate CPP are required"
Decompressive craniectomy for the treatment of intracranial hypertension	Level III	"Decompressive craniectomy with duraplasty … may be considered for pediatric patients … showing early signs of neurologic deterioration or herniation or are developing intracranial hypertension refractory to medical management…"

(continued on next page)

Table 2 *(continued)*		
Topic	Level of Evidence	Recommendation
Hyperventilation	Level III	"Avoidance of prophylactic severe hyperventilation to a $Paco_2$ <30 mm Hg may be considered within the first 48 h … If hyperventilation is used … advanced neuromonitoring for evaluation of cerebral ischemia may be considered"
Corticosteroids	Level II	"The use of corticosteroids is not recommended to improve outcome or lower ICP…"
Glucose and nutrition	Level II	"The evidence does not support the use of an immune-modulating diet … to improve outcome"
	Level III	"…glycemic control … should be left to the treating physician"
Antiseizure prophylaxis	Level III	"Prophylactic treatment with phenytoin may be considered to reduce the incidence of early posttraumatic seizures…"

Abbreviations: CPP, cerebral perfusion pressure (mean arterial blood pressure minus intracranial pressure); CSF, cerebrospinal fluid; CT, computed tomography; ICP, intracranial pressure.

Data from Kochanek PK, et al. Guidelines for the acute medical management of severe traumatic brain injury in infants, children, and adolescents: second edition. Pediatr Crit Care Med 2012;13(Suppl 1):S1–82.

that this form of immune-modulated diet could not be recommended at this time. Moreover, the fourth Class II recommendation regarded the avoidance of corticosteroids to improve outcome or reduce ICP that were described in the previous guideline.

Several of the optional therapies from the previous guideline were included in the new version as Class III evidence, including the indication for ICP monitoring, threshold for ICP treatment, threshold for CPP, utility of barbiturates, and decompressive surgery for intracranial hypertension. However, several new Class III recommendations were also generated. Within the new topic of advanced neuromonitoring, a Class III recommendation was generated, based on studies from the groups of Figaji and Narotam[44,45] establishing that a threshold of 10 mm Hg may be considered when brain-tissue oxygen partial pressure (PbO_2) is used. For neuroimaging, Figg and colleagues[46] found that repeated computed tomography scans without neurologic deterioration were not fruitful in an observational cohort from a single center performed over a decade. For antiseizure prophylaxis, a retrospective study of 31 children demonstrated that prophylactic administration of phenytoin reduced the incidence of posttraumatic seizures, leading to the Class III recommendation.[47] For a variety of other topics, including glycemic control, cerebrospinal fluid drainage, and analgesics/sedatives/neuromuscular blockade, definitive recommendations could not be made based on the available literature.

In their totality, the newest version of the Guidelines represents a synthesis of a body of literature spanning more than 40 years into a workable document to guide clinical practice and research protocols. Literature of the highest quality in these topics is desirable for a condition that is responsible for the largest number of deaths of children every year in the United States, and the pediatric neurotrauma community is frustrated by the lack of definitive evidence to generate high-level recommendations. In this version of the Guidelines, suggestions for future studies are made at the end of each topic in an effort to spur the pediatric neurotrauma community to add to the existing foundation of the literature. It is only with new data that better and more comprehensive recommendations can be generated.

NEW STEPS FORWARD: COMMON DATA ELEMENTS FOR PEDIATRIC TBI

A reasonable conclusion to reach after reviewing the Guidelines is that there is insufficient high-quality evidence to make specific treatment plans for children with severe TBI. One reason for this is the inadequate sample sizes of clinical studies, likely because of both the relatively recent focus on pediatric neurocritical care and the relatively small numbers of severe patients seen at individual institutions. As an example, there were 8 randomized controlled trials outlined within the revised Guidelines that included only 469 children. The small sample sizes of these trials obviously hinder the statistical power to prove their primary hypothesis (especially if it is related to overall outcomes) as well as the performance of secondary analyses. Combining data derived from these trials and, possibly, adding other data from well-performed observational studies, might prove valuable in increasing the sample size so that other analyses of secondary hypotheses might be possible. A tremendous impediment to this possibility is the lack of firm criteria identifying data elements that are essential for clinical trials in pediatric TBI.

An effort to identify such key data elements for children with severe TBI was initiated for just this purpose by the National Institute of Neurological Disorders and Stroke (NINDS) in 2009, and completed in 2012. Panels of experts in pediatric TBI were convened to determine data elements essential for (1) demographics and clinical assessment, (2) neurologic imaging, (3) outcome assessments, and (4) biomarkers.[48–51] These panels worked via e-mail, phone conferences, and an in-person meeting to identify which elements were essential to all TBI studies (core elements), elements that might be useful in a subset of TBI studies (supplemental elements), and those that may have some future use (emerging elements). In the demographics and clinical assessment effort, 44 separate data elements were identified and precisely defined, while the neuroimaging group identified several overlapping elements along with stressing the "proper age-dependent interpretation" of radiologic findings as a necessary next step in the process. Meanwhile, the outcomes group painstakingly reviewed the potential outcome tests within the literature and determined age-specific tests within 18 different domains of functioning after TBI, and the biomarker group made recommendations regarding how biological samples from children with TBI should be processed and analyzed. The work done by these panels of experts will need to be implemented into new trials and then undoubtedly revised into newer versions of these important data points, to ultimately allow comparison and recombining of TBI studies to expand data sets with common definitions and completeness of data. For adult TBI studies, this process has ultimately led to electronic data-collection forms that can be used for all studies, ultimately allowing thousands of subjects to be integrated into a common database. More information regarding this constantly evolving effort can be found at the Web site of the Federal Interagency Traumatic Brain Injury Research (FITBIR) (http://fitbir.nih.gov).

SUMMARY

By any measure, there has been an enormous effort within the pediatric neurotrauma community to identify the optimal practices that can lead to improved outcomes for

TBI, a disorder that is the leading killer of children. It is equally obvious that the current state of TBI literature is such that a wide variety of clinical approaches can fall "within" the guidelines because of the lack of data regarding the superiority of clinical decisions made every day for children with severe injuries. With the development of common data elements, it is possible that some of these questions may be answered by combining clinical trials in the future for secondary analyses. Alternatively, the time may be right for an observational study of pediatric TBI that uses novel statistical methods to compare the effectiveness of these commonly used TBI therapies as they are currently used in clinical practice.

REFERENCES

1. Adelson PD, Bratton SL, Carney NA, et al. Guidelines for the acute medical management of severe traumatic brain injury in infants, children, and adolescents. Chapter 3. Prehospital airway management. Pediatr Crit Care Med 2003; 4(Suppl 3):S9–11.
2. Adelson PD, Clyde B, Kochanek PM, et al. Guidelines for the acute medical management of severe traumatic brain injury in infants, children, and adolescents. Chapter 4. Resuscitation of blood pressure and oxygenation and prehospital brain-specific therapies for the severe pediatric traumatic brain injury patient. Pediatr Crit Care Med 2003;4(Suppl 3):S12–8.
3. Adelson PD, Bratton SL, Carney NA, et al. Guidelines for the acute medical management of severe traumatic brain injury in infants, children, and adolescents. Chapter 18. Nutritional support. Pediatr Crit Care Med 2003;4(Suppl 3):S68–71.
4. Adelson PD, Bratton SL, Carney NA, et al. Guidelines for the acute medical management of severe traumatic brain injury in infants, children, and adolescents. Chapter 16. The use of corticosteroids in the treatment of severe pediatric traumatic brain injury. Pediatr Crit Care Med 2003;4(Suppl 3):S60–4.
5. Adelson PD, Bratton SL, Carney NA, et al. Guidelines for the acute medical management of severe traumatic brain injury in infants, children, and adolescents. Chapter 15. Surgical treatment of pediatric intracranial hypertension. Pediatr Crit Care Med 2003;4(Suppl 3):S56–9.
6. Adelson PD, Bratton SL, Carney NA, et al. Guidelines for the acute medical management of severe traumatic brain injury in infants, children, and adolescents. Chapter 14. The role of temperature control following severe pediatric traumatic brain injury. Pediatr Crit Care Med 2003;4(Suppl 3):S53–5.
7. Adelson PD, Bratton SL, Carney NA, et al. Guidelines for the acute medical management of severe traumatic brain injury in infants, children, and adolescents. Chapter 13. The use of barbiturates in the control of intracranial hypertension in severe pediatric traumatic brain injury. Pediatr Crit Care Med 2003; 4(Suppl 3):S49–52.
8. Adelson PD, Bratton SL, Carney NA, et al. Guidelines for the acute medical management of severe traumatic brain injury in infants, children, and adolescents. Chapter 12. Use of hyperventilation in the acute management of severe pediatric traumatic brain injury. Pediatr Crit Care Med 2003;4(Suppl 3):S45–8.
9. Adelson PD, Bratton SL, Carney NA, et al. Guidelines for the acute medical management of severe traumatic brain injury in infants, children, and adolescents. Chapter 11. Use of hyperosmolar therapy in the management of severe pediatric traumatic brain injury. Pediatr Crit Care Med 2003;4(Suppl 3):S40–4.
10. Adelson PD, Bratton SL, Carney NA, et al. Guidelines for the acute medical management of severe traumatic brain injury in infants, children, and

adolescents. Chapter 10. The role of cerebrospinal fluid drainage in the treatment of severe pediatric traumatic brain injury. Pediatr Crit Care Med 2003;4(Suppl 3): S38–9.

11. Adelson PD, Bratton SL, Carney NA, et al. Guidelines for the acute medical management of severe traumatic brain injury in infants, children, and adolescents. Chapter 9. Use of sedation and neuromuscular blockade in the treatment of severe pediatric traumatic brain injury. Pediatr Crit Care Med 2003;4(Suppl 3): S34–7.

12. Adelson PD, Bratton SL, Carney NA, et al. Guidelines for the acute medical management of severe traumatic brain injury in infants, children, and adolescents. Chapter 8. Cerebral perfusion pressure. Pediatr Crit Care Med 2003; 4(Suppl 3):S31–3.

13. Adelson PD, Bratton SL, Carney NA, et al. Guidelines for the acute medical management of severe traumatic brain injury in infants, children, and adolescents. Chapter 7. Intracranial pressure monitoring technology. Pediatr Crit Care Med 2003;4(Suppl 3):S28–30.

14. Adelson PD, Bratton SL, Carney NA, et al. Guidelines for the acute medical management of severe traumatic brain injury in infants, children, and adolescents. Chapter 6. Threshold for treatment of intracranial hypertension. Pediatr Crit Care Med 2003;4(Suppl 3):S25–7.

15. Adelson PD, Bratton SL, Carney NA, et al. Guidelines for the acute medical management of severe traumatic brain injury in infants, children, and adolescents. Chapter 5. Indications for intracranial pressure monitoring in pediatric patients with severe traumatic brain injury. Pediatr Crit Care Med 2003;4(Suppl 3):S19–24.

16. Adelson PD, Bratton SL, Carney NA, et al. Guidelines for the acute medical management of severe traumatic brain injury in infants, children, and adolescents. Chapter 2: trauma systems, pediatric trauma centers, and the neurosurgeon. Pediatr Crit Care Med 2003;4(Suppl 3):S5–8.

17. Adelson PD, Bratton SL, Carney NA, et al. Guidelines for the acute medical management of severe traumatic brain injury in infants, children, and adolescents. Chapter 1: introduction. Pediatr Crit Care Med 2003;4(Suppl 3):S2–4.

18. Adelson PD, Bratton SL, Carney NA, et al. Guidelines for the acute medical management of severe traumatic brain injury in infants, children, and adolescents. Chapter 17. Critical pathway for the treatment of established intracranial hypertension in pediatric traumatic brain injury. Pediatr Crit Care Med 2003; 4(Suppl 3):S65–7.

19. Adelson PD, Bratton SL, Carney NA, et al. Guidelines for the acute medical management of severe traumatic brain injury in infants, children, and adolescents. Chapter 19. The role of anti-antiseizure prophylaxis following severe pediatric traumatic brain injury. Pediatr Crit Care Med 2003;4(Suppl 3):S72–5.

20. Bullock R, Chesnut RM, Clifton G, et al. Guidelines for the management of severe head injury. Brain Trauma Foundation. Eur J Emerg Med 1996;3(2):109–27.

21. Johnson DL, Krishnamurthy S. Send severely head-injured children to a pediatric trauma center. Pediatr Neurosurg 1996;25(6):309–14.

22. Hulka F, Mullins RJ, Mann NC, et al. Influence of a statewide trauma system on pediatric hospitalization and outcome. J Trauma 1997;42(3):514–9.

23. Potoka DA, Schall LC, Gardner MJ, et al. Impact of pediatric trauma centers on mortality in a statewide system. J Trauma 2000;49(2):237–45.

24. Cooper A, DiScala C, Foltin G, et al. Prehospital endotracheal intubation for severe head injury in children: a reappraisal. Semin Pediatr Surg 2001; 10(1):3–6.

25. Gausche M, Lewis RJ, Stratton SJ, et al. Effect of out-of-hospital pediatric endotracheal intubation on survival and neurological outcome: a controlled clinical trial. JAMA 2000;283(6):783–90.

26. Murray JA, Demetriades D, Berne TV, et al. Prehospital intubation in patients with severe head injury. J Trauma 2000;49(6):1065–70.

27. Nakayama DK, Gardner MJ, Rowe MI. Emergency endotracheal intubation in pediatric trauma. Ann Surg 1990;211(2):218–23.

28. Luerssen TG, Klauber MR, Marshall LF. Outcome from head injury related to patient's age. A longitudinal prospective study of adult and pediatric head injury. J Neurosurg 1988;68(3):409–16.

29. Michaud LJ, Rivara FP, Longstreth WT, et al. Predictors of survival and severity of disability after severe brain injury in children. Neurosurgery 1992;31(2):254–64.

30. Pigula FA, Wald SL, Shackford SR, et al. The effect of hypotension and hypoxia on children with severe head injuries. J Pediatr Surg 1993;28(3):310–4 [discussion: 315–6].

31. Ong L, Selladurai BM, Dhillon MK, et al. The prognostic value of the Glasgow Coma Scale, hypoxia and computerised tomography in outcome prediction of pediatric head injury. Pediatr Neurosurg 1996;24(6):285–91.

32. Downard C, Hulka F, Mullins RJ, et al. Relationship of cerebral perfusion pressure and survival in pediatric brain-injured patients. J Trauma 2000;49(4):654–8 [discussion: 658–9].

33. Fanconi S, Meuli M, Zaugg H, et al. Dexamethasone therapy and endogenous cortisol production in severe pediatric head injury. Intensive Care Med 1988; 14(2):163–6.

34. Kloti J, Fanconi S, Zachmann M, et al. Dexamethasone therapy and cortisol excretion in severe pediatric head injury. Childs Nerv Syst 1987;3(2):103–5.

35. Skippen P, Seear M, Poskitt K, et al. Effect of hyperventilation on regional cerebral blood flow in head-injured children. Crit Care Med 1997;25(8):1402–9.

36. Stringer WA, Choi SC, Fatouros P, et al. Hyperventilation-induced cerebral ischemia in patients with acute brain lesions: demonstration by xenon-enhanced CT. AJNR Am J Neuroradiol 1993;14(2):475–84.

37. Kochanek PM, Carney N, Adelson PD, et al. Guidelines for the acute medical management of severe traumatic brain injury in infants, children and adolescents: second Edition. Pediatr Crit Care Med 2012;13(Suppl 1):S1–82.

38. Owens DK, Lohr KN, Atkins D, et al. AHRQ series paper 5: grading the strength of a body of evidence when comparing medical interventions–agency for healthcare research and quality and the effective health-care program. J Clin Epidemiol 2010; 63(5):513–23.

39. Fisher B, Thomas D, Peterson B. Hypertonic saline lowers raised intracranial pressure in children after head trauma. J Neurosurg Anesthesiol 1992;4(1):4–10.

40. Simma B, Burger R, Falk M, et al. A prospective, randomized, and controlled study of fluid management in children with severe head injury: lactated Ringer's solution versus hypertonic saline. Crit Care Med 1998;26(7):1265–70.

41. Hutchison JS, Ward RE, Lacroix J, et al. Hypothermia therapy after traumatic brain injury in children. N Engl J Med 2008;358(23):2447–56.

42. Adelson PD. Phase II clinical trial of moderate hypothermia after severe traumatic brain injury in children. Neurosurgery 2005;56(4):740–54 [discussion: 740–54].

43. Briassoulis G, Filippou O, Kanariou M, et al. Temporal nutritional and inflammatory changes in children with severe head injury fed a regular or an immune-enhancing diet: a randomized, controlled trial. Pediatr Crit Care Med 2006;7(1): 56–62.

44. Figaji AA, Zwane E, Thompson C, et al. Brain tissue oxygen tension monitoring in pediatric severe traumatic brain injury. Part 1: relationship with outcome. Childs Nerv Syst 2009;25(10):1325–33.

45. Narotam PK, Burjonrappa SC, Raynor SC, et al. Cerebral oxygenation in major pediatric trauma: its relevance to trauma severity and outcome. J Pediatr Surg 2006;41(3):505–13.

46. Figg RE, Stouffer CW, Vander Kolk WE, et al. Clinical efficacy of serial computed tomographic scanning in pediatric severe traumatic brain injury. Pediatr Surg Int 2006;22(3):215–8.

47. Lewis RJ, Yee L, Inkelis SH, et al. Clinical predictors of post-traumatic seizures in children with head trauma. Ann Emerg Med 1993;22(7):1114–8.

48. Adelson PD, Pineda J, Bell MJ, et al. Common data elements for pediatric traumatic brain injury: recommendations from the working group on demographics and clinical assessment. J Neurotrauma 2012;29(4):639–53.

49. Berger RP, Goyal A, Carter M, et al. Common data elements for pediatric traumatic brain injury: recommendations from the biospecimens and biomarkers workgroup. J Neurotrauma 2012;29(4):672–7.

50. Duhaime AC, Berger RP, Beers SR, et al. Common data elements for neuroimaging of traumatic brain injury: pediatric considerations. J Neurotrauma 2012;29(4):629–33.

51. McCauley SR, Wilde EW, Miller ER, et al. Recommendations for the use of common outcome measures in pediatric traumatic brain injury research. J Neurotrauma 2012;29(4):678–705.

Pediatric Intensive Care Treatment of Uncontrolled Status Epilepticus

Ryan Wilkes, MD[a], Robert C. Tasker, MBBS, MD[a,b],*

KEYWORDS

• Status epilepticus • Super-refractory • FIRES epilepsy • Anesthesia • Pediatric

KEY POINTS

- Impending status epilepticus (SE) is defined as continuous seizures lasting more than 5 minutes, or intermittent clinical or electroencephalographic (EEG) seizures lasting more than 15 minutes without full recovery of consciousness between seizures.
- Refractory SE is a state whereby clinical or EEG seizures last longer than 60 minutes despite treatment with at least 1 first-line (ie, benzodiazepine) and 1 second-line (ie, phenytoin, phenobarbital, or valproate) anticonvulsant drug.
- Super-refractory SE is a stage of refractory SE characterized by unresponsiveness to initial anesthetic therapy, and is defined as SE that continues or recurs 24 hours or more after the onset of general anesthesia, including those cases in which SE recurs on the reduction or withdrawal of anesthesia.
- The evidence base from randomized controlled trials on which anticonvulsant drug strategy should be used to treat SE in the intensive care unit is inadequate.
- There is increasing experience with using high-dose midazolam, barbiturate anesthesia, and volatile anesthetics for uncontrolled SE.

INTRODUCTION

The pediatric critical care physician is usually involved in the treatment of children presenting with a prolonged seizure after the fact. The child has had emergency treatment during prehospital transport, or in the emergency department. The physician is then faced with 3 possible clinical pathways:

1. The previously well child now requires endotracheal intubation and mechanical ventilation because of respiratory depression complicating treatment or the acute disease that has produced the seizure.

Disclosures: The authors have no conflicts of interest and no disclosures to make.
[a] Division of Critical Care, Department of Anesthesia, Pain and Perioperative Medicine, Boston Children's Hospital, 300 Longwood Avenue, Boston, MA 02115, USA; [b] Department of Neurology, Boston Children's Hospital, 300 Longwood Avenue, Boston, MA 02115, USA
* Corresponding author.
E-mail address: robert.tasker@childrens.harvard.edu

Crit Care Clin 29 (2013) 239–257
http://dx.doi.org/10.1016/j.ccc.2012.11.007
0749-0704/13/$ – see front matter © 2013 Elsevier Inc. All rights reserved.

criticalcare.theclinics.com

2. For the child with a known seizure disorder on multiple antiepileptic drugs (AED), AED pharmacokinetics need to be checked and optimized.
3. The child who is mechanically ventilated with ongoing seizures that are refractory to any treatment; the pathway for this group is the focus of this article.

In the modern era, a protocol-driven approach to acute seizure care[1] of children in the first 2 pathways now means that the classic end stage of status epilepticus (SE) with disruption in systemic physiology and metabolism leading to hyperpyrexia, exhaustion, and death is no longer seen.[2–5] However, there is a risk that rather than too little medication being given too infrequently, the morbidity of emergency seizure treatment may now exceed the morbidity of the SE itself.[6]

It is assumed that the reader is familiar with standard emergency department guidelines for acute care and the respiratory management of children in the first 2 pathways (**Fig. 1**). Hence, the focus of this article is how to approach seizure control for children

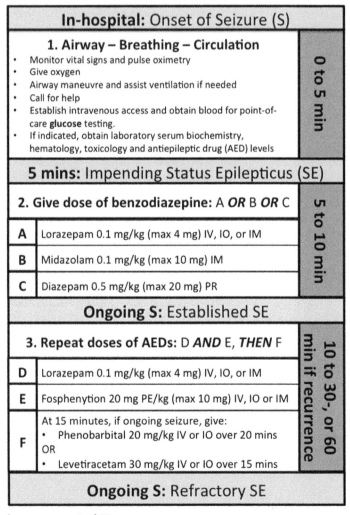

Fig. 1. Early management of SE.

in the third pathway, during admission to the pediatric intensive care unit (PICU). The approach to the finding of nonconvulsive SE in PICU patients undergoing EEG monitoring is not dealt with in this review, because that topic is beyond the scope of this article.

DEFINITIONS

The point in time at which a prolonged seizure becomes an episode of SE has changed over the last 20 years.[7] There is no consensus on when usual seizure duration has been surpassed and the transition to a state whereby there is failure in intrinsic mechanisms that bring about seizure cessation has been reached (ie, onset of SE). SE was once defined as seizure activity, either continuous or episodic without complete recovery of consciousness, lasting for at least 30 to 60 minutes. In PICU practice, we now use an operational definition starting with 5 minutes of seizure activity, and think of episodes in relation to their response to therapy. Hence terms such as impending SE, refractory SE, and super-refractory SE are now frequently used in the literature.

Impending SE

One proposal for the definition of convulsive tonic-clonic SE is seizure activity lasting at least 5 minutes.[8,9] In adults, this definition is based on videotape-telemetry studies that show a mean duration of generalized convulsive seizures range from 62.2 seconds (n = 120) to 52.9 $\pm$ 14 seconds (n = 50) for the behavioral manifestations and 59.9 $\pm$ 12 seconds for the electroencephalographic (EEG) manifestations.[10,11] Because none of these seizures lasted 2 minutes, an operational definition of SE as 5 minutes of continuous generalized convulsive activity would reflect an episode lasting some 20 standard deviations (SD) more than the norm, making it a rare event. However, it might be even more appropriate to terminate an episode with intravenous AEDs after 4 to 5 SDs more than the norm (ie, after 2 minutes).[10]

In emergency practice in children, there is little difference between 2 and 5 minutes because it takes at least 5 minutes to administer an intravenous AED.[12] Hence, a definition of 5 minutes of continuous seizure activity is a pragmatic solution to the question of definition of SE: it uses a duration that is consistent with practice in the emergency department; and it places the definition of SE far outside the norm for seizure duration. Some investigators have chosen to call these 5-minute episodes impending SE, because a significant proportion of patients stop seizing spontaneously in the next few minutes.[13] Therefore, impending SE is defined as "continuous seizures lasting more than 5 minutes, or intermittent clinical or EEG seizures lasting more than 15 minutes without full recovery of consciousness between seizures."[14] This definition recognizes the need to treat such patients with intravenous AEDs and applies to adults and children more than 5 years of age. Separating impending SE from other definitions of SE also helps to better define subpopulations for morbidity and mortality statistics, outcome measures, and clinical trials of AEDs.

Another approach to making a decision about when a seizure episode has become SE is to consider the form of the seizure. This approach is often used in the PICU in patients with epilepsy. Typically, at baseline, these individuals may have several seizures each day. It is counterproductive to their ongoing management and return to baseline care to use the seizure protocol shown in **Fig. 1** every time a 5-minute event occurs. In this instance, the clinical question is "how likely is it that this new seizure will extend into SE?" **Table 1** provides a summary of the different forms of seizure types and SE. There is some evidence in adults that seizure duration differs

Table 1
Forms of seizures in SE

Forms	Seizure	Behavior and Autonomic	Medication
Convulsive			
Generalized tonic-clonic (GTC)	Increased seizures in epilepsy Duration of each seizure shortens May have abnormal cranial nerve examination	Obtunded Salivation, bradypnea Cyanosis, hypotension	First: lorazepam Second: fosphenytoin
Generalized clonic	Waxing and waning for hours Postictal hemiplegia	Variable behaviors Consciousness preserved Less autonomic than GTC	First: lorazepam Second: fosphenytoin
Generalized tonic	Serial tonic episodes In epilepsy precipitated by benzodiazepines May last days with serial seizures	Increased bronchial secretions and respiratory irregularity Eye deviation	First: lorazepam Second: fosphenytoin
Focal motor	Epileptic disorder or acute insult (AI) AI developing secondary GTC seizures Restricted distribution in epilepsy	Some impairment of consciousness Some autonomic features	First: lorazepam Second: fosphenytoin
Myoclonic	Repetitive myoclonic jerks AI and epilepsy	Seen postanoxia in coma	First: lorazepam Second: fosphenytoin or valproate
Nonconvulsive			
Absence	Petit mal SE	Variable impaired consciousness Complex automatisms	First: lorazepam Second: valproate
Complex partial seizure (CPS)	Psychomotor SE Can present with recurring partial seizures	Cycling from unresponsive to partial response Reactive automatisms	First: lorazepam Second: fosphenytoin
Classic form and SE in coma	Prolonged altered in consciousness or CPS EEG changes from preseizure state to ictal state Improved EEG/state with treatment	Seen in epilepsy (Landau-Kleffner) A form occurs in coma/AI	First: lorazepam Second: fosphenytoin or anesthesia

for the various seizure types. For example, in a study of 599 seizures in 159 adults, seizures with partial onset spreading to both hemispheres had the longest duration.[15] Secondarily generalized tonic-clonic seizures lasted longer than complex partial seizures, which lasted longer than simple partial seizures. Secondarily generalized tonic-clonic seizures were unlikely to last more than 11 minutes, complex partial seizures more than 10 minutes, and simple partial seizures more than 4 minutes. This gradation is likely related to activation of different neuronal networks at the onset and during propagation of seizures. So, from a practical perspective, a working definition of SE based on these limits in timings has been proposed for patients with a seizure disorder.

Refractory SE

Over the last 10 years, there has been increasing use of the term refractory SE as a description of an episode of SE that persists despite treatment with adequate doses of multiple AEDs. There are many definitions in the literature and there is considerable variation in the duration required for an episode to reach so-called refractoriness.[16] In contrast to the definition used to describe impending SE, the features used to characterize refractory SE are duration as well as response to AEDs and EEG features. The latter is particularly important because there is both experimental and clinical evidence to show that the EEG during the course of generalized convulsive SE in adults follows a predictable sequence with 5 identifiable patterns: I, discrete seizures; II, merging seizures with waxing and waning amplitude and frequency of EEG rhythms; III, continuous ictal activity; IV, continuous ictal activity punctuated by low-voltage flat periods; and V, periodic epileptiform discharges on a flat background.[17,18] The significance of this staging is apparent when duration and seizure response to treatment are examined in the experimental model. Stage I EEG represents a treatment-responsive state to combination therapy with diazepam and phenobarbital, whereas stage III is a treatment-refractory state even though there is overlap in absolute duration of SE in both patterns.[19] When diazepam alone is used to treat seizures, stage I EEG again represents a treatment-responsive state, whereas treatment in stages II to V has increasing likelihood of conversion to subclinical nonconvulsive SE or EEG SE.[17]

A commonly used definition for refractory SE is a state that meets the following criteria: clinical or EEG seizure lasting longer than 60 minutes despite treatment with at least 1 first-line AED (ie, benzodiazepine) and 1 second-line AED (ie, phenytoin, phenobarbital, or valproate).[16,20] In children, such episodes are frequent and occur in 25% to 50% of patients in case series of SE.[20–22] In 1 study of 154 children with SE, 45% of the cases of refractory SE had nonconvulsive SE,[22] which is much higher than the 27% seen in adults.[16] One possible explanation for the refractoriness is that in contrast to seizures that rapidly generalize and stop spontaneously, seizures that do not readily generalize and involve the motor cortex may be associated with more severe underlying brain pathology, and hence may be more refractory to therapy. As discussed earlier, the EEG is a vital sign in those patients who do not arouse after acute control of motor seizures, particularly in those patients with acute structural lesions and at higher risk for nonconvulsive episodes.

Super-refractory SE

Super-refractory SE is a new descriptive term in the literature, first appearing in 2011 in the summary of the Third London-Innsbruck Colloquium on SE.[23] Super-refractory SE is not a new entity; the condition was seen before 2011, but giving it a name helps to clarify an approach to therapy in this difficult clinical situation. Super-refractory SE is a stage of refractory SE characterized by unresponsiveness to initial anesthetic therapy, and is defined as "SE that continues or recurs 24 hours or more after the onset of general anesthesia, including those cases in which SE recurs on the reduction or withdrawal of anesthesia." In adults, it is generally seen in 2 distinctive clinical situations: in patients with severe acute brain injury; and, in previously healthy patients who have no apparent cause for SE, so-called new-onset refractory SE (NORSE).[24]

The pattern of presentation is similar in children, but rather than talking about NORSE, investigators have focused on specific age at occurrence and fever as an apparent triggering factor for the second entity. Fever might even have preceded the onset of neurologic symptoms and no longer be present at the time of presentation. Two conditions have been described in younger age groups: in school-aged children, febrile infection-related epilepsy syndrome (FIRES)[25]; and, in infants, idiopathic hemiconvulsion-hemiplegia syndrome (IHHS).[26] Whether the diagnosis of NORSE, FIRES, and IHHS represents distinct pathophysiologies or a spectrum of acute encephalopathy with inflammation-mediated and immunology-mediated SE, or some genetic or acquired channelopathy is unknown at present.[27,28]

SECOND-TIER ANTICONVULSANTS FOR REFRACTORY SE

The hierarchy in escalation of AED treatment should be considered in relation to the continuum in time that starts with the recognition of impending SE (5 minutes), to the determination of refractory SE (60 minutes), and later super-refractory SE (after 24 hours). The protocol for treating impending SE is shown in **Fig. 1** and occurs long before arrival at the PICU. The second-tier AEDs include some combination of fosphenytoin and phenobarbital, although levetiracetam and valproic acid are also frequently given. In recent years, matching the continuum in seizure duration with escalation to high-dose midazolam has become an option.

Fosphenytoin

Fosphenytoin is the water-soluble prodrug of phenytoin and is used preferentially in the United States. Phenytoin is associated with a higher risk of arrhythmias, hypotension, and, because it is dissolved in propylene glycol and ethanol (pH 12), it can cause a severe extravasation injury, purple glove syndrome. Fosphenytoin slows the rate of recovery of voltage-activated sodium channels and causes an activity-dependent inhibition of action potential firing. Doses are calculated as phenytoin equivalents and typical intravenous boluses are 15 to 20 mg/kg over 20 minutes. Continuous cardiac monitoring is recommended even though arrhythmias and hypotension are far less common with fosphenytoin than with phenytoin. Peak levels are not reached until 20 minutes after the infusion because of the time required for conversion of fosphenytoin to phenytoin, but it is not uncommon for seizures to stop some time before the infusion has finished. With regard to AED monitoring, it is important to follow free phenytoin levels because phenytoin is highly protein bound; and in patients with hypoalbuminemia or those on valproic acid (which displaces phenytoin from albumin), the free level may be high with prolonged use.

Several studies report that using fosphenytoin after a benzodiazepine is successful in seizure control, with rates of 89% to 100%.[29,30] Its relative lack of respiratory depression also makes this agent useful.

Phenobarbital

Phenobarbital is a long-acting barbiturate that is considered to have greater intrinsic antiepileptic properties than other barbiturates (see discussion on pentobarbital). It is commonly used after 2 doses of a benzodiazepine and a dose of fosphenytoin. Its mechanism of action is via the γ-aminobutyric acid (GABA) receptor at a different binding site to that of the benzodiazepines, and so, theoretically, it is useful during treatment of prolonged seizures. Phenobarbital has slow entry into the brain but during seizure activity, cerebral uptake is increased and the drug may be concentrated near seizure foci.[31]

The typical dose of phenobarbital is 15 to 20 mg/kg, infused at a rate of 2 mg/kg/min for children less than 40 kg and 100 mg/min for those more than 40 kg.[32] Repeat dosing of 5 mg/kg is given if seizures persist. (Some investigators have recommended a high-dose strategy with repeated boluses of 10 mg/kg every 30 minutes until seizures stop[33]; although in our experience this dosing is likely to induce coma.) The onset of drug action is within 5 minutes; peak levels occur at 15 minutes. However, a course of intravenous doses can result in prolonged somnolence and recovery because of the elimination half-life of 50 to 150 hours.

Thus, phenobarbital is an effective AED. Its main drawback is respiratory depression and hypotension. In brain-injured patients, endotracheal intubation and mechanical ventilation should be anticipated if previous doses of benzodiazepines have been given, with or without the addition of fosphenytoin. It is the frequent need for airway and hemodynamic intervention that has led to the use of other agents with much lower rates of respiratory depression and hypotension (eg, valproic acid and levetiracetam).

Valproic Acid

Valproic acid works by modulation of sodium and calcium currents along with activating the GABA receptor.[34] The main advantages of valproate are its efficacy against a wide variety of seizure types and an almost complete lack of significant cardiopulmonary depression. It has been used as adjunctive therapy in adults and children with refractory SE[35] and it may be particularly helpful in patients with myoclonic SE, absence SE, or Lennox-Gastaut syndrome. The dose is 20 to 40 mg/kg (infused at a rate of 6 mg/kg/min) followed by a continuous infusion at 1 to 5 mg/kg/h.

The main disadvantages of valproate are hepatotoxicity and hyperammonemia. Among children less than 2 years of age, 1 in 500 develop hepatotoxicity[36]; the risk is much higher in those with an inborn error in metabolism. Therefore, transaminase levels and liver function should be monitored. The other complications include pancreatitis, thrombocytopenia, and coagulation disorders; the latter is possibly caused by decreased hepatic production of clotting factors.

Levetiracetam

Levetiracetam acts at glutamate and GABA receptors as well as calcium channels,[34] but its exact mechanism of action is unknown. It is unique as an AED because of its linear pharmacokinetics, minimal drug-drug interactions, and minimal metabolism. The antiepileptic effects of levetiracetam start within 24 hours of administration and in refractory SE its most attractive potential feature, like that of valproic acid, is the lack of cardiopulmonary depression. But, unlike valproic acid, levetiracetam does not have significant end-organ toxicity and drug-to-drug interactions.[36]

Bolus dosing of levetiracetam ranges from 30 to 60 mg/kg in children and 500 to 2000 mg in adults. Its role in refractory SE is unclear with only small case series being reported. Compared with phenytoin and valproic acid, it seems less effective.

High-Dose Midazolam

There is no evidence that one particular AED is better than any other in the treatment of refractory SE. Therefore, the risks and benefits of each agent must be assessed in a given clinical situation. Patients who are hemodynamically unstable have responded well to benzodiazepines; patients with a relatively benign cause may be candidates for high-dose midazolam by continuous infusion.

The use of midazolam for refractory SE in children is a relatively new practice; the initial PICU experiences were reported in the early 1990s.[37] This imidazobenzodiazepine has a short elimination half-life of 1.5 to 3.5 hours, and little accumulation. These favorable pharmacokinetics allow for repeat bolus dosing, aggressive titration of an infusion, and relatively fast recovery time. It causes little hypotension, and vasopressors are usually only needed when high doses of midazolam are used. Midazolam is soluble at pH less than 4 and undergoes a structural change at the body's physiologic pH. This structural change creates a highly lipophilic structure accounting for its rapid penetration into the brain and rapid onset of action. However, the acidic diluent can cause metabolic acidosis with high infusion rates. Midazolam shares anxiolytic, muscle-relaxant, hypnotic, and anticonvulsant actions with other benzodiazepines. Yet, given these similarities, an obvious question is: Why should it be effective when other GABA agonists (eg, phenobarbitone and diazepam) have failed to control refractory SE?

A recent PICU experience of using midazolam for refractory SE shows that high loading doses (0.50 mg/kg) and infusion rates (mean 0.63 mg/kg/h, maximum 1.92 mg/kg/h) can be given safely.[38] Breakthrough seizures occur frequently even when using infusion rates of 1.44 mg/kg/h after a bolus dose (see earlier discussion), but higher dosing up to 1.92 mg/kg/h can be effective with negligible hemodynamic embarassment. EEG burst suppression is rarely achieved with these doses and should not be the therapeutic goal. A seizure-free period of 24 to 48 hours should be the target before a trial of weaning the infusion (**Table 2**).

GENERAL ANESTHESIA FOR REFRACTORY SE

If seizures persist despite second-tier and third-tier AEDs, then most protocols end with the phrase "refer to anesthesiologist for anesthesia." In the PICU, there are 2 choices: intravenous pentobarbital, a short-acting barbiturate, or an inhalational anesthetic such as isoflurane. Propofol has been used increasingly in the adult population in the last 10 years. However, the risk of propofol infusion syndrome in children is unacceptable and therefore propofol is not recommended for use in the PICU in several countries.

Pentobarbital

Pentobarbital penetrates the central nervous system rapidly, allowing for rapid titration to EEG burst suppression. It has multiple actions: activation of the GABA receptor in a way that is different to the benzodiazepines; inhibition of N-methyl-D-aspartate (NMDA) receptors; and, alteration in the conductance of chloride, potassium, and calcium ion channels. These multiple mechanisms of action explain the drug's potential effectiveness in refractory SE that is resistant to benzodiazepine therapy.[39] Prolonged infusion of pentobarbital results in a transition from the usual first-order elimination kinetics seen with bolus doses to the unpredictable zero-order kinetics and a prolonged elimination half-life because of distribution in lipid. This phenomenon makes recovery time prolonged and the drug effect can last days, even with short infusion periods of 12 to 24 hours.[40]

Pentobarbital causes a reduction in cerebral metabolic rate for oxygen ($CMRO_2$) and, to a lesser degree, a matched decrease in cerebral blood flow (CBF). A consequence of the decrease in CBF is a reduction in the level of intracranial pressure (ICP), which may be an advantage in patients with cerebral swelling.[41] Theoretically, pentobarbital may also be neuroprotective because of its inhibition of NMDA receptors and reduction in $CMRO_2$.

Dosing of pentobarbital

Anesthesia is induced by giving a bolus dose (range 5–15 mg/kg), usually over 30 minutes to 1 hour. The onset of drug action is within a few minutes and the peak effect

Table 2
Strategy for high-dose intravenous midazolam in refractory SE

Timing from Start of this Strategy	Midazolam Dosing	Steps
0 min: initial bolus	Give 0.5 mg/kg	A
0 min: start continuous infusion	Start at 2 μg/kg/min (0.12 mg/kg/h)	B
5 min: if seizure persists 5 min after bolus (step A)	Give 0.5 mg/kg Increase infusion to 4 μg/kg/min (0.24 mg/kg/h)	C
10 min: if seizure persists or recurs 5 min after step C	Give 0.1 mg/kg Increase infusion by 4 μg/kg/min (0.24 mg/kg/h)	D
15 min: if seizure persists or recurs 5 min after step D	Repeat step D	E
20–45 min: if seizure persists or recurs 5 min after step E, then continue to repeat step D every 5 min until a maximum infusion rate is achieved	Maximum infusion rate of 36 μg/kg/min (1.92 mg/kg/h)	F (5 cycles of D-to-E may be needed)
45 min: by the completion of step F an EEG should be available to confirm seizure control or otherwise. If seizure is not controlled then consider this episode as treatment failure and move to step H	Maintain dose of continuous infusion that achieves clinical and EEG seizure control and 24–48 h later move to step I	G
45–60 min: treatment failure	Discontinue midazolam infusion and start general anesthesia with pentobarbital or isoflurane	H
24–48 h: if patient is free of clinical and EEG seizures then start to wean the infusion	Reduce infusion by 4 μg/kg/min every 6–8 h	I
48–84 h: continued EEG monitoring to observe for breakthrough seizures	Plan to discontinue infusion after optimizing other AEDs. If seizures recur then consider step K for weaning failure; alternatively this episode may be in the category of super-refractory SE	J
Weaning failure	Consider rebolus of 0.1 mg/kg and increase infusion by 4 μg/kg/min and/or Consider alternative AEDs	K

is seen within 15 minutes. To achieve EEG burst suppression in a timely manner, it is best to repeat small (5 mg/kg) boluses while monitoring EEG and the hemodynamic state.[42–44] Simply giving a single bolus and adjusting the infusion typically causes an unnecessary delay in achieving therapeutic goals.[43,44] The continuous infusion rate that many investigators use is 1 to 5 mg/kg/h. However, PICU reports show that most patients achieve EEG burst suppression at steady-state infusion rates of 1 mg/kg/h.[42] When patients receive prolonged treatment with pentobarbital, they develop tolerance to the sedative effect, but tolerance to the anticonvulsant effect should not occur, which explains why tachyphylaxis is less common with pentobarbital than with midazolam infusions.[39]

Complications

Hypotension should be anticipated in all patients receiving pentobarbital.[42] It is caused by drug-related dilation of venous capacitance vessels, which results in reduced cardiac preload and output. The total systemic vascular resistance changes little, and there should be no myocardial depression. One use of continuous EEG monitoring is to ensure that the minimum infusion rate of pentobarbital necessary to induce burst suppression is given, thereby avoiding overtreatment and the hemodynamic risks. It is also advisable to make sure that the patient has adequate preload and that vasopressors are readily available.[45]

Pentobarbital also causes white blood cell dysfunction and it is associated with an increased rate of nosocomial infection, especially pneumonia. Patients may also be at risk of significant abdominal complications because these patients invariably develop ileus.[46]

Treatment strategy

Despite the undesirable pharmacokinetics and side effects of pentobarbital, it remains a reliable drug for inducing anesthesia and stopping refractory SE.[47] Burst suppression is usually maintained for 24 to 48 hours, although some investigators argue that longer periods are associated with lower rates of recurrent seizures.[43,44,48] Despite its tissue accumulation and long elimination half-life, breakthrough seizures can occur from abrupt discontinuation of the infusion, and so tapering the dose during weaning is recommended.[49]

Inhaled Anesthetics

The inhaled anesthetic isoflurane has been used for the treatment of refractory SE for more than 20 years. More recently, desflurane has also been used. Unlike other therapies for refractory SE (eg, high-dose midazolam or pentobarbital), inhaled anesthetics provide almost immediate control of seizure activity regardless of seizure chronicity or type. These medications are considered a last line of therapy because there are technical difficulties with safe administration outside the operating room and concerns about potential toxicity with long-term use. The mechanism by which the inhaled anesthetics control seizure activity likely involves multiple receptors including GABA, nicotinic, and glycine receptors, and potassium-gated ion channels.

Dosing of anesthesia

Isoflurane and desflurane produce a powerful dose-dependent suppression of EEG activity. Typically, volatile anesthetic potency is described in minimum alveolar concentration (MAC) units. The MAC is defined as the concentration of vapor in the lungs at 1 atm that prevents the reaction to a standard surgical stimulus in 50% of patients. When comparing vapors, the unit is actually a median value and a lower MAC represents a more potent volatile anesthetic. Isoflurane has a MAC of 1.15. Other uses of MAC terminology include MAC-BAR (1.7–2.0 MAC), which is the concentration required to block autonomic reflexes to nociceptive stimuli, and MAC-awake (0.3–0.5 MAC), the concentration required to block voluntary reflexes and control perceptive awareness. The MAC value for EEG burst suppression is 1.5 to 2.0. This potency of central nervous system depression means that induction of burst suppression and control of refractory SE occurs at doses used in the operating room, and normally under the supervision of an anesthesiologist.

Isoflurane is given via an anesthetic machine with end-tidal monitoring of isoflurane concentration. Initially, the concentration of the anesthetic is gradually increased until adequate suppression of the seizure and background EEG activity has occurred, and this dose is maintained. Then, at regular intervals, the minimum dose of anesthetic needed to achieve EEG burst suppression should be determined. We also follow the total anesthetic exposure by calculating the MAC-hours of treatment (ie, the hourly end-tidal percentage concentration of isoflurane divided by 1.15 is summed for each hour of treatment).

The use of volatile anesthetics for refractory SE is limited to small case series and reports.[50–52] The largest series is of 9 adults and children receiving isoflurane after, on average, 25 days of refractory SE.[50] The outcome was poor (6 of 9 patients died) but this study showed that the agent could stop long-standing and super-refractory SE. More recently, Mirsatarri and colleagues[51] reported 7 patients (aged 17–71 years) anesthetized for up to 55 days. EEG burst suppression was achieved within minutes in all patients. Vasopressors were used in all patients and there was no evidence of organ toxicity, even with prolonged use.

Complications

The anesthetic agents cause nonlinear decrease in $CMRO_2$ and once burst suppression occurs, there is no further decrease in cerebral metabolism. Hence, there is little value in going beyond EEG burst suppression and inducing electrocerebral silence. It also means that monitoring continuous EEG is the only technique by which to recognize that minimum necessary anesthetic dosing is being given. The anesthetic agents also decrease cerebrovascular resistance, thereby causing increase in CBF and, potentially, ICP; this complication is seen with isoflurane and, to a lesser degree, with desflurane. This increase in ICP is typically mild, transient, and of major significance only in patients with evidence of preexisting intracranial hypertension.[41,50]

Both isoflurane and desflurane produce a dose-dependent predictable decrease in arterial blood pressure via lowering of systemic vascular resistance and, to a much lesser degree, negative inotropy. As a consequence, a compensatory increase in heart rate is frequently seen when starting these agents. Occasionally, rapid changes in the delivery of the anesthetics cause an increase in heart rate and blood pressure secondary to sympathetic stimulation.

There are some concerns that the volatile anesthetics may be neurotoxic when used for prolonged periods in the treatment of SE.[52] The first cases of adverse neurologic effects of prolonged isoflurane in PICU patients was reported in 1993 by Arnold and colleagues.[53] Isoflurane was used for sedation and bronchodilation and it proved to be effective, without significant cardiovascular, hepatic, or renal toxicity. However, 5 of 10 patients developed a syndrome of extreme agitation and nonpurposeful movements after stopping the isoflurane. All 5 patients were less than 5 years old and received at least 70 MAC-hours of volatile anesthetic. Other reports reflect a similar experience of psychomotor disturbances after stopping the anesthetic abruptly.[54–57] Therefore, it is unclear whether these symptoms are the result of a withdrawal syndrome or a direct neurologic insult, but typically the symptoms are transient and self-resolving.

Treatment strategy

It is difficult to determine what role the volatile anesthetics should have in the treatment of refractory SE and super-refractory SE. Many protocols mention the use of these agents as a last resort. However, at this stage, permanent neurologic damage is likely to have already occurred and advocates argue that initiation sooner would yield better outcomes. The anesthetics are a reliable method for controlling seizures and inducing EEG burst suppression. These therapeutic goals are achieved within minutes, breakthrough seizures are rare, and hypotension is almost never dose limiting. The inhalational anesthetics can be readily titrated in a way that intravenous pentobarbital cannot. In PICU practice, this means that long-term AEDs can be started and blood levels optimized while the patient is in EEG burst suppression. However, each PICU should decide who is able to initiate, supervise, and monitor such therapy.

GENERAL ANESTHESIA FOR SUPER-REFRACTORY SE

General anesthesia allows us to control seizure activity and maintain a patient's homeostasis. This state, however, is not an end in itself. It provides an opportunity to develop a strategy for mid-term to long-term management and AED therapy, for example, by establishing the cause of the episode of refractory or super-refractory SE by following a protocol for investigation (**Box 1**). In the PICU, this process is exemplified in the approach to FIRES that leads to immunotherapy (see later discussion) and the approach to potential small-vessel central nervous system vasculitis[58,59] or

---

Box 1
Diagnostic considerations in patients presenting with refractory SE

Diagnostic steps

1. Clinical assessment

    a. General assessment

        i. Acute cause: meningoencephalitis, sepsis, FIRES, electrolyte disorder, hypoglycemia, stroke, demyelinating disease, trauma, intoxication

    b. Detailed neurologic assessment

        i. Nonacute cause: cortical malformation, neurocutaneous syndromes, brain tumor, autoimmune disorder, monogenic epileptic encephalopathies, chromosomal abnormalities, metabolic disease

2. Laboratory testing to consider

    a. Complete blood count and differential; coagulation work-up

    b. Inflammatory markers: C-reactive protein, erythrocyte sedimentation rate, von Willebrand factor antigen

    c. Infectious work-up: bacteria, fungal, and viral cultures and serology

    d. Testing for oligoclonal banding

    e. Testing for antibodies, including neuronal and ion-channel antibodies

3. Neuroimaging

    a. Brain magnetic resonance imaging with gadolinium, fluid attenuation inversion recovery sequences, diffusion-weighted imaging, and angiography

    b. Conventional angiogram for microvasculitis

4. Lumbar puncture and cerebrospinal fluid (CSF) analysis

    a. Measurement of opening pressure

    b. CSF cell count and differential, protein and glucose levels

    c. Bacterial, fungal, and viral cultures and serology

    d. Testing for oligoclonal bands

    e. Testing for neuronal and ion-channel antibodies

5. Brain biopsy

    a. Consider if normal angiogram as diagnostic of microvascular vasculitis

type II focal cortical dysplasia[60–62] that leads to diagnostic brain biopsy. Concurrent with this investigational process, there is also the need to optimize AED therapy (ie, rationalizing the choice of new and old medications) and their blood levels.

General anesthesia provides a period when transitions can be performed. It is not magic and should not be considered as therapy that is successful or unsuccessful; what is considered successful is whether the choices of long-term AEDs bring about control or not, or whether appropriate and effective immune therapy has been used. The approach to these choices is multidisciplinary and often there is little in the way of evidence-based information to help inform decision making (**Fig. 2**). However, new ideas are being developed and clinical trials are needed in this area of intensive care. For example, there is an association between prolonged SE and increased drug

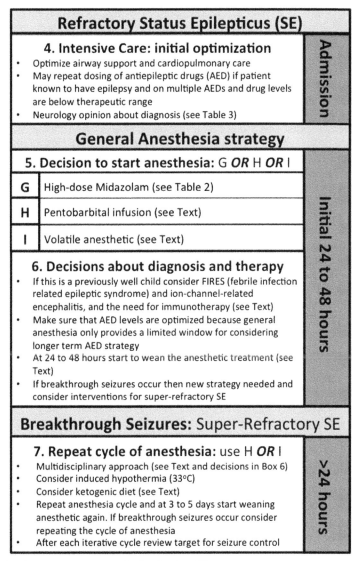

Fig. 2. Intensive care management of refractory SE.

resistance. This phenomenon may be related to increased expression of drug-efflux reporter genes and proteins (eg, P-glycoprotein [P-gp] and multidrug-resistance proteins).[63–65] Early in the episode, expression of efflux transporter genes is low because of down-modulation by increased levels of proinflammatory cytokines, but later this relationship is reversed and drug resistance occurs. Verapamil can act as a P-gp inhibitor and there are 2 case reports of its use in patients with refractory SE.[66,67] Further basic research and clinical trials are need to prove the effectiveness of P-gp inhibition by coadministration of verapamil during AED therapy for SE.

Duration of Anesthesia

Having induced anesthesia and achieved steady-state EEG burst suppression with the minimum dose necessary, how long should the patient remain in this state? There is no evidence-based answer to this question. However, if categorization of super-refractory SE is considered important, then at 24 hours after starting anesthesia, it should be lightened to ascertain whether breakthrough seizures occur or not. Abrupt weaning may lead to breakthrough seizures and so weaning should occur slowly. Weaning should be longer with intravenous anesthesia (pentobarbital) than volatile anesthetics, and it is reasonable to wean over 24 hours (but may be much longer with pentobarbital). In our practice, patients are initially maintained in an anesthetized EEG burst suppression state for 48 hours and then the depth of anesthesia is lightened over a further 24 hours. This 3-day interval allows us time to make choices about AEDs and optimize drug levels. If seizures recur, then a repeat cycle of anesthesia is reestablished and the duration of individual cycles of anesthesia is increased, often for 3 to 5 days. There is no limit on the time or the number of cycles of general anesthesia. The limit comes down to setting goals and deciding at what point the therapeutic target should change from total seizure control to accepting a particular seizure frequency in a patient. For example, in the literature there is an example of an 18-year-old patient with a flulike prodrome and super-refractory SE who had pentobarbital-induced EEG burst suppression for more than 7 weeks while other AEDs were tried.[68] In our practice, the choice of AEDs, the duration of drug-induced coma, and setting realistic therapeutic targets is a multidisciplinary process between the PICU, anesthesiology, and epileptology/neurology teams.

Other Medications and Approaches During Anesthesia

The other AEDs that have been used for control of refractory SE and super-refractory SE include propofol, ketamine, and topiramate. There are too few data to make an evidence-based assessment about such treatment and prolonged propofol infusion is not recommended in PICU practice in many countries because of the risk of propofol infusion syndrome. Some patients may benefit from surgical corpus callosotomy, lobar resection, or hemispherectomy for discrete, localized seizure foci.[69] This approach is only available in epilepsy surgery centers. The other therapies that have been used or tried include ketogenic diet, hypothermia, and immunomodulation.[70]

FEVER-INDUCED REFRACTORY EPILEPTIC ENCEPHALOPATHY AND FIRES

This group of conditions have multiple labels in the literature including FIRES, fever-induced refractory epileptic encephalopathy in school-aged children, IHHS, acute encephalopathy with inflammation-mediated status epilepticus (AEIMSE), acute encephalitis with refractory repetitive partial seizures (AERRPS), NORSE, and devastating epilepsy in school-age children (DESC).[24–28] In the following text, these conditions are grouped together because the diagnostic evaluation fails to show any specific cause. From the non-AED management perspective, it is critical to establish whether the condition is consistent with autoimmune disease (eg, glutamate-receptor subunit R3 antibodies, NMDA-receptor antibodies, voltage-gated potassium channel antibodies) because early plasmapheresis and immunomodulation may have a role.

General Anesthesia

First-tier and second-tier AEDs are universally ineffective at providing sustained seizure control in cases of FIRES,[71] and the results of barbiturate anesthesia also seem to be disappointing.[72] For example, in a series of 77 patients with FIRES, 46 underwent drug-induced EEG burst suppression for a median duration of 7 days (mean 14.3 days). Nine patients died, and 66 of 68 survivors developed severe refractory epilepsy.[71] The investigators found that induction of EEG burst suppression was not associated with an increased risk of death, but a longer duration of this state was associated with worse long-term cognitive outcome.[72] However, it is also possible that these patients had more severe disease.[73]

In a multicenter report of AERRPS, Sakuma and colleagues[74] described their experience with pentobarbital and midazolam in 29 patients aged 1 to 14 years. Of the 22 patients treated with intravenous barbiturates, 13 had a complete response, 3 had an excellent response, and 4 had a good response. None of the patients had a poor response. The maximum dose of pentobarbital was 4.98 ± 2.06 mg/kg/h and the mean duration of infusion was 52 ± 72.6 days. Midazolam was given to 25 patients and only 3 had complete seizure control; 5 others had a good response and 17 were judged to be poor responders. The maximum midazolam infusion dose rate was 0.47 ± 0.33 mg/kg/h, which is not as high as the high-dose strategy described by Morrison and colleagues[37,38] (see earlier discussion). These findings suggest that midazolam, at least at the doses used in this study, is inadequate to produce enough neuronal suppression in this malignant process.

Other Therapies for FIRES

Immunomodulatory therapy does not seem to work in cases of FIRES.[25–27,70–73] A ketogenic diet, however, may have some role. For example, Nabbout and colleagues[75] reported on 9 children who received a diet with a ratio of fat to combined protein and carbohydrate ketogenic diet of 4:1. The diet was started between 4 and 55 days after presentation with FIRES. In 7 of 8 patients reaching ketonuria (1 patient was unable to reach ketonuria because of use of steroids), seizure activity stopped within 2 to 4 days of reaching ketonuria, and within 4 to 6 days of starting the diet. One of the 7 responders was taken off the diet and experienced abrupt return of refractory SE, and died 10 days later. For the 6 responders who were kept on the diet, isolated seizures returned within a few months. These seizures were considered mild, with a frequency of up to 2 seizures per week.

SUMMARY

When a child with ongoing SE is admitted to the PICU, the evidence base from randomized controlled trials on what AED strategy should be used is inadequate. To date, therapy has been based on case series with a dearth of open data, and this lack of information compromises optimal therapy. The presentation of information in the tables and figures is one approach and this review represents progress from our previous report.[1] However, because cases of truly refractory SE and super-refractory SE are seen infrequently at any given institution, the first way to improve the quality of evidence is to develop national and multinational case registries of existing practices.

REFERENCES

1. Tasker RC. Emergency treatment of acute seizures and status epilepticus. Arch Dis Child 1998;79:78–83.
2. Meldrum BS, Horton RW. Physiology of status epilepticus in primates. Arch Neurol 1973;28:1–9.
3. Meldrum BS, Brierley JB. Prolonged epileptic seizures in primates. Arch Neurol 1973;28:10–7.
4. Meldrum BS, Vigouroux RA, Brierley JB. Systemic factors and epileptic brain damage. Prolonged seizures in paralyzed, artificially ventilated baboons. Arch Neurol 1973;29:82–7.
5. Lothman E. The biochemical basis and pathophysiology of status epilepticus. Neurology 1990;40(Suppl 2):13–23.
6. Freeman JM. Status epilepticus: it's not what we've thought or taught. Pediatrics 1989;83:444–5.
7. Guidelines for epidemiologic studies on epilepsy. Commission on Epidemiology and Prognosis, International League Against Epilepsy. Epilepsia 1993;34:592–6.
8. Lowenstein DH, Bleck T, Macdonald RL. It's time to revise the definition of status epilepticus. Epilepsia 1999;40:120–2.
9. Shinnar S, Berg AT, Moshe SL, et al. How long do new-onset seizures in children last? Ann Neurol 2001;49:659–64.
10. Kramer R, Levisohn P. The duration of secondarily generalized tonic-clonic seizures [abstract]. Epilepsia 1992;33:68.
11. Theodore W, Porter R, Albert P, et al. The secondarily generalized tonic-clonic seizure: a videotape analysis. Neurology 1994;44:1403–7.
12. Lahat E, Goldman M, Barr J, et al. Comparison of intranasal midazolam with intravenous diazepam for treating febrile seizures in children: prospective randomized study. BMJ 2000;321:83–6.
13. Smith RA, Martland T, Lowry MF. Children with seizures presenting to accident and emergency. J Accid Emerg Med 1996;13:54–8.
14. Wasterlain CG, Chen JW. Definition and classification of status epilepticus. In: Wasterlain CG, Treiman DM, editors. Status epilepticus: mechanisms and management. Cambridge (MA): MIT Press; 2006. p. 11–6.
15. Jenssen S, Gracely EJ, Sperling MR. How long do most seizures last? A systematic comparison of seizures recorded in the epilepsy monitoring unit. Epilepsia 2006;47:1499–503.
16. Mayer SA, Claassen J, Lokin J, et al. Refractory status epilepticus: frequency, risk factors, and impact on outcome. Arch Neurol 2002;59:205–10.
17. Walton NY, Treiman DM. Response of status epilepticus induced by lithium and pilocarpine to treatment with diazepam. Exp Neurol 1988;101:267–75.
18. Treiman DM, Walton NY, Kendrick C. A progressive sequence of electroencephalographic changes during generalized convulsive status epilepticus. Epilepsy Res 1990;5:49–60.
19. Wang NC, Good LB, Marsh ST, et al. EEG stages predict treatment response in experimental status epilepticus. Epilepsia 2009;50:949–52.
20. Sahin M, Menache CC, Holmes GL, et al. Outcome of severe refractory status epilepticus in children. Epilepsia 2001;42:1461–7.
21. Koul R, Chacko A, Javed H, et al. Eight-year study of childhood status epilepticus: midazolam infusion in management and outcome. J Child Neurol 2002;17:908–10.
22. Lambrechtsen FA, Buchhalter JR. Aborted and refractory status epilepticus in children: a comparative analysis. Epilepsia 2008;49:615–25.

23. Shorvon S. Super-refractory status epilepticus: an approach to therapy in this difficult clinical situation. Epilepsia 2011;52(Suppl 8):53–6.
24. Wilder-Smith EP, Lim EC, Teoh HL, et al. The NORSE (new-onset refractory status epilepticus) syndrome: defining a disease entity. Ann Acad Med Singapore 2005; 34:417–20.
25. Van Baalen A, Stephani U, Kluger G, et al. FIRES: febrile infection responsive epileptic (FIRE) encephalopathies of school age. Brain Dev 2009;31:92–3.
26. Chauvel P, Dravet C. The HHE syndrome. In: Roger J, Bureau M, Dravet C, et al, editors. Epileptic syndromes in infancy, childhood and adolescence. 4th edition. London: J Libbey; 2005. p. 277–93.
27. Nabbout R, Vezzani A, Dulac O, et al. Acute encephalopathy with inflammation-mediated status epilepticus. Lancet Neurol 2011;10:99–108.
28. Ismail FY, Kossoff EH. AERRPS, DESC, NORSE, FIRES: multi-labeling or distinct epileptic entities? Epilepsia 2011;52:e185–9.
29. Brevoord JC, Joosten KF, Arts WF, et al. Status epilepticus: clinical analysis of a treatment protocol based on midazolam and phenytoin. J Child Neurol 2005; 20:476–81.
30. Sreenath TG, Gupta P, Sharma KK, et al. Lorazepam versus diazepam-phenytoin combination in the treatment of convulsive status epilepticus in children: a randomized controlled trial. Eur J Paediatr Neurol 2010;14:162–8.
31. Walton NY, Treiman DM. Phenobarbital treatment of status epilepticus in a rodent model. Epilepsy Res 1989;4:216–21.
32. Abend NS, Marsh E. Convulsive and nonconvulsive status epilepticus in children. Curr Treat Options Neurol 2009;11:262–72.
33. Crawford TO, Mitchell WG, Fishman LS, et al. Very-high-dose phenobarbital for refractory status epilepticus in children. Neurology 1988;38:1035–40.
34. Rogawski MA, Losher W. The neurobiology of antiepileptic drugs. Nat Rev Neurosci 2004;5:553–64.
35. Saunders PA, Ho IK. Barbiturates and GABA$_A$ receptor complex. Prog Drug Res 1990;34:261–86.
36. Abend NS, Dlugos DJ. Treatment of refractory status epilepticus: literature review and a proposed protocol. Pediatr Neurol 2008;38:377–90.
37. Tasker RC. Midazolam for refractory status epilepticus: higher dosing and more rapid and effective control. Intensive Care Med 2006;32:1935–6.
38. Morrison G, Gibbons E, Whitehouse WP. High-dose midazolam therapy for refractory status epilepticus in children. Intensive Care Med 2006;32:2070–6.
39. Rossetti AO. Which anesthetic should be used in the treatment of refractory status epilepticus? Epilepsia 2007;48(Suppl 8):52–5.
40. Owens J. Medical management of refractory status epilepticus. Semin Pediatr Neurol 2010;17:176–81.
41. Stullken EH, Milde JH, Michenfelder JD, et al. The nonlinear responses of cerebral metabolism to low concentrations of halothane, enflurane, isoflurane, and thiopental. Anesthesiology 1977;46:28–34.
42. Barberio M, Reiter PD, Kaufman J, et al. Continuous infusion pentobarbital for refractory status epilepticus in children. J Child Neurol 2012;27:721–6.
43. Krishnamurthy KB, Drislane FW. Depth of EEG suppression and outcome in barbiturate anesthetic for refractory status epilepticus. Epilepsia 1999;40:759–62.
44. Schreiber JM, Gaillard WD. Treatment of refractory status epilepticus in childhood. Curr Neurol Neurosci Rep 2011;11:195–204.
45. Schmutzhard E, Pfausler B. Complications of the management of status epilepticus in the intensive care unit. Epilepsia 2011;52(Suppl 8):39–41.

46. Holmes GL, Riviello JJ Jr. Midazolam and pentobarbital for refractory status epilepticus. Pediatr Neurol 1999;20:259–64.
47. Claassen J, Hirsch LJ, Emerson RG, et al. Treatment of refractory status epilepticus with pentobarbital, propofol, or midazolam: a systematic review. Epilepsia 2002;43:146–53.
48. Rossetti AO, Logroscino G, Bromfield EB. Refractory status epilepticus: effect of treatment aggressiveness on prognosis. Arch Neurol 2005;62:1698–702.
49. Kim SJ, Lee DY, Kim JS. Neurologic outcomes of pediatric epileptic patients with pentobarbital coma. Pediatr Neurol 2001;25:217–20.
50. Kofke WA, Snider MT, Young RS, et al. Prolonged low flow isoflurane anesthesia for status epilepticus. Anesthesiology 1989;71:653–9.
51. Mirsattari SM, Sharpe MD, Young GB. Treatment of refractory status epilepticus with inhalational anesthetic agents isoflurane and desflurane. Arch Neurol 2004;61:1254–9.
52. Fugate JE, Burns JD, Wijdicks EFM, et al. Prolonged high-dose isoflurane for refractory status epilepticus: is it safe? Anesth Analg 2010;111:1520–4.
53. Arnold JH, Truog RD, Rice SA. Prolonged administration of isoflurane to pediatric patients during mechanical ventilation. Anesth Analg 1993;76:520–6.
54. Kelsall AW, Ross-Russell R, Herrick MJ. Reversible neurologic dysfunction following isoflurane sedation in pediatric intensive care. Crit Care Med 1994;22:1032–4.
55. McBeth C, Watkins TG. Isoflurane for sedation in a case of congenital myasthenia gravis. Br J Anaesth 1996;77:672–4.
56. Hughes J, Leach HJ, Choonara I. Hallucinations on withdrawal of isoflurane used as sedation. Acta Paediatr 1993;82:885–6.
57. Shankar V, Churchwell KB, Deshpande JK. Isoflurane therapy for severe refractory status asthmaticus in children. Intensive Care Med 2006;32:927–33.
58. Cellucci T, Benseler SM. Diagnosing central nervous system vasculitis in children. Curr Opin Pediatr 2010;22:731–8.
59. Elbers J, Halliday W, Hawkins C, et al. Brain biopsy in children with primary small-vessel central nervous system vasculitis. Ann Neurol 2010;68:602–10.
60. Moritani T, Smoker WR, Leee HK, et al. Differential diagnosis of cerebral hemispheric pathology. Clin Neuroradiol 2011;21:53–63.
61. Chassoux F, Landre E, Mellerio C, et al. Type II focal cortical dysplasia: electro-clinical phenotype and surgical outcome related to imaging. Epilepsia 2012;53:349–58.
62. Aronica E, Becker AJ, Spreafico R. Malformations of cortical development. Brain Pathol 2012;22:380–401.
63. Loscher W, Potschka H. Drug resistance in brain diseases and the role of drug efflux transporters. Nat Rev Neurosci 2005;6:591–602.
64. Kuteykin-Teplyakov K, Brandt C, Hoffmann K, et al. Complex time-dependent alterations in the brain expression of different drug efflux transporter genes after status epilepticus. Epilepsia 2009;50:887–97.
65. Bankstahl JP, Bankstahl M, Kuntner C, et al. A novel emission tomography imaging protocol identifies seizure-induced regional overactivity of P-glycoprotein at the blood brain barrier. J Neurosci 2011;31:8803–11.
66. Iannetti P, Spalice A, Parisi P. Calcium-channel blocker verapamil administration in prolonged and refractory status epilepticus. Epilepsia 2005;46:967–9.
67. Schmitt FC, Dehnicke C, Merschhemke M, et al. Verapamil attenuates the malignant treatment course in recurrent status epilepticus. Epilepsy Behav 2010;17:565–8.

68. Mirski M, Williams M, Hanley DF. Prolonged pentobarbital and phenobarbital coma for refractory generalized status epilepticus. Crit Care Med 1995;23:400–4.
69. Greiner HM, Tillema J-M, Hallinan BE, et al. Corpus callosotomy for treatment of pediatric refractory status epilepticus. Seizure 2012;21:307–9.
70. Wheless JW. Treatment of refractory convulsive status epilepticus in children: other therapies. Semin Pediatr Neurol 2010;17:190–4.
71. Kramer U, Chi CS, Lin KL, et al. Febrile infection-related epilepsy syndrome (FIRES): pathogenesis, treatment, and outcome: a multicenter study on 77 children. Epilepsia 2011;52:1956–65.
72. Kramer U, Chi CS, Lin KL, et al. Febrile infection-related epilepsy syndrome (FIRES): does duration of anesthesia affect outcome? Epilepsia 2011;52(Suppl 8):28–30.
73. Howell KB, Katanyuwong K, Mackay MT, et al. Long-term follow-up febrile infection-related epilepsy syndrome. Epilepsia 2012;53:101–10.
74. Sakuma H, Awaya Y, Shiomi M, et al. Acute encephalitis with refractory, repetitive partial seizures (AERRPS): a peculiar form of childhood encephalitis. Acta Neurol Scand 2010;121:251–6.
75. Nabbout R, Mazzuca M, Hubert P, et al. Efficacy of ketogenic diet in severe refractory status epilepticus initiating fever induced refractory epileptic encephalopathy in school age children (FIRES). Epilepsia 2010;51:2033–7.

Acute Encephalitis

Dennis W. Simon, MD[a], Yong Sing Da Silva, MD[a],
Giulio Zuccoli, MD[b], Robert S.B. Clark, MD[c,d],*

KEYWORDS

- Acute disseminated encephalomyelitis • Altered mental status • Encephalitis
- Encephalopathy • Seizure

KEY POINTS

- Encephalitis is an inflammation of the brain parenchyma that presents with fever, alterations in consciousness, seizure, and focal neurologic signs. It should be distinguished from bacterial meningitis and conditions causing encephalopathy.
- Despite an extensive work-up, the cause of encephalitis is often not identified. Electroencephalography and magnetic resonance imaging can assist in diagnosis and management.
- Treatment of encephalitis should focus on prompt initiation of antibiotics and antivirals until infectious causes and bacterial meningitis can be excluded.
- There is limited evidence to guide the management of critical neurologic sequelae, such as seizures, intracranial hypertension, cerebral ischemia, and irreversible brain tissue damage.
- Noninfectious causes are being discovered, such as N-methyl-D-aspartate receptor antibodies, which are treated with immunotherapy.

Fly blind • *Feel one's way, proceed by guesswork.*
—From The American Heritage Dictionary of Idioms.

INTRODUCTION

The evaluation and management of critically ill children with acute encephalitis is complicated by diagnostic challenges and a lack of successfully trialed therapeutic options. Encephalitis is strictly a pathologic diagnosis, in which neuroinflammation,

[a] Department of Critical Care Medicine, The Children's Hospital of Pittsburgh of UPMC, University of Pittsburgh School of Medicine, 4401 Penn Avenue, Pittsburgh, PA 15224, USA; [b] Department of Radiology, The Children's Hospital of Pittsburgh of UPMC, University of Pittsburgh School of Medicine, 4401 Penn Avenue, Pittsburgh, PA 15224, USA; [c] Departments of Critical Care Medicine and Pediatrics, The Children's Hospital of Pittsburgh of UPMC, University of Pittsburgh School of Medicine, 4401 Penn Avenue, Pittsburgh, PA 15224, USA; [d] Safar Center for Resuscitation Research, University of Pittsburgh, 3434 Fifth Avenue, Pittsburgh, PA 15260, USA
* Corresponding author. Pediatric Critical Care Medicine, The Children's Hospital of Pittsburgh, 4401 Penn Avenue, Pittsburgh, PA 15224.
E-mail address: clarkrs@upmc.edu

Crit Care Clin 29 (2013) 259–277
http://dx.doi.org/10.1016/j.ccc.2013.01.001
0749-0704/13/$ – see front matter © 2013 Elsevier Inc. All rights reserved.
criticalcare.theclinics.com

brain tissue damage, and a pathogen are detected. In clinical practice, a diagnosis is made presumptively based on a constellation of clinical findings that often includes fever and neurologic dysfunction, coupled with clinical testing including electroencephalogram (EEG) and neuroimaging findings (eg, magnetic resonance imaging [MRI]), with or without cerebrospinal fluid (CSF) studies. Despite an extensive work-up, it is often not possible to identify the cause of these symptoms. Population-based studies, such as the California Encephalitis Project (CEP), have shown how limited the current diagnostic methods can be. A 2007 CEP database review found that a confirmed or probable agent was identified in only 16% of cases.[1] Fifty-eight percent of the patients enrolled were admitted to an intensive care unit (ICU). In addition to highlighting the many cases without a known cause, these studies have led to further understanding the role of *Mycoplasma pneumoniae* and noninfectious causes such as *N*-methyl-D-aspartate receptor (NMDAR) antibodies as a cause of encephalitis.

Overall, encephalitis results in high mortality and often severe morbidity for survivors. These patients frequently have a rapidly progressive course and require admission to an ICU for the management of altered mental status, seizures including status epilepticus, respiratory failure, hemodynamic instability, and/or electrolyte disturbances. This evidence-based review provides a framework for pediatric intensivists to guide the initial approach to diagnosis, management, and treatment of patients presenting with symptoms of encephalitis. An in-depth review is presented of the most common and recently identified causes of encephalitis in children. The objective is to promote early recognition, appropriate testing and empiric treatment, and management of the expected complications of acute encephalitis.

CAUSES

Viruses are the infectious agents most commonly associated with encephalitis. Recent studies have highlighted 2 points:

1. The confirmed or probable cause is only identified in 37% to 70% of patients.[1–3]
2. Bacterial and immune-mediated causes are being recognized more frequently.

Box 1 lists causes of encephalitis in infants and children. Between 1998 and 2005, the CEP enrolled 1570 patients 6 months old or older (median 23 years) with altered mental status and at least 1 of the following: fever, seizure, focal neurologic signs, CSF pleocytosis, abnormal EEG, or neuroimaging findings consistent with encephalitis. Patient data including exposures, laboratory data, clinical data, and demographics were collected. Testing for a battery of 16 infectious causes was performed on available CSF, brain, respiratory, acute-phase, and convalescent-phase serum samples; in addition, an additional 24 infectious causes were screened based on epidemiologic factors. Despite this thorough work-up, a confirmed or probable infectious cause was identified in only 244/1570 (16%) patients and a noninfectious cause was identified in 122/1570 (8%). A 2-year prospective study of children (mean age 6 years) admitted with encephalitis to a large tertiary-care children's hospital had similar results. Fifty children underwent a comprehensive infectious work-up and a confirmed or probable agent was detected in 20/50 (40%) cases: *M pneumoniae* (9 cases), *M pneumoniae* and enterovirus (2 cases), and herpes simplex virus (4 cases) were the most common.[3]

Noninfectious or postinfectious causes of encephalitis include acute disseminated encephalomyelitis (ADEM), also referred to as postinfectious encephalomyelitis, and anti-NMDAR encephalitis. Beginning in 2007, the CEP began testing subjects for anti-NMDAR antibodies and found this cause to be more frequent than encephalitis caused by HSV-1, enterovirus, West Nile virus (WNV), and varicella zoster virus

Box 1
Causes of encephalitis

Infectious

Viral	HSV-1/2, VZV, EBV, CMV, HHV-6, EV, WNV, EEE, other arboviruses, rabies, LCM, influenza, adenovirus, mumps, measles
Bacterial	*Rickettsia* spp, *Ehrlichia* spp, *Borrelia burgdorferi*, *Mycoplasma* spp, *Bartonella* spp, *Mycobacterium* spp, *Treponema pallidum*
Protozoa	*Baylisascaris procynosis*, *Balamuthia mandrillaris*
Fungi	*Aspergillus fumigatus*, *Blastomyces dermatitidis*, *Candida* spp, *Cryptococcus neoformans*, *Coccidioides immitis*, *Histoplasma capsulatum*
Parasites	*Acanthamoeba*, *Naegleria fowleri*, *Entamoeba histolytica*, *Plasmodium falciparum*, *Toxoplasma gondii*

Autoimmune

ADEM	Coronavirus, Coxsackie virus, EV, HSV, CMV, EBV, HHV-6, hepatitis A, influenza A/B, parainfluenza, measles, rubella, VXV, WNV, Rotavirus, *M pneumoniae*, *Borellia burgdorferi*, *Bartonella henselae*, *Chlamydia*, *Leptospira*, *Rickettsia*, *Streptococcus*
Autoantibodies	αNMDAR, αVGKC, αAMPAR, αGABABR, αGAD

Abbreviations: αAMPAR, AMPA receptor antibody; αGABABR, gamma-aminobutyric acid B receptor antibody; αNMDAR, NMDAR antibody; αVGKC, voltage-gated potassium channel complex antibody; ADEM, acute disseminated encephalomyelitis; CMV, cytomegalovirus; EBV, Epstein-Barr virus; EEE, eastern equine encephalitis virus; EV, enterovirus; HHV-6, human herpesvirus type 6; HSV, herpes simplex virus; LCM, lymphocytic choriomeningitis; VZV, Varicella zoster virus; WNV, West Nile virus.

(VZV).[4] These patients often require ICU-level care and the management of these conditions differs significantly from acute infectious encephalitis. Critical care physicians should therefore be aware of the clinical features that aid in making this diagnosis, and each of these conditions is discussed in detail later.

CLINICAL SYMPTOMS

The clinical features of encephalitis may vary by causal agent, degree of parenchymal involvement, and various host factors. Many conditions affect more than 1 location of the central nervous system (CNS), and symptoms can be used to help distinguish the site(s) of CNS involvement (**Box 2**). In a study of children 1 month to 18 years old with encephalitis, 80% presented with fever (temperature 38C), 78% had seizures (21% generalized, 79% focal), 47% had Glasgow Coma Scale (GCS) score less than 14, and 78% had focal neurologic signs.[3]

Encephalitis also tends to present differently based on the age of the patient. In neonates, encephalitis may present with nonspecific symptoms of fever, shock,

Box 2
Symptoms associated with site of CNS involvement

Brain: encephalitis	Fever, altered mental status, headache, nausea, vomiting, seizure, focal neurologic signs
Meninges: meningitis	Fever, neck stiffness, photophobia, headache, nausea, vomiting
Brainstem: rhombencephalitis	Fever, cranial nerve palsy, myoclonus, tremor, ataxia, apnea, coma
Spinal cord: myelitis	Weakness or paralysis, paresthesia, synesthesia, hyporeflexia

lethargy, irritability, poor feeding, seizures, or apnea. Again, a high index of suspicion is required to make a timely diagnosis in these cases.

INITIAL MANAGEMENT

Although there are many causes of acute encephalitis, the initial management of these patients should proceed similarly to other causes of acute brain injury: identify and treat the primary cause of injury and avoid/prevent secondary brain injury. Patients may present to the ICU with altered mental status for a variety of reasons including shock, hypoxia, metabolic derangements, intoxication, trauma, and CNS infections (**Box 3**). Therefore, in cases of encephalitis, a high index of suspicion is required to initiate timely therapy. On arrival, the initial evaluation should begin with assessment of airway, breathing, and circulation. Hypoxia, hypotension, fever, and seizures should be promptly treated to reduce the likelihood of secondary brain injury. If there is coma (GCS≤8) or loss of airway protective reflexes, a definitive airway should be obtained with endotracheal intubation. Following the initial resuscitation, a focused history and physical examination should be performed. The history is often obtained from caregivers because of the age of the patient and/or encephalopathy. The physician should be alert to any preceding symptoms, underlying medical conditions, and exposures that may assist in diagnosis (**Box 4**). A physical examination should then be performed with particular attention to level of consciousness, airway protective reflexes, seizure activity, and physical clues that may point to a particular cause. Although not validated in patients with nontraumatic brain injury, the GCS can be performed quickly and is helpful to standardize examinations, quantify the degree of neurologic dysfunction, and monitor for clinical deterioration or improvement. Bacterial meningitis may present with encephalitic symptoms and is unlikely to be excluded until the results of laboratory CSF studies and cultures are available.

In the presence of coma or obtundation, the authors think that imaging is warranted and that lumbar puncture should be delayed in patients with suspected CNS infection. Because of the morbidity and mortality associated with delayed antimicrobial therapy in cases with bacterial meningitis or herpes encephalitis, we also recommend that broad-spectrum antibiotics and acyclovir be administered empirically without delay

---

Box 3
Differential diagnosis of acute encephalopathy

Acute encephalitis	Hepatic encephalopathy
Bacterial meningitis	Uremic encephalopathy
Brain abscess	Hypoglycemia
Cerebral malaria	Hyposmolar or hyperosmolar states
Tuberculous meningitis	Inborn errors of metabolism
Trauma	Shigellosis
Intracranial hemorrhage	*Salmonella*
Intracranial thrombosis	Pertussis
Benign intracranial hypertension	Toxic ingestion
Nonconvulsive status epilepticus	Lead encephalopathy
Intracranial tumor	Carbon monoxide poisoning
Acute confusional migraine	Lupus cerebritis/vasculitis
Hypoglycemia	Psychosis

Data from Singhi PD. Central nervous system infections. In: Rogers' Textbook of Pediatric Intensive Care. Philadelphia, PA: Lippincott Williams & Wilkins 2008; p. 1372.

Box 4
Causal agents based on epidemiologic clues

Age
Neonates   HSV-2, Enterovirus, CMV, *Listeria monocytogenes, T pallidum, T gondii*
Children   HSV-1, Enterovirus, *M pneumoniae*, Arbovirus, influenza, VZV, EBV, CMV,
                HHV-6, adenovirus, measles, mumps, Rotavirus, *B henselae*, ADEM,
                αNMDAR
Insect/Animal Contact
Mosquito   Arbovirus
Tick   *Rickettsia rickettsii, Ehrlichia chaffeenis, Anaplasma phagocytophilium,*
                B burgdorferi, tick-borne encephalitis virus, Powassan virus
Bat   Rabies
Cat   Rabies, *Coxiella burnetti, B henselae, T gondii*
Dog   Rabies
Raccoon   Rabies
Immunocompromise
                VZV, CMV, HHV-6, WNV, HIV, JC virus, *L monocytogenes, Mycobacterium*
                tuberculosis, C neoformans, Coccidioides spp, *H capsulatum, T gondii*
Transplantation and Transfusion
                CMV, EBV, WNV, HIV
Person-to-person Transmission
                HSV (neonatal), VZV, Enterovirus (nonpolio), measles, mumps, EBV, HHV-6,
                influenza, *M pneumoniae, M tuberculosis*
Season
Summer/Fall   Mosquito and tick transmission (see earlier), Enterovirus
Winter   Influenza
Recent Vaccination
                ADEM
Unvaccinated
                VZV, Japanese encephalitis virus, measles, mumps, rubella, polio
Travel
Africa   *P falciparum, Trypanosoma brucei gambiense, T brucei rhodesiense*, rabies
Asia   Japanese encephalitis virus, tick-borne encephalitis, Nipah virus
South America   Rabies virus, EEE, WNV, Venezuelan equine encephalitis virus, St Louis
                encephalitis virus, *R rickettsii, P falciparum, Taenia solium*

Abbreviation: HIV, human immunodeficiency virus.
Adapted from Tunkel AR, Glaser CA, Bloch KC, et al. The management of encephalitis: clinical
practice guidelines by the Infectious Diseases Society of America. Clin Infect Dis 2008;47:303–27;
with permission.

---

for results of CSF analysis or imaging in critically ill children (**Fig. 1**).[5,6] During the
appropriate season, if the patient presents with exposure or clinical features of rickett-
sial or ehrlichial infection, empiric antibacterial treatment should also include
doxycycline.

DIAGNOSIS

In patients presenting with encephalitis, there is a core group of diagnostic studies that
should be performed in almost all patients: (1) complete blood cell count; (2) complete
metabolic profile; (3) coagulation studies; (4) blood culture; (5) CSF for cell count,
glucose, protein, cultures, and HSV polymerase chain reaction (PCR); (6) MRI or
computed tomography (CT) with and without contrast; and (7) EEG.

Although a lumbar puncture may be crucial to making an accurate diagnosis, we
recommend caution in the timing of the procedure in critically ill patients with

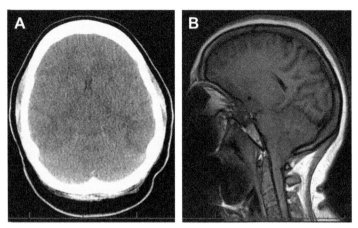

Fig. 1. Adolescent with altered level of consciousness and suspected viral encephalitis found to have bacterial meningitis. (*A*) Axial computed tomography image after lumbar puncture showing decreased extra-axial space and slitlike lateral ventricles. (*B*) Sagittal MRI after lumbar puncture showing effacement of fourth ventricle and quadrigeminal cistern and tonsillar herniation.

suspected encephalitis. Lumbar puncture is contraindicated in patients with space-occupying lesions, evidence of increased ICP seen on neuroimaging, or coagulopathy. Our recommendation is to avoid lumbar puncture in patients with altered mental status, because this may reflect intracranial hypertension (compression of both cerebral hemispheres and/or the reticular activating system). Even after acquiring imaging studies, we recommend deferring lumbar puncture, because neuroimaging studies are insensitive in detecting intracranial hypertension in patients with meningoencephalitis. The insensitivity of CT scans in the detection of increased intracranial pressure (ICP) may be related to globally high pressures within all intracranial CSF compartments, in contrast with external compression from mass lesions, for instance, that result in compression of cisterns. Furthermore, lumbar puncture in the presence of increased ICP increases the pressure gradient from within the skull to the spine, even after removal of the needle, because CSF can leak into soft tissues after penetration of the dura. We also recommend delaying lumbar puncture in patients with hemodynamic instability or respiratory compromise until these issues can be corrected.

Once safe to perform, CSF obtained via lumbar puncture will generally be clear and colorless (in contrast with CSF from patients with bacterial meningitis or subarachnoid hemorrhage). Opening pressure should be obtained to document ICP and may be normal or increased. CSF mononuclear pleocytosis (>5 WBC/μL) is present in most cases; the median level was 23 cells/μL reported in the CEP (range 0–13,000). If sampled early in the course of illness, a polymorphonuclear predominance may be seen. A persistent neutrophilic predominance can be seen in patients with West Nile encephalitis or eastern equine encephalitis. CSF protein and glucose are generally normal, with mean values of 57 mg/dL and 64 mg/dL respectively reported in the CEP. Although bacterial culture of the CSF can be helpful, primarily to rule out bacterial meningitis, viral culture of CSF has low yield. A review of 22,394 viral cultures of CSF found that less than 0.1% recovered a nonenterovirus, non-Herpesviridae species.[7]

MRI is the preferred imaging modality in patients with encephalitis, although CT scan with intravenous contrast may be adequate in cases in which MRI is contraindicated or not available (**Fig. 2**). Initial neuroimaging is abnormal in up to half of patients with encephalitis and therefore cannot be used to exclude the diagnosis.[1,3] In the case of acute viral encephalitis, a study of 18 patients by Kiroğlu and colleagues[8] found diffusion-weighted imaging (DWI) to be superior to conventional MRI in the detection of early lesions and depiction of lesion borders. A study by Teixeira and colleagues[9] of children with herpes encephalitis found that DWI detected additional lesions or, in 1 case in which conventional MRI was normal, showed acute infection. In addition to added sensitivity, there are characteristic neuroimaging patterns that may point to a particular cause. For example, HSV encephalitis may show edema or hemorrhage localized to the temporal lobes and bilateral temporal lobe involvement is nearly pathognomonic for HSV encephalitis, but this tends to be a late finding. Enterovirus 71 (EV71), a virus known to cause a poliolike rhombencephalitis, may

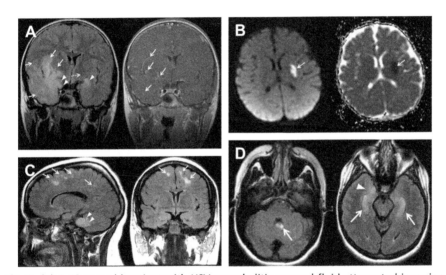

Fig. 2. (*A*) A 12-year-old patient with HSV encephalitis; coronal fluid-attenuated inversion recovery (FLAIR) image (*left*) shows extensive infection-related edema involving the right temporal lobe, right insular lobe, and right temporofrontal junction (*arrows*) with uncal herniation noted (*double arrowheads*). There is also involvement of the left temporal lobe (*arrowhead*). Mild shift to the left of the midline structures is identified (*dashed arrow*). Postcontrast coronal T1-weighted image (*right*) shows enhancement consistent with leptomeningitis over the right frontal temporal region (*arrows*). (*B*) A 12-month-old patient with H1N1 influenza A infection and seizures. A focus of increased signal identified in the left posterior putamen on diffusion-weighted image (*left, arrow*) is consistent with restricted diffusion (cytotoxic edema), as shown on the apparent diffusion coefficient map (*right, arrow*). This lesion may result from direct brain viral entry as well as from H1N1-related vasculitides in the territory supplied by the perforating arteries. (*C*) A 16-year-old patient affected by ADEM. Sagittal (*left*) and coronal (*right*) FLAIR images show confluent T2-FLAIR hyperintense lesions in the subcortical white matter of the cerebral hemispheres bilaterally (*arrows*). A tumorlike ADEM lesion of the left middle cerebellar peduncle extending to the cerebellar white matter is also identified (*arrowheads*). (*D*) A 26-year-old patient with NMDAR encephalitis and ovarian teratoma. Axial FLAIR images show hyperintensity of the vermis of the cerebellum (*left, arrow*), and bilateral alterations in the hippocampus (*right, arrows*) and right temporal uncus (*right, arrrowhead*).

cause lesions seen with T2-weighted imaging and DWI within the brainstem and spinal cord. Eastern equine and Flavivirus (WNV, St Louis encephalitis virus [SEV], Japanese encephalitis virus [JEV]) encephalitis also characteristically show lesions in the brainstem. MRI can also be helpful to make the diagnosis of ADEM, which is characterized by multifocal subcortical and central white matter areas of T2 or fluid-attenuated inversion recovery (FLAIR) signal abnormality in the subcortical and central white matter.[10]

EEG should be performed routinely as part of the diagnostic work-up. Although nonspecific in most cases, EEG is a sensitive marker for brain dysfunction and is abnormal in 87% to 96% of children with encephalitis.[1,3] Cases of HSV encephalitis often have a temporal focus and may show periodic lateral epileptiform discharges (PLED), although PLED can be seen in other disease processes as well. EEG may also be used to monitor for seizure activity or to differentiate encephalitis from nonconvulsive status epilepticus in patients who are confused, obtunded, or comatose.

Following the initial work-up and neuroimaging, the diagnostic evaluation of a patient with encephalitis should then be individualized and guided by the history, examination, screening laboratory data, and epidemiologic factors (see **Box 4**). Identification of a particular cause is important for several reasons:

- Certain causes require specific therapy and outcome may be improved with early treatment.
- Empiric therapies have dose-dependent toxicity and can be stopped if another cause is found.
- Identification of a specific cause may be useful for purposes of prognosis, prophylaxis, and public health interventions.[11]

An expert panel of the Infectious Diseases Society of America published guidelines in 2008 for the diagnosis and treatment of encephalitis.[11] Consultation with a specialist in pediatric infectious disease is useful to guide further work-up. If a brain biopsy is considered, neuroimaging can be used to guide neurosurgery to a noneloquent area of abnormality. Tissue samples should be sent for pathology, PCR, immunofluorescence, and electron microscopy.

ICU MANAGEMENT

Children with encephalitis can have a rapidly progressive course and therefore should be monitored closely in an ICU. In general, broad-spectrum antibiotics and acyclovir should have already been administered emergently, with additional empiric coverage based on epidemiologic risk factors. To highlight the urgency of early antibiotics, in a retrospective study of adult patients with HSV encephalitis diagnosed by PCR, the 2 factors in a multivariate analysis that were independently associated with outcome were severity of illness on presentation and a delay of more than 2 days between hospital admission and initiation of acyclovir.[12] Once a cause is identified, or excluded, therapy can be adjusted accordingly. Choice of empiric antibiotic therapy may be guided by the National Institute for Health and Clinical Excellence guidelines for the management of bacterial meningitis in children younger than 16 years.[13] These guidelines suggest parenteral ceftriaxone at the earliest opportunity for patients older than 3 months presenting to a hospital; for prehospital empiric therapy, benzylpenicillin is recommended. For patients less than 3 months old, empiric ampicillin and cefotaxime are suggested. Addition of vancomycin is indicated if patients have had a history of recent overseas travel or have had a recent prolonged antibiotic course or multiple antibiotic exposures.

The second goal of therapy should be to avoid/prevent secondary brain injury. Patients with encephalitis may develop:

- Airway compromise or hypoventilation caused by depressed mental status that can lead to hypoxemia and/or hypercarbia
- Hypotension caused by systemic inflammatory response or autonomic instability
- Fever
- Seizures
- Increased ICP

These complications should be anticipated and managed aggressively. The management of seizure and increased ICP secondary to encephalitis is discussed later.

Status Epilepticus

Patients with encephalitis are at risk for seizure, which may cause hypoxemia, hyperthermia, and acidosis, and increase the metabolic demand and ICP in an already compromised brain. The use of empiric antiepileptic drugs in children with encephalitis has not been thoroughly studied. In a retrospective review of 46 children admitted to an ICU with encephalitis complicated by status epilepticus, 20/46 (43%) went on to develop refractory status epilepticus defined as seizure lasting more than 2 hours despite treatment with therapeutic dosage of benzodiazepines, phenobarbital, and phenytoin. Patients who developed refractory status epilepticus were more likely to have a generalized or multifocal pattern on their initial EEG and more likely to have poor neurologic outcome at 6 months on Glasgow Outcome Scale score and medically refractory epilepsy.[14] In the CEP, 56% of patients had seizure(s) responsive to standard medical therapy, whereas only 4% developed refractory seizures and required induced coma for management. In this cohort, patients with refractory status epilepticus were more likely to be young (median age 10 years); have fever (93%), prodromal respiratory illness (57%), or gastrointestinal illness (64%); and less likely to have a CSF pleocytosis (47%) or abnormal imaging (16%). The median interval from onset of status epilepticus to induced coma was 4 days (range 0–41 days) and patients were kept in coma for a median of 15 days (range 2–76 days). In-hospital mortality was 21% in patients with refractory seizures versus 9% in patients without seizure. At 2 years follow-up in the patients with refractory seizures, 28% had died and 56% were neurologically impaired or undergoing rehabilitation.[15]

Given the high morbidity and mortality associated with refractory status epilepticus and the effects of seizure duration on outcome, we practice aggressive management of clinical or electrographic seizures. In general, a seizing patient is treated emergently with lorazepam or diazepam, followed by maintenance therapy with fosphenytoin. If a patient in status epilepticus fails to respond to initial dose(s) of benzodiazepines, it is unlikely that the next agent in protocols (phenobarbital, phenytoin) will be effective. In The Veteran Affairs Cooperative Study by Treiman and colleagues,[16] a randomized double-blind clinical trial of 4 intravenous treatment options for status epilepticus, the first antiepileptic drug administered failed to resolve status epilepticus in 45% of cases; in cases of nonconvulsive status epilepticus, the first agent failed in 85% of cases. Second and third agents were successful less than 10% of the time. To effectively treat status epilepticus in pediatric patients, clinicians should consider high-dose continuous infusions of midazolam or pentobarbital to produce medically induced coma. Patients receiving this therapy require endotracheal intubation for airway protection and ventilatory support and often require hemodynamic support in the form of fluid boluses or vasopressors. EEG should be used to monitor and titrate the midazolam or pentobarbital infusion, with typical targets being suppression of seizures or burst-suppression pattern.[17] It is our practice to titrate our therapy to burst-suppression with interburst interval of 10 seconds for 24 hours followed by a taper over 24 to 48 hours monitoring for recurrence of seizure activity. In adults with refractory status epilepticus, propofol infusion with or without midazolam may also be used to induce coma. However, because of the risk of propofol infusion syndrome (cardiovascular collapse, lactic acidosis, hypertriglyceridemia, and rhabdomyolysis), particularly in prolonged infusions and in children, we caution against its use in pediatric patients for treatment of refractory status epilepticus.

Increased ICP

The true incidence of increased ICP in patients with encephalitis is unknown. In cases of encephalitis, altered level of consciousness (often a marker of increased ICP in other causes of brain injury) may be caused by global cerebral or brainstem dysfunction. CT scan has been shown to be an insensitive marker of increased ICP. Therefore, it is unclear which patients may benefit from ICP monitoring. More importantly, if ICP monitors are placed, it is unclear that therapy directed by ICP or cerebral perfusion pressure (CPP) influences outcome in patients with encephalitis.

In a prospective study of patients (93% children) with JEV admitted to an infectious disease referral hospital, increased opening pressure was found in 52% of patients who had lumbar puncture performed. Of the 17 patients who died in this study, 15 had clinical signs of transtentorial herniation as the proximate cause of death.[18] In a French cohort of 13 patients with encephalitis and GCS less than 8 who received ICP monitoring, 6/13 (46%) had a maximum ICP greater than 20, although none of the patients had an initial ICP greater than 20, suggesting an alternate cause for their coma.[19] In addition, Shetty and colleagues[20] published a feasibility study of a CPP-guided approach in children with CNS infection and GCS less than 8. In this study, the physicians targeted a CPP greater than 70 mm Hg in children 2 years old or older and greater than 60 mm Hg in children less than 2 years old. Their protocol called for a fluid bolus when CPP was less than threshold and central venous pressure (CVP) was less than 10 mm Hg. If CPP was less than threshold and CVP adequate, a dopamine infusion was added followed by epinephrine if necessary. Once on vasopressors, if CPP remained less than threshold as a consequence of ICP greater than 20 mm Hg, then boluses of mannitol were given every 4 to 6 hours, with urinary losses replaced with isotonic fluid. The mortality in patients with encephalitis was 6/14 (42%); in 4 of these cases, death was attributed to refractory intracranial hypertension. A comparison of the survivors without neurologic sequelae, survivors with sequelae, and children who died found no significant difference across these groups in terms of initial CPP or ICP and mean CPP and ICP over the first 48 hours. GCS and minimum recorded CPP were lower in patients who died ($P = .01$).

The use of osmolar therapies for treatment of children with acute encephalopathy was reviewed in a meta-analysis of articles published between 1966 and 2009.[21] Four randomized controlled trials (RCTs), 3 prospective studies, 2 retrospective studies, and 1 case report were analyzed with reduction of ICP as primary outcome and resolution of coma and clinical outcome as secondary outcomes. Hypertonic saline achieved a greater reduction in ICP compared with mannitol, normal saline, or Ringer s lactate with a longer sustained effect when given as a continuous infusion rather than as boluses. However, there was no significant difference in mean ICP between the groups. Boluses of glycerol and mannitol induced a transient reduction in ICP. For children with cerebral malaria, mannitol boluses had a dose-response effect in moderately increased ICP (ICP>20 mm Hg, CPP<50 mm Hg), but not with severely increased ICP (ICP>40 mm Hg, CPP<40 mm Hg). For pediatric patients with bacterial meningitis, oral glycerol both alone and in combination with dexamethasone was associated with lower mortality and less severe neurologic sequelae compared with placebo. No difference in time to resolution of coma was found in comparison of mannitol versus placebo for cerebral malaria patients. For patients with nontraumatic encephalopathies, hypertonic saline was associated with lower mortality compared with mannitol; however, data from the 4 RCTs were heterogenous in relation to interventions used and could not be pooled for meta-analysis.

Based on the available data and our clinical experience, we posit that ICP monitoring in patients with encephalitis and GCS less than 8 would be valuable toward a stepwise approach to goal-directed therapy, similar to the traumatic brain injury guidelines targeting ICP less than 20 mm Hg and age-adjusted normal CPP. However, there are insufficient data at this point to make a stronger recommendation and the patient's management should be individualized and made in discussion with consulting services such as neurology, neurosurgery, and infectious diseases. As an alternative, empiric ICP-targeted therapy (**Table 1**) may be instituted in patients with coma (GCS≤8) with the duration based on the predicted phase of maximal brain swelling.

SELECT INFECTIOUS CAUSES
HSV Type 1

In children and adults, HSV-1 is commonly identified as a cause of encephalitis. Studies have found that it accounts for 19% to 33% of cases with a confirmed or probable pathogen identified.[2,22] HSV-1 encephalitis is a particularly severe infection, with 70% mortality in untreated cases and 9% in patients treated with acyclovir. In survivors who receive acyclovir, 39% develop normally and 61% have moderate to severe neurologic sequelae. Early treatment is crucial because delays in the administration of

Table 1 Empiric management of suspected or documented intracranial hypertension used at the Children's Hospital of Pittsburgh	
Therapy/Intervention	**Comments**
Mannitol 250 mg/kg every 6 h	Place Foley catheter Avoid hypovolemia Monitor serum osmolality and hold dose if >320 mOsm
Hypertonic saline	Desired range serum Na^+ >135 and <150 mEq/L Deliver centrally
Arterial and central venous lines for continuous monitoring of blood pressure and CVP, respectively	Prevent and aggressively treat hypotension
Mechanical ventilation	Maintain $Paco_2$ 35–40 mm Hg Maintain Pao_2 >90 mm Hg
Temperature control	Prevent and treat hyperthermia Consider hypothermia for refractory status epilepticus
Seizure prophylaxis (refer to text for management of documented seizures)	Consider fosphenytoin or levetiracetam
Glucose management	Prevent and/or aggressively treat hypoglycemia

acyclovir have been associated with increased morbidity and mortality.[23] If encephalitis is considered in the differential diagnosis of a patient, acyclovir should be added empirically until the results of confirmatory tests are available.

Studies by Nahmias and colleagues[24] have determined that one-third of cases are caused by primary infection caused by retrograde spread of virus via the olfactory nerves. In the other two-thirds of patients, reactivation of latent infection from the trigeminal nerve ganglion is suspected but only 10% have a history of recurrent herpes labialis. Patients typically present with fever, headache, and altered mental status. The PCR assay for HSV DNA in CSF performed in most clinical laboratories has excellent test characteristics: 94% sensitivity and 98% specificity for the diagnosis of encephalitis in published reports. However, false negatives may occur, especially within the first 72 hours of illness. If clinical suspicion is high, diffusion-weighted MRI may show abnormalities earlier than PCR, and CSF should be re-sampled in 1 to 3 days.[25,26] If a diagnostic lumbar puncture cannot be performed early in the patient's course, HSV DNA persists in 80% of patients despite adequate antiviral therapy and HSV antibodies can also be tested.

Given the poor outcome for many patients treated with acyclovir, studies have been performed to find adjunctive treatments for these patients. Because of their immunosuppressive effects, controversy currently exists regarding the use of adjunctive steroids in the treatment of deteriorating patients with HSV-1 infection. In vitro studies have shown viral replication may increase in cells treated with steroids; however, when steroid treatment and viral infection occur simultaneously, viral yield is unchanged.[27] Studies using a rodent model of herpes encephalitis show that animals treated with dexamethasone in addition to acyclovir have no change in viral load and a significant improvement in long-term MRI findings. In human subjects, case reports are available but randomized studies have not been performed.

H1N1 Influenza A

Although influenza viral infection predominantly causes respiratory illness, severe neurologic complications may occur. Influenza is detected in 4% to 7% of cases of childhood encephalitis, with most patients being less than 5 years old.[3,28,29] In these children, greater than 90% have a prodromal respiratory illness with neurologic symptoms that develop concomitantly or soon thereafter. Influenza viruses do not seem to have a tropism for the CNS and the pathophysiology of influenza-associated neurologic disease is under investigation.

Following the 2009 influenza A (H1N1) pandemic, our institution reported neurologic sequelae of 4 children admitted to the pediatric ICU (PICU) with H1N1 infection, altered level of consciousness (GCS<10), and abnormal EEG. In our cohort, all children survived, but 2 of the children had neurologic deficits at the time of discharge.[30] Glaser and colleagues[31] evaluated 2069 patients with severe (treated in an ICU) or fatal H1N1 infection and found that 1.4% were classified with influenza-associated encephalopathy or encephalitis. Almost all of these patients presented with fever (90%) and respiratory symptoms (86%). One-quarter developed seizures and required intubation, primarily for airway protection. Lumbar puncture and neuroimaging was normal in most patients and most had returned to baseline mental status before discharge. In a multicenter review of PICU admissions for 2009 H1N1 in the Pediatric Acute Lung Injury and Sepsis Investigators (PALISI) network, encephalitis was an independent risk factor for mortality (relative risk 3.3; 95% confidence interval 1.4–7.8, $P = .02$).[32]

A case report was recently published of 5 children with 2009 H1N1 influenza evaluated for late-onset delirium (>3 days after fever). Brain MRI was normal in all 5 children and EEG was normal in 4/5 children. All patients had mildly increased NMDAR antibodies in CSF or serum that normalized in the 3 patients who had follow-up levels.[33]

M pneumoniae

M pneumoniae is the most common infection diagnosed in a series of 50 children with encephalitis who underwent standardized infectious work-up, as well as the 1570 patients referred to the CEP; of reported cases in which M pneumoniae was directly detected in brain tissue or CSF, 70% were in children.[1,34] However, because Mycoplasma is a common infection in the general population and does not have a strong tropism for the CNS, most studies label it as a coinfection rather than a cause of encephalitis. More recent evidence, such as case reports of patients in whom the organism is cultured from brain parenchyma and detected by PCR in the CSF, support M pneumoniae as a cause of encephalitis. As opposed to bacterial or viral CNS infections, in which interferon-gamma and tumor necrosis factor alpha are increased, increased CSF levels of interleukin (IL) 6 and IL-8 (neutrophil chemotactic factor) have been measured.[35] These findings are consistent with the neutrophilic infiltrate seen on histology after fatal cases.[36]

Mycoplasma sp can be detected by serology, specialized culture, and PCR methods. To improve diagnostic accuracy, a combination of these methods should be used on available specimens (**Box 5**).[34] In their guidelines for treatment of encephalitis, The Infectious Diseases Society of America states that poor evidence exists to support a recommendation for treatment of M pneumoniae when detected in cases of encephalitis. Options for treatment include azithromycin, doxycycline, and fluoroquinolones.[14] Children diagnosed with encephalitis and acute M pneumoniae infections are at high risk for refractory status epilepticus (defined as seizures lasting >2 hours despite treatment with conventional antiepileptic drugs) and postencephalitic epilepsy.

Box 5
Diagnosis of *M pneumoniae* encephalitis

Probable	Detection of *M pneumoniae* in CSF (PCR, culture, or both)
	Or
	Detection of *M pneumoniae* in throat (PCR, culture, or both) with confirmatory results of serologic tests (seroconversion and/or >4× change in antibody titers)
Possible	Serologic evidence of *M pneumoniae* infection
	Negative results of culture and PCR of throat and CSF, and absence of convincing evidence for other possible causal agents
	Or
	Detection of *M pneumoniae* in throat (PCR, culture or both)
	Without confirmatory results of serologic tests
Indeterminate	Serologic evidence of *M pneumoniae* infection, with negative results of culture and PCR of throat and CSF, and convincing evidence that implicated at least 1 other pathogen
	Or
	Limited serology of an acute *M pneumoniae* infection

Adapted from Tunkel AR, Glaser CA, Bloch KC, et al. The management of encephalitis: clinical practice guidelines by the Infectious Diseases Society of America. Clin Infect Dis 2008;47:303–27; with permission.

ACUTE DISSEMINATED ENCEPHALOMYELITIS

The International Pediatric MS Study Group defines ADEM as a "first clinical event with a presumed inflammatory or demyelinating cause, with acute or subacute onset that affects multifocal areas of the CNS." Patients typically present with encephalopathy, multifocal neurologic deficits (**Table 2**), and asymmetric white matter lesions on MRI (see **Fig. 2**). Patients often have a preceding infection (93%) or vaccination (5%), but this is not required to make the diagnosis. The median age of 27 children with ADEM admitted to a PICU in the UK Pediatric Intensive Care Audit Network (PICANet) was 4.8 years (range 1.0–13.8 years). Twenty-one patients (78%) required mechanical ventilation (median of 3 days).[37] The average hospitalization is 9 days, with 50% to 80% of patients showing complete recovery and an additional 19% with mild motor or behavioral deficits.[38]

Like other demyelinating conditions, patients with ADEM typically have increased levels of CSF protein and a mild lymphocytic CSF pleocytosis; oligoclonal bands are rarely detected. T2-weighted and FLAIR MRI sequences may show multiple large ($\geq$1–2 cm) hyperintense lesions in the supratentorial and infratentorial white matter. Gray matter involvement may be seen, particularly in the thalamus and basal ganglia. Meningeal enhancement is not commonly seen and there are variable findings on T1-weighted postcontrast imaging.[39]

ADEM is likely an immune-mediated process triggered by antigenic stimulation following an infection or other trigger. As a result, first-line therapy recommended for the treatment of ADEM is high-dose intravenous corticosteroids, usually methylprednisolone 10 to 30 mg/kg for 3 to 5 days, followed by an oral taper over 4 to 6 weeks.[40] There are no case-control studies or randomized clinical trials of steroids for the treatment of ADEM. A retrospective study of 84 children with ADEM found that children treated with methylprednisolone had improved disability scores compared with children who received dexamethasone.[41] A taper greater than 3 weeks is associated with decreased rate of relapse.[42] Intravenous immunoglobulin (IVIG), either alone or in combination with steroids, at a dose of 2 g/kg divided over 2 to 5 days may be used. The successful use of plasmapheresis has been reported in a small number of pediatric cases, typically when steroid treatment has failed.[43,44] A double-blind,

Table 2 Presenting features of acute disseminated encephalomyelitis	
Feature/Symptom	Prevalence (%)
Unilateral or bilateral pyramidal signs	60–95
Acute hemiplegia	76
Ataxia	18–65
Cranial nerve palsies	22–45
Optic neuritis	7–23
Seizure	13–35
Spinal cord involvement	24
Impaired speech	5–21
Hemiparesthesia	2–3
Respiratory failure (caused by brainstem involvement or severely impaired consciousness)	11–16

Data from Tenembaum S, Chitnis T, Ness J, et al. Acute disseminated encephalomyelitis. Neurology 2007;68:S24.

sham-controlled RCT of patients with acute demyelination that had failed to respond to 5 days of high-dose steroids showed a response rate of 42% in treated patients versus 6% in controls. In fulminant cases with severe cerebral edema not responding to medical therapy, successful decompressive craniectomy has been reported in adults and children.[45–47]

ANTI-NMDAR ENCEPHALITIS

In 2007, Dalmau and colleagues[48] reported on 12 women with ovarian or mediastinal teratoma treated for paraneoplastic encephalitis caused by antibodies that reacted to the NR2B subunit of the NMDAR and antagonize gamma-aminobutyric acid (GABA) transmission. These women had prominent psychiatric symptoms, amnesia, dyskinesias, seizures, autonomic dysfunction, and often required ventilatory support because of decreased levels of consciousness. Resection of the tumor and immunotherapy was curative. More recent studies have established anti-NMDAR encephalitis as the cause for many cases of idiopathic encephalitis, encephalitis of unclear cause, and even patients diagnosed with psychiatric disorders admitted to the ICU.[4,49,50] In population-based studies from California and the United Kingdom, NMDAR antibodies were identified in 4% of patients with encephalitis.[4,22] This finding makes NMDAR encephalitis the second most common immune-mediated cause, behind ADEM, and 4 times more common than HSV-1, WNV, or VZV. In a review of 32 patients 18 years old or younger with NMDAR encephalitis, 77% were female and 31% of those girls had an ovarian teratoma. None of the male patients had a tumor identified.[51]

Many children with NMDAR encephalitis require ICU management as the symptoms progress from psychiatric/behavioral disturbances to include seizure (77%), autonomic instability (86%), and hypoventilation (23%).[51] The diagnosis is suggested by clinical history that includes a prodrome of fever, headache, and gastrointestinal or respiratory symptoms followed by psychiatric symptoms, language deficits, progressing to the decreased level of consciousness, dyskinesia, seizure, autonomic disturbance, and hypoventilation. MRI is normal in 50% of patients but may show T2 or FLAIR signal in the hippocampus, frontotemporal region, and insular region of cortex, basal ganglia, brainstem, or spinal cord.[48] EEG tracings are generally slow and disorganized and may show seizure activity. Initial lumbar puncture typically shows a moderate lymphocytic pleocytosis, normal or mildly increased protein, and may show oligoclonal bands. The diagnosis is made by serum and CSF detection of NMDAR antibodies. All patients should be tested for an underlying ovarian teratoma or testicular germ cell tumor; in some cases, microscopic tumors can cause severe neurologic symptoms.[52]

Treatments consists of tumor removal and immunotherapy, typically methylprednisolone and IVIG or plasmapheresis. If there is poor response to treatment, rituximab, cyclophosphamide, or both are added,[53] which is usually required in patients without a tumor or with delays in diagnosis. Approximately 75% of patients have full or substantial recovery; the remaining patients all have severe neurologic sequelae or die.[51] Many patients have a prolonged hospitalization and require months of physical and behavioral rehabilitation after discharge.

SUMMARY

Acute encephalitis remains one of the contemporary challenges of critical care medicine. Not only is the diagnosis difficult and sometimes unconfirmed, but encephalitis remains a disease without clear evidence-based therapies or even therapeutic goals to strive for toward the prevention of unacceptably high neurologic sequelae. In essence, acute encephalitis remains one of the few diseases where one can feel as though they are "flying blind". Management should focus on initial stabilization, identification of cause, and treatment and/or prevention of primary and secondary brain injury. Clinical seizures should be emergently treated and may require medically induced coma for refractory status epilepticus. A stepwise approach to therapy guided by ICP/CPP may be used to treat intracranial hypertension. If increased ICP is suspected in comatose patients without ICP monitoring, ICP-targeted therapy is an option. Causes such as H1N1 influenza, *M pneumoniae*, and anti-NMDAR encephalitis have been diagnosed more frequently in recent years because of outbreaks (H1N1) or improved understanding of the pathophysiology affecting these patients (*M pneumoniae*, anti-NMDAR). Future studies should evaluate ICU management of these patients to determine the value of invasive monitoring and neuroprotective treatment strategies.

ACKNOWLEDGMENTS

With heartfelt recognition of our critically ill patients: past, present, and future.

REFERENCES

1. Glaser CA, Honarmand S, Anderson LJ, et al. Beyond viruses: clinical profiles and etiologies associated with encephalitis. Clin Infect Dis 2006;43:1565–77.
2. Glaser CA, Gilliam S, Schnurr D, et al. In search of encephalitis etiologies: diagnostic challenges in the California Encephalitis Project, 1998-2000. Clin Infect Dis 2003;36:731–42.
3. Kolski H, Ford-Jones EL, Richardson S, et al. Etiology of acute childhood encephalitis at The Hospital for Sick Children, Toronto, 1994-1995. Clin Infect Dis 1998; 26:398–409.
4. Gable MS, Sheriff H, Dalmau J, et al. The frequency of autoimmune N-methyl-D-aspartate receptor encephalitis surpasses that of individual viral etiologies in young individuals enrolled in the California Encephalitis Project. Clin Infect Dis 2012;54:899–904.
5. Aronin SI, Peduzzi P, Quagliarello VJ. Community-acquired bacterial meningitis: risk stratification for adverse clinical outcome and effect of antibiotic timing. Ann Intern Med 1998;129:862–9.
6. Auburtin M, Wolff M, Charpentier J, et al. Detrimental role of delayed antibiotic administration and penicillin-nonsusceptible strains in adult intensive care unit patients with pneumococcal meningitis: the PNEUMOREA prospective multicenter study. Crit Care Med 2006;34:2758–65.
7. Polage CR, Petti CA. Assessment of the utility of viral culture of cerebrospinal fluid. Clin Infect Dis 2006;43:1578–9.
8. Kiroğlu Y, Calli C, Yunten N, et al. Diffusion-weighted MR imaging of viral encephalitis. Neuroradiology 2006;48:875–80.
9. Teixeira J, Zimmerman RA, Haselgrove JC, et al. Diffusion imaging in pediatric central nervous system infections. Neuroradiology 2001;43:1031–9.
10. Maschke M, Kastrup O, Forsting M, et al. Update on neuroimaging in infectious central nervous system disease. Curr Opin Neurol 2004;17:475–80.
11. Tunkel AR, Glaser CA, Bloch KC, et al. The management of encephalitis: clinical practice guidelines by the Infectious Diseases Society of America. Clin Infect Dis 2008;47:303–27.

12. Raschilas F, Wolff M, Delatour F, et al. Outcome of and prognostic factors for herpes simplex encephalitis in adult patients: results of a multicenter study. Clin Infect Dis 2002;35:254–60.

13. NICE. Bacterial meningitis and meningococcal septicaemia: management of bacterial meningitis and meningococcal septicaemia in children and young people younger than 16 years in primary and secondary care. Clinical guideline 102. London: National Institute for Health and Clinical Excellence; 2010.

14. Lin JJ, Lin KL, Wang HS, et al. Analysis of status epilepticus related presumed encephalitis in children. Europ J Paediatr Neurol 2008;12:32–7.

15. Glaser CA, Gilliam S, Honarmand S, et al. Refractory status epilepticus in suspect encephalitis. Neurocrit Care 2008;9:74–82.

16. Treiman DM, Meyers PD, Walton NY, et al. A comparison of four treatments for generalized convulsive status epilepticus. Veterans Affairs Status Epilepticus Cooperative Study Group. N Engl J Med 1998;339:792–8.

17. Rossetti AO, Lowenstein DH. Management of refractory status epilepticus in adults: still more questions than answers. Lancet Neurol 2011;10:922–30.

18. Solomon T, Dung NM, Kneen R, et al. Seizures and raised intracranial pressure in Vietnamese patients with Japanese encephalitis. Brain 2002;125:1084–93.

19. Rebaud P, Berthier JC, Hartemann E, et al. Intracranial pressure in childhood central nervous system infections. Intensive Care Med 1988;14:522–5.

20. Shetty R, Singhi S, Singhi P, et al. Cerebral perfusion pressure–targeted approach in children with central nervous system infections and raised intracranial pressure: is it feasible? J Child Neurol 2008;23:192–8.

21. Gwer S, Gatakaa H, Mwai L, et al. The role for osmotic agents in children with acute encephalopathies: a systematic review. BMC Pediatr 2010;10:23.

22. Granerod J, Ambrose HE, Davies NW, et al. Causes of encephalitis and differences in their clinical presentations in England: a multicentre, population-based prospective study. Lancet Infect Dis 2010;10:835–44.

23. Poissy J, Wolff M, Dewilde A, et al. Factors associated with delay to acyclovir administration in 184 patients with herpes simplex virus encephalitis. Clin Microbiol Infect 2009;15:560–4.

24. Nahmias AJ, Whitley RJ, Visintine AN, et al. Herpes simplex virus encephalitis: laboratory evaluations and their diagnostic significance. J Infect Dis 1982;145:829–36.

25. Weil AA, Glaser CA, Amad Z, et al. Patients with suspected herpes simplex encephalitis: rethinking an initial negative polymerase chain reaction result. J Infect Dis 2002;34:1154–7.

26. Akyldz BN, Gumus H, Kumandas S, et al. Diffusion-weighted magnetic resonance is better than polymerase chain reaction for early diagnosis of herpes simplex encephalitis: a case report. Pediatr Emerg Care 2008;24:377–9.

27. Erlandsson AC, Bladh LG, Stierna P, et al. Herpes simplex virus type 1 infection and glucocorticoid treatment regulate viral yield, glucocorticoid receptor and NF-kappaB levels. J Endocrinol 2002;175:165–76.

28. Amin R, Ford-Jones E, Richardson SE, et al. Acute childhood encephalitis and encephalopathy associated with influenza: a prospective 11-year review. Pediatr Infect Dis J 2008;27:390–5.

29. Bhat N, Wright JG, Broder KR, et al. Influenza-associated deaths among children in the United States, 2003-2004. N Engl J Med 2005;353:2559–67.

30. Baltagi SA, Shoykhet M, Felmet K, et al. Neurological sequelae of 2009 influenza A (H1N1) in children: a case series observed during a pandemic. Pediatr Crit Care Med 2010;11:179–84.

31. Glaser CA, Winter K, DuBray K, et al. A population-based study of neurologic manifestations of severe influenza A(H1N1)pdm09 in California. Clin Infect Dis 2012;55:514–20.

32. Randolph AG, Vaughn F, Sullivan R, et al. Critically ill children during the 2009–2010 influenza pandemic in the United States. Pediatrics 2011;128: e1450–8.

33. Takanashi J, Takahashi Y, Imamura A, et al. Late delirious behavior with 2009 H1N1 influenza: mild autoimmune-mediated encephalitis? Pediatrics 2012;129: e1068–71.

34. Bitnun A, Richardson SE. *Mycoplasma pneumoniae*: innocent bystander or a true cause of central nervous system disease? Curr Infect Dis Rep 2010;12:282–90.

35. Narita M. Pathogenesis of neurologic manifestations of *Mycoplasma pneumoniae* infection. Pediatr Neurol 2009;41:159–66.

36. Stamm B, Moschopulos M, Hungerbuehler H, et al. Neuroinvasion by *Mycoplasma pneumoniae* in acute disseminated encephalomyelitis. Emerg Infect Dis 2008;14:641–3.

37. Absoud M, Parslow RC, Wassmer E, et al. Severe acute disseminated encephalomyelitis: a paediatric intensive care population-based study. Mult Scler 2011; 17:1258–61.

38. Tenembaum S, Chitnis T, Ness J, et al. Acute disseminated encephalomyelitis. Neurology 2007;68:S23–36.

39. Parrish JB, Yeh EA. Acute disseminated encephalomyelitis. Adv Exp Med Biol 2012;724:1–14.

40. Pohl D, Tenembaum S. Treatment of acute disseminated encephalomyelitis. Curr Treat Options Neurol 2012;14:264–75.

41. Tenembaum S, Chamoles N, Fejerman N. Acute disseminated encephalomyelitis: a long-term follow-up study of 84 pediatric patients. Neurology 2002;59:1224–31.

42. Anlar B, Basaran C, Kose G, et al. Acute disseminated encephalomyelitis in children: outcome and prognosis. Neuropediatrics 2003;34:194–9.

43. Keegan M, Pineda AA, McClelland RL, et al. Plasma exchange for severe attacks of CNS demyelination: predictors of response. Neurology 2002;58:143–6.

44. RamachandranNair R, Rafeequ M, Girija AS. Plasmapheresis in childhood acute disseminated encephalomyelitis. Indian Pediatr 2005;42:479–82.

45. von Stuckrad-Barre S, Klippel E, Foerch C, et al. Hemicraniectomy as a successful treatment of mass effect in acute disseminated encephalomyelitis. Neurology 2003;61:420–1.

46. Ahmed AI, Eynon CA, Kinton L, et al. Decompressive craniectomy for acute disseminated encephalomyelitis. Neurocrit Care 2010;13:393–5.

47. Dombrowski KE, Mehta AI, Turner DA, et al. Life-saving hemicraniectomy for fulminant acute disseminated encephalomyelitis. Br J Neurosurg 2011;25: 249–52.

48. Dalmau J, Tuzun E, Wu HY, et al. Paraneoplastic anti-*N*-methyl-D-aspartate receptor encephalitis associated with ovarian teratoma. Ann Neurol 2007;61: 25–36.

49. Pruss H, Dalmau J, Harms L, et al. Retrospective analysis of NMDA receptor antibodies in encephalitis of unknown origin. Neurology 2010;75:1735–9.

50. Davies G, Irani SR, Coltart C, et al. Anti-*N*-methyl-D-aspartate receptor antibodies: a potentially treatable cause of encephalitis in the intensive care unit. Crit Care Med 2010;38:679–82.

51. Florance NR, Davis RL, Lam C, et al. Anti-*N*-methyl-D-aspartate receptor (NMDAR) encephalitis in children and adolescents. Ann Neurol 2009;66:11–8.

52. Johnson N, Henry C, Fessler AJ, et al. Anti-NMDA receptor encephalitis causing prolonged nonconvulsive status epilepticus. Neurology 2010;75:1480–2.
53. Dalmau J, Lancaster E, Martinez-Hernandez E, et al. Clinical experience and laboratory investigations in patients with anti-NMDAR encephalitis. Lancet Neurol 2011;10:63–74.

Renal Complications and Therapy in the PICU

Hypertension, CKD, AKI, and RRT

Rodney C. Daniels, MD[a],*, Timothy E. Bunchman, MD[b]

KEYWORDS

- Pediatric • Critical care • Hypertension • Chronic kidney failure • Acute kidney injury
- Renal replacement therapy

KEY POINTS

- Hypertension in children is a relatively uncommon problem, with only about 4% of children 8 to 12 years old meeting criteria for hypertension.
- CKDs in children are from a variety of disorders and may not be initially well recognized.
- It is essential that AKI is identified as early as possible in a patient's course, with close attention paid to potential sources of renal injury.
- The choice of RRT modality is best decided on local expertise.

This article provides the bedside clinician an overview of the unique renal complications that are seen commonly in the pediatric intensive care unit (PICU). The sections are purposely succinct to give a quick guide to the clinician for the care of these children. We have identified four major areas that should result in discussion and cooperative care between intensive care physicians and nephrologists for the care of these children: (1) hypertension, (2) chronic kidney disease (CKD), (3) acute kidney injury (AKI), and (4) renal replacement therapy (RRT).

HYPERTENSIVE EMERGENCIES

Hypertension in children is a relatively uncommon problem, with only about 4% of children 8 to 12 years old meeting criteria for hypertension in a National Health and Nutrition Examination Study, although rates are increasing with the growing prevalence of childhood obesity.[1] Given the low prevalence of hypertension, hypertensive emergencies are even more uncommon, but can cause lasting injury if not treated appropriately. In

[a] Pediatric Critical Care and Biomedical Engineering, Children's Hospital of Richmond, Virginia Commonwealth University, 1001 East Marshall Street, PO Box 980530, Richmond, VA 23298, USA; [b] Pediatric Nephrology, Children's Hospital of Richmond, Virginia Commonwealth University, 1112 East Clay Street, Richmond, VA 23298, USA
* Corresponding author.
E-mail address: rdaniels@mcvh-vcu.edu

Crit Care Clin 29 (2013) 279–299
http://dx.doi.org/10.1016/j.ccc.2013.01.002   criticalcare.theclinics.com
0749-0704/13/$ – see front matter © 2013 Elsevier Inc. All rights reserved.

adults hypertensive crisis occurs in only about 1% of the hypertensive population and is defined as an acute, severe elevation of blood pressure (BP) above 180/120 mm Hg, with further classification into subcategories based on evidence of end-organ dysfunction. Those with signs of end-organ dysfunction are classified as hypertensive emergency, whereas those with hypertensive crisis but no sign of end-organ dysfunction are defined as hypertensive urgency.[2]

In children, the only definitions for hypertension include four stages: (1) normal, (2) prehypertension, (3) stage I hypertension, and (4) stage II hypertension. The highest level (stage II) is defined as systolic or diastolic BP greater than or equal to the 99th percentile plus 5 mm Hg. Unfortunately, there is no definition for hypertensive crisis in children, and thus unclear parameters for defining hypertensive urgency or emergency. However, general consensus exists that if a child presents with stage II hypertension or higher, then prompt treatment is required. Along these lines, if a child has at least stage II hypertension and also presents with evidence of end-organ dysfunction, then it is reasonable for the clinician to consider it hypertensive emergency and treat appropriately.

The most common causes for hypertension in children vary by age groups and are wide ranging, involving multiple organ systems. In addition, medications, toxins, and clinical interventions may be a source for the hypertension and must be considered (**Table 1**). Interestingly, neonates who are diagnosed with failure to thrive and have concurrent congestive heart failure often may have normal BP initially, but then progress to hypertensive crisis/stage II hypertension on the administration of diuretics, and are a unique class of patients who develop hypertensive emergency. Overall, renal, cardiovascular, neurologic, and ophthalmologic organ systems are most commonly involved. **Table 2** gives a list of some clinical presentations for hypertensive emergency based on the organ system involved.

Because of the variety of organs potentially affected, the initial clinical evaluation must include a complete medical history and physical examination. This includes past medical history (prematurity, intrauterine growth restriction, frequent urinary tract infections, headache, palpitations, joint pain, rashes, and so forth); family history (diabetes, obesity, stroke, autoimmune disorders, hypertension, and so forth); social history (drug abuse, alcohol, smoking, and pregnancy risk); and medication history. Furthermore, a complete physical examination must be performed paying close attention for evidence of clinical features associated with underlying causes of hypertension, such as edema, rashes, thyroid enlargement, abdominal mass, hepatomegaly, and cushingoid features. In addition, four-extremity BP in lying and sitting positions should be performed on all patients, as should an electrocardiogram. Initial laboratory evaluation should include a complete blood count; basic metabolic panel with magnesium and phosphorus; chest radiograph; electrocardiogram; serum uric acid; renal ultrasound; urinalysis with microscopic evaluation; urine electrolytes (including creatinine [Cr] and protein); and urine cultures. An echocardiogram should also be considered if indicated based on the initial work-up. Further work-up may also be required depending on the cause and may include an endocrine or rheumatoid evaluation and imaging studies (see **Table 2**).

Regarding the medical treatment of hypertensive emergencies in children, there have been no studies directly comparing different antihypertensive classes and few studying these drugs in children overall. Most classes of antihypertensives have shown benefit in lowering BP effectively in children, but very few have been evaluated in the setting of hypertensive emergency. There was a recent systemic review performed in adult patients comparing nicardipine versus labetalol for the management of hypertensive crisis, and although both showed comparable efficacy and safety,

Table 1
Causes of hypertension by age groups and organ systems

Group	Causes	
Age range		
Neonates	Renal vascular thrombosis	
	Renal artery stenosis	
	Congenital renal anomalies	
	Coarctation of the aorta	
	Bronchopulmonary dysplasia	
Childhood (infant to 6 y)	Renal parenchymal disease	
	Renal vascular disease	
	Wilms tumor/neuroblastoma	
	Coarctation of the aorta	
School age (6–12 y)	Renal parenchymal disease	
	Renal vascular disease	
	Endocrine disorders	
	Essential hypertension	
Adolescence (12–18 y)	Essential hypertension	
	Renal parenchymal disease	
	Endocrine disorders	
Organ system		
Renal	Congenital dysplastic kidneys	ATN
	Multicystic/polycystic kidney disease	HUS
		Obstructive uropathy
	Renal artery stenosis	Wilms tumor
	Renal vascular thrombosis	Diabetic nephropathy
	Hydronephrosis	Pyelonephritis
	Glomerulonephritis	
Cardiovascular	Coarctation of the aorta	Moyamoya disease
	Takayasu arteritis	(essential hypertension)
Endocrine/autoimmune	Cushing syndrome	Systemic lupus erythematosis
	Hyperthyroidism	Goodpasture syndrome
	Hyperparathyroidism	Wegener disease
	Congenital adrenal hyperplasia	Mixed connective tissue
	Pheochromocytoma	Polyarteritis nodosa
	Obesity	Rheumatoid arthritis
Central nervous system	Brain tumors	Autonomic dysfunction
	Intracranial hemorrhage	Neuroblastoma
	TBI/increased ICP	Encephalitis
Medications/toxins	Corticosteroids	Anabolic steroids
	Tacrolimus/cyclosporine	Amphetamines
	Erythropoietin	Cocaine
	Oral contraceptives	Alcohol
	Vitamin D toxication	Smoking
	Drug withdraw (including clonidine, β-blockers)	Phencyclidine
		Lead, thallium, mercury toxicity
Genetic disorders	Gordon syndrome	Friedreich ataxia
	Liddle syndrome	TS/neurofibromatosis
	Turner syndrome	Von Hippel-Lindau disease
	Williams syndrome	Multiple endocrine neoplasms
Other causes	Pregnancy	Umbilical artery catheterization
	Hypervolemia	Hypercalcemia
	Pain	IUGR

Abbreviations: ATN, acute tubular necrosis; HUS, hemolytic-uremic syndrome; ICP, intracranial pressure; IUGR, intrauterine growth restriction; TBI, traumatic brain injury; TS, tuberous sclerosis.

Data from Singh D, Akingbola O, Yosypiv I, et al. Emergency management of hypertension in children. Int J Nephrol 2012;2012:420247; and Gavrilovici C, Boiculese LV, Brumariu O, et al. [Etiology and blood pressure patterns in secondary hypertension in children]. Rev Med Chir Soc Med Nat Iasi 2007;111(1):70–81. [in Romanian].

Table 2
Objective evidence and clinical symptoms of end-organ damage by organ systems

Organ System	Evidence/Symptom of End-organ Damage
Renal	
Objective evidence	Hematuria
	Oliguria
	Increased microalbuminuria
	Decreased GFR
Clinical symptoms	Flank pain
	Decreased urine output
Cardiovascular	
Objective evidence	Left ventricular hypertrophy
	Left ventricular dysfunction
	Increase in carotid intima media thickness
	Congestive heart failure with FTT (neonates)
Clinical symptoms	Increased work of breathing/SOB
	Chest pain
	Palpitations
	Apnea/irritability/poor feeding (neonates)
Neurologic	
Objective evidence	Posterior reversible encephalopathy syndrome
	Increased ICP
	Focal neurologic deficits
	Seizure
	Facial palsy
	Hemiplegia
Clinical symptoms	Headache (most common)
	Altered mental status
	Nausea/vomiting
Ophthalmologic	
Objective evidence	Hypertensive retinopathy (usually mild)
	Papilledema
	Retinal bleeding
	Acute ischemic optic neuropathy
	Cortical blindness
Clinical symptoms	Loss of visual acuity

Abbreviations: FTT, failure to thrive; GFR, glomerular filtration rate; ICP, intracranial pressure; SOB, shortness of breath.

BP control with nicardipine was more consistent and predictable.[3] However, choosing the primary agent for treating hypertensive emergency in children should be based on the clinical scenario and safety of the agent used (**Table 3**). For example, in a patient with AKI or CKD, nitroprusside and enalaprilat are relatively contraindicated, whereas esmolol should not be used if there is suspicion of substance abuse, especially if cocaine is suspected. Nicardipine often requires a significant volume to be infused, and hydralazine is given in multiple doses, but not as a continuous infusion. Given these considerations, nicardipine is often the best first choice because of its relative safety, but the choice of agent must be considered in light of the underlying cause. If no intravenous (IV) access is available and urgent treatment is required, the clinician may choose to use a nitroglycerin patch for initial control until IV access is established.

The primary goal for treatment of hypertensive emergencies is to reduce the BP to less than the 95th percentile in all patients if possible, and less than the 90th percentile

Table 3
Antihypertensive medications

Medication	Dose Range (all IV)	Mechanism of Action	Duration of Effect	Important Points
Nitroprusside	0.5–10 μg/kg/min	Release of nitric oxide and peripheral vasodilation	1–2 min	Thiocyanate in formulation can lead to cyanide toxicity (especially in AKI) Thiosulfate can be added to nitroprusside infusion to decrease risk of cyanide toxicity Risk of methemoglobinemia Relative contraindication in AKI/CKD
Nicardipine	0.5–3 μg/kg/min	Calcium channel blocker	15–30 min, can last up to 4 h	May require larger volume infused Can contribute to peripheral edema May cause flushing
Esmolol	125–500 μg/kg/min	β-blocker	10–20 min	Contraindicated in cocaine toxicity (unopposed alpha affect) Caution in asthma, congestive heart failure May cause hyperkalemia in AKI May cause bradycardia, bronchospasm, and Reynaud phenomenon
Labetalol	0.25–3 mg/kg/h	α- and β-blockade	Up to 4 h	May cause bradycardia, arteriovenous conduction abnormalities, and bronchospasm
Hydralazine	0.1–0.6 mg/kg/dose Every 4–6 h	Direct vasodilatation of arterioles	1–4 h	May cause arthralgias, systemic lupus erythematosis-like syndrome (including positive antinuclear antibodies) May cause peripheral neuropathy May cause flushing
Enalaprilat	5–10 μg/kg/dose Every 8–24 h	Angiotensin-converting enzyme inhibitor	4–6 h	Relative contraindication in AKI Relative contraindication in suprarenal aortic stenosis and renal artery stenosis May cause rash or angioedema May cause neutropenia and hepatic necrosis (rare) Contraindicated in pregnancy
Nitroglycerin	0.5–1 stamp/kg (patch)	Peripheral vasodilation by increase in cAMP	3–15 min	Allow 10–12 h per day of drug-free time to avoid nitrate tolerance May cause headache or flushing Caution if using with phosphodiesterase inhibitors (eg, sildenafil)

Data from Singh D, Akingbola O, Yosypiv I, et al. Emergency management of hypertension in children. Int J Nephrol 2012;2012:420247.

in patients with comorbid conditions, such as diabetes, cardiac, or renal disease. However, the mean arterial pressure should not be reduced by more than 25% in the first 1 to 2 hours of treatment, and a gradual reduction to goal BP should be pursued over the next 24 hours. Reducing the BP gradually is especially important in the setting of long-term hypertension because cerebral vascular autoregulatory mechanisms can be overwhelmed with acute changes in systemic BP. If the BP is decreased too rapidly, compensatory mechanisms cannot compensate causing serious neurologic injury. Special consideration must also be made for those patients presenting with stroke based on the underlying cause (ischemic vs hemorrhagic), but unfortunately no guidelines currently exist to direct therapy. Therefore, best clinical judgment must be practiced in these cases. Any patient being treated for hypertensive emergency with a continuous IV infusion requires continual monitoring and care to identify any evidence of clinical deterioration caused by changes in systemic BP. As with AKI, the underlying cause for the hypertensive emergency must also be identified and corrected or treated timely and appropriately.

CHRONIC KIDNEY FAILURE IN THE PICU

CKD in children is from a variety of disorders and may not be initially well recognized. It is best to think about these patients either as having polyuric CKD or oliguric CKD. Up to 70% of children with CKD are polyuric, therefore making their renal dysfunction less obvious at first evaluation.[4] This points out that the urine output and solute clearance may be discrepant with each other.

Often polyuric CKD salt and water wasting. This, in turn, may cause hypovolemia with secondary hyperkalemia. These children have a concentration defect; therefore, when a urinalysis is done the specific gravity may never be above 1.010. It is not unusual that these children require one to two times "maintenance" fluids to maintain euvolemia. Further avoidance of potassium-containing fluid may be in order. In contrast, oliguric acute CKD is associated with what one more commonly would expect with AKI. This could be associated with salt and water retention, hypertension, and edema.

CKD is staged from a CKD 1 to 4 scale, correlating with the glomerular filtration rate (GFR) of the child. As the CKD staging deteriorates to CKD stage 3 or higher, metabolic complications of CKD become more evident (**Table 4**).

Whether one has polyuric or oliguric CKD the metabolic complications that occur include a metabolic acidosis, calcium phosphorus disruption, anemia, and additional problems of dehydration and/or hypertension.[5] Metabolic acidosis is related to bicarbonate wasting and lack of acid clearance. In a patient in the critical care unit who may have some degree of respiratory compromise, it is not unusual for these patients to have a mixed respiratory and a metabolic acidosis. In the short term, the treatment of metabolic acidosis is not critical unless there is associated hyperkalemia, but in

| Table 4 | |
CKD staging	
CKD Staging	GFR (mL/min/1.73 m²)
I	>90
II	60–90
III[a]	30–60
IV	15–30
V	<15

[a] Point in time that metabolic consequence of CKD manifest.

the long term management as an outpatient requires correction of metabolic acidosis corrected because of the risk of bone disease. Because one treats the metabolic acidosis with buffer, a drop in the serum potassium and the ionized calcium may occur.

Calcium phosphorus disruption occurs commonly in patients with CKD. Since 1997, the chemistry panels that are commonly used in hospitals in the United States do not measure phosphorus. Therefore, one needs to make an active effort to measure phosphorus in these patients. In CKD phosphorus retention occurs causing secondary hypocalcemia, which in turn stimulates parathyroid overproduction. To correct this phenomena one needs to monitor the phosphorus, normalize it either by phosphorus reduction or by blinding within a nonaluminum-containing product, and adding an active forms of vitamin D for normalization of the calcium. Some of these patients require calcium supplementation in addition to the vitamin D. There are three forms of oral calcium supplementation: (1) calcium carbonate, (2) calcium glubionate, and (3) calcium gluconate. The latter two are better absorbed with fewer effects if binding phosphorus, whereas the former is less absorbed with better chance of binding phosphorus. Therefore, the form of calcium and the timing related to the dietary phosphorus intake should be considered.

Anemia in CKD is related to the lack of adequate iron stores and the lack of natural erythropoiesis. Use of short-acting erythropoietic agents (Epogen) or long-acting (Aranesp) is a style of practice, although kinetically in outpatient children in end-stage renal disease the longer-acting form seems more effective.[6] These medications have been used for more than two decades in patients with CKD and end-stage renal disease.

These agents only work if there are adequate iron stores. Measurement of iron stores can be done by looking at total iron and iron-binding capacity or at ferritin. Ferritin may be elevated, especially in the critical care setting if there is any other inflammation. Therefore, elevation of ferritin by itself is not a good indication of iron stores. Causes of Epogen or Aranesp nonresponsiveness include inadequate iron stores, or inflammation, or secondary hyperparathyroidism, which may be a secondary form of inflammation. Use of these agents may take 2 to 3 weeks to become affective, but may not work in an ICU setting with inflammation.

Another risk of patients with CKD in the ICU is related to drug dosing. One often looks at urine output and assumes there is adequate renal function. Furthermore, patients with CKD have a tendency to be poorly grown resulting in a poor muscle mass that may affect (lower) the baseline serum Cr (sCr). It is important that nephrotoxic agents, such as nonsteroidal anti-inflammatory drugs (NSAIDs), aminoglycosides, and the use of vancomycin be monitored appropriately. NSAIDs should be avoided if there is any question of CKD. Furthermore, contrast agents for computed tomography scans or Intravenous Pyelogram (IVP) or gadolinium for magnetic resonance imaging should be avoided in patients with CKD unless there is an absolute indication for these medications.

In general, the care of the child with CKD is a cooperative effort between the ICU and nephrology and it should be easy to avoid unexpected complications if attention is paid to details.

ACUTE KIDNEY INJURY

Pediatric AKI (pAKI) presents early in the PICU course, most often within the first week of admission, and is associated with increased mortality and increased ICU length of stay.[7] Based on the data obtained in the development of Pediatric Risk, Injury, Failure, Loss, and End-Stage (pRIFLE) criteria, if a patient does not develop AKI by Day 7, they are much less likely to develop it later.[8] However, it is essential that AKI is identified as early as possible in a patient's course, with close attention paid to potential sources of renal injury. There is evidence that even small changes in sCr may indicate significant kidney injury and may be associated with poor outcomes.[9] Preventive strategies for averting future AKI is the best practice, but if prevention is not possible, timely therapies and interventions, as indicated, must then be initiated to provide the best opportunity for recovery. If RRT is the first therapeutic intervention attempted, then it is likely that risk factors for AKI, clinical evidence of renal dysfunction, or earlier therapeutic opportunities were missed.

To discuss pAKI, one should first discuss an established definition of AKI. Unfortunately, no consensus definition exists and clinicians and researchers have used varying criteria for defining pAKI. To date, there are four systems that define AKI (**Tables 5** and **6**): (1) Acute Kidney Injury Network staging, (2) RIFLE criteria, (3) pRIFLE criteria, and (4) Kidney Disease Improving Global Outcomes criteria. Although pRIFLE is considered the best system for defining AKI in the pediatric population, within this system the clinician can choose to define risk, injury, or failure in terms of change in estimated Cr clearance (eCCl) or urine output criteria, which continues to cause inconsistency in pAKI definitions used between centers. eCCl was used in the pRIFLE criteria to account for variations in sCr caused by variations in body mass among patients. Optimally, eCCl and urine output parameters should be used together when possible. Using eCCl criteria alone may give the clinician a fairly accurate viewpoint based on pRIFLE, but we discourage using solely the urine output criteria of pRIFLE for classifying pAKI.

Overall, the incidence of pAKI continues to increase, and is most often multifactorial in cause with complex mechanisms taking place involving endothelial injury, the release of vasoactive substances and cytokines, and alterations in oxygen homeostasis, among others. The most common causes for AKI in the critical care setting are hypoxic/ischemic injury, sepsis/septic shock, and nephrotoxic injury, with primary renal

Table 5
Comparison of pRIFLE and RIFLE definitions of AKI

	pRIFLE		RIFLE	
	eCCl Criteria	UOP Criteria	GFR Criteria	UOP Criteria
RIFLE stage				
Risk	eCCl[a] ↓ by 25%	<0.5 mL/kg/h × 8 h	Cr ↑ × 1.5 or GFR[b] ↓ >25%	<0.5 mL/kg/h × 6 h
Injury	eCCl ↓ by 50%	<0.5 mL/kg/h × 16 h	Cr ↑ × 2 or GFR ↓ >50%	<0.5 mL/kg/h × 12 h
Failure	eCCl ↓ by 75% or eCCl <35 mL/min/ 1.73 m²	<0.5 mL/kg/h × 24 h or anuria × 12 h	Cr ↑ × 3 or GFR ↓ >75% or Cr ≥4 with acute rise ≥0.5	<0.3 mL/kg/h × 24 h or anuria × 12 h
Loss	Persistent failure for >4 wk	RRT or dialysis required	Persistent loss of renal function >4 wk (require RRT/dialysis >4 wk)	
End-stage	Persistent failure for >3 mo (end- stage renal disease)		End-stage renal disease (dialysis required for >3 mo)	

Abbreviations: eCCl, estimated creatinine clearance; UOP, urine output.
    [a] eCCl estimated by the Schwartz formula. If no baseline is available, then use 100 mL/min/1.73 m².
    [b] GFR estimated by the Modification for Diet in Renal Disease formula. If no baseline is available, then use 75 mL/min.

Table 6
Comparison of AKIN and KDIGO definitions of AKI

	AKIN		KDIGO		
	GFR Criteria	UOP Criteria	GFR Criteria	UOP Criteria	
AKIN stage					KDIGO Stage
I	Cr ↑ × 1.5 or ≥0.3 mg/dL	<0.5 mL/kg/h × 6 h	1.5–1.9 × baseline or ≥0.3 mg/dL increase	<0.5 mL/kg/h for 6–12 h	1
II	Cr ↑ × 2	<0.5 mL/kg/h × 12 h	2–2 × baseline	<0.5 mL/kg/h for ≥12 h	2
III	Cr ↑ × 3 or Cr ≥4 with acute rise ≥0.5	<0.3 mL/kg/h × 24 h or anuria × 12 h	3 × baseline or ↑ Cr to ≥4 mg/dl or initiation of RRT or ↓ in GFR to <35 mL/min/1.73 m²	<0.3 mL/kg/h for ≥24 h or Anuria for ≥12 h	3
	(patients who require RRT/ dialysis are considered stage III regardless of their stage before initiation of RRT/ dialysis)				

Abbreviations: AKIN, Acute Kidney Injury Network; KDIGO, Kidney Disease Improving Global Outcomes; UOP, urine output.

disease making up a much smaller portion of pAKI. Given these common causes of AKI, it is no surprise that multiple studies have shown the patients at highest risk for developing AKI are patients on mechanical ventilation with one or more vasoactive medications, patients with heart failure, patients who have undergone cardiopulmonary bypass, patients who are status-post (s/p) hematopoietic stem cell transplantation, and those with sepsis or septic shock.

When AKI is suspected, the clinician should perform a careful review of the record, including medications and therapeutic interventions performed to identify any sources for the AKI and potentially reversible causes. Often, nephrotoxic medications contribute to the developing AKI, if not cause it outright. A list of the most common offenders with mechanism of injury is given in **Table 7**. Of note, a few medications (eg, cimetidine and trimethoprim) may increase sCr, but do not affect GFR and therefore are thought not likely to affect kidney function.

Although drugs often contribute to AKI, the initial evaluation generally requires a determination of whether the injury is caused by prerenal, intrinsic renal, or postrenal mechanisms. The most common causes for each are given in **Table 8**. Recently, the idea of "fluid-responsive" or "fluid nonresponsive" AKI has also been presented as a way to classify AKI,[10] and this makes sense in many ways because hypovolemic/prerenal AKI can often be rapidly reversed with appropriate fluid resuscitation and hemodynamic management, with prerenal and intrinsic renal components often contributing to overall AKI. However, for the purposes of this article the classic terms of prerenal, intrinsic renal, and postrenal are used.

Knowing definitions, classifications, and causes for AKI is helpful, but a plan must be formulated to identify, treat, monitor, and when possible prevent AKI. Prevention can be difficult, and clinicians currently do not have adequate tools by which to predict

Medication	Mechanism of Renal Damage
Table 7	
Most common nephrotoxic medications and their renal effects	
Antibiotics	
Aminoglycosides[a]	Tubular cell toxicity by lysosomal dysfunction of the proximal tubules leading to ATN (reversible)
Vancomycin[a]	Acute interstitial nephritis
Amphotericin B (lipid form has less nephrotoxicity)[a]	Tubular cell toxicity including direct cell membrane damage (reversible)
Acyclovir (IV form)[a]	Acute interstitial nephritis Crystal-induced nephropathy
β-Lactams (ie, penicillin family)[a]	Acute interstitial nephritis
Gancyclovir	Crystal-induced nephropathy
Quinolones	Acute interstitial nephritis Crystal-induced nephropathy
Sulfonamides	Acute interstitial nephritis Crystal-induced nephropathy
Rifampin	Acute interstitial nephritis
Pentamidine	Tubular cell toxicity
Foscarnet	Tubular cell toxicity
Chemotherapy and immunosuppressants	
Cisplatin[a]	Tubular cell toxicity Renal microvascular vasoconstriction Proinflammatory effects
Ifosphamide[a]	Tubular cell toxicity
Methotrexate[a]	Crystal-induced nephropathy
Cyclosporine	Chronic interstitial nephritis Thrombotic microangiopathy
Contrast (radiographic)[a]	Tubular cell toxicity, ATN
NSAIDs[a]	Glomerulonephritis Acute and chronic interstitial nephritis
Angiotensin-converting enzyme inhibitors	Interference with autoregulation of GFR Altered renal vascular regulation
Aspirin/acetaminophen	Chronic interstitial nephritis
Lithium	Glomerulonephritis Chronic interstitial nephritis Rhabdomyolysis

Abbreviation: ATN, acute tubular necrosis.
[a] Indicates most common causes of nephrotoxicity.

AKI; however, one can work to ensure an atmosphere that is the least catalytic for the development of AKI. The best way to do this is to ensure the following:

- Identify those at risk for AKI and perform close monitoring of their clinical progression, including regular surveillance of urine output, electrolytes, and renal function.
- Prevent the use of nephrotoxic medications when possible and discontinue these medications when not essential to treatment. Verify appropriate medication dosing.
- Ensure adequate but not excessive volume resuscitation and fluid balance.

Table 8	
AKI categories with associated causes	
AKI Categories	**Causes**
Prerenal	Intravascular volume depletion (can occur in relative fluid overload [ie, congestive heart failure/third spacing])

Intrinsic renal injury	Acute tubular necrosis
	  Hypoxic/ischemic injury
	  Drug induced
	  Toxin mediated
	    Endogenous (eg, myoglobin)
	    Exogenous (eg, ethylene glycol/methanol)
	Interstitial nephritis
	  Drug induced
	  Idiopathic
	Sepsis/multiple organ dysfunction syndrome
	Glomerulonephritis
	Hemolytic uremic syndrome
	Vascular lesions
	  Vascular thrombosis
	  Cortical necrosis
	Cortical hypoplasia/dysplasia
	Tumor lysis syndrome/uric acid nephropathy

Postrenal (obstructive)	Ureteral obstruction Urethral obstruction Obstruction of solitary kidney

Data from Andreoli SP. Acute kidney injury in children. Pediatr Nephrol 2009;24:253–6; and Basu RK, Devarajan P, Wong H, et al. An update and review of acute kidney injury in pediatrics. Pediatr Crit Care Med 2011;12:339–47.

- Ensure adequate and optimal nutrition, including the use of a metabolic cart as appropriate, and minimize overall catabolism.[11]
- Identify the underlying disorder or source of AKI as early as possible and treat the underlying condition.
- Avoid significant increases in blood glucose (>215) when possible, but also protect from hypoglycemia, keeping blood glucose greater than 125 during acute phase of kidney injury.

In addition to this list, a special category of patients in which prevention is possible are those who are scheduled to receive contrast for imaging procedures. Avoidance is optimal if practical, but most often this is not the case, and even with preemptive treatment contrast-induced nephropathy (CIN) cannot always be prevented. Concurrent use of nephrotoxic drugs, intravascular volume depletion, hemodynamic instability (especially hypotension), diabetes, and the presence of underlying CKD all contribute to the risk for CIN. In the end, there is conflicting evidence on suggested therapies for avoiding CIN. The best evidence supports the following:

- When possible, use low-volume, nonionic, low-osmolar, or iso-osmolar contrast formulations.
- Use isotonic crystalloid (with or without bicarbonate, because there is equivocal evidence regarding the benefits of bicarbonate) for volume expansion preexposure and postexposure to contrast. In general, approximately 20 mL/kg pre-exposure and postexposure (depending on fluid status of the patient).
- Avoid concurrent administration of nephrotoxic medications precontrast and postcontrast (eg, NSAIDs).

- Optimize hemodynamics, avoiding hypotension.
- Although there is conflicting evidence for the use of N-acetylcysteine before contrast exposure, there is very little risk in its use. Therefore, the decision to use this medication to prevent CIN is left to the individual practitioner.
- Theophylline has also been suggested as a therapy for preventing CIN, but the evidence is inconsistent; therefore, its use is left to the discretion of the practitioner.
- Fenoldopam has shown to be of no benefit compared with saline or N-acetylcysteine and is therefore not recommended for the prevention of CIN.

Just as fluid management is of upmost importance in a patient receiving contrast, the overall volume status of any patient at risk for AKI must be monitored closely, and any fluid overload identified early in the course. Adult data have shown a correlation between fluid overload and mortality in AKI,[12] whereas available pediatric data have demonstrated increased mortality in patients with increased fluid administration requiring RRT.[13] Although sometimes difficult to obtain in the ICU setting, a good way to monitor daily fluid/volume status is with daily weights, although the electronic medical record has improved the ability to assess fluid inputs and outputs and fluid balance overall. If reliable input and output fluid volumes are available, then a percent fluid overload can be calculated by the following: $[(\Sigma \, Fluid_{Input} - \Sigma \, Fluid_{Output})/Admit \, Wt_{kg}] \times 100$.[14] In general, fluid overload of 10% to 15% should prompt discussion of the patient's clinical condition and the potential need for interventions to reduce this overload, such as RRT. If RRT is not thought to be indicated at the time, diuretics are often the therapy of choice to manage mild fluid overload. Although it is appropriate to attempt to use diuretics to control volume overload, diuretics have not been shown to reduce the duration of AKI, improve mortality, reduce the need for RRT, or improve renal recovery,[15,16] and should not be used solely with the goal of "converting" an oliguric state to a nonoliguric state in a patient with underlying AKI. Furthermore, the clinician must pay careful attention not to delay RRT in critically ill patients with AKI and fluid overload, especially in the setting of escalating diuretic therapy or other negative metabolic consequences related to solute clearance. In addition, close attention must be paid to serum electrolytes throughout the course of diuretic therapy, with ongoing replacement as needed.

While monitoring fluid status, clinicians must also make every attempt to identify the underlying source of AKI; many tools have been put forth to aid in this evaluation. Among them, and often one of the first indices evaluated to determine prerenal versus intrinsic renal dysfunction, is the fractional excretion of sodium (FeNa), or fractional excretion of urea (FeUr), with each reflecting the tubular reabsorption capacity. Results of less than 1% indicate prerenal causes for AKI, with results greater than 2% indicating a higher risk for intrinsic renal disease, such as acute tubular necrosis. However, care must be taken because the FeNa is inaccurate in patients who have received diuretics or in patients with CKD. The FeUr is more accurate in patients who have received diuretics, but again must be used in caution in patients with any underlying kidney disease. Along with these indices, laboratory results and clinical data must be evaluated paying close attention to serum electrolytes, blood urea nitrogen (BUN), sCr, urine output, urinalysis with sediment evaluation, and urine electrolytes. From these measurements, the clinician can then derive additional clinical data that may be useful, including eCCl, BUN/Cr ratio, protein loss, and electrolyte clearance, along with an evaluation of pRIFLE stage. **Table 9** lists common equations used in the evaluation of AKI, including GFR, FeNa, FeUr, and Cr clearance.

In addition to the clinical indices noted previously, evaluating the urine by urine microscopy can provide vital information to the clinician by identifying the presence or absence of casts, cells, eosinophils, and other sediments that can point to the

Table 9
Equations used in the evaluation of AKI

Equation	Formula
Equations for GFR (mL/min/1.73 m^2)	
Schwartz formula (use for children and for pRIFLE criteria)	$eGFR = [0.413 \times height(cm)]/S_{cr}$
Modification of Diet in Renal Disease formula (use for adults and for RIFLE criteria)	$eGFR = 175 \times (S_{cr})^{-1.154} \times (age)^{-0.203} \times (0.742$ if female$) \times (1.212$ if African American$)$
FeNa/FeUr	
FeNa (unreliable with diuretics or CKD)	$FeNa = (Ur_{Na} \times S_{Cr})/(S_{Na} \times Ur_{Cr}) \times 100$ If <1% = likely prerenal source, but also found in acute glomerulonephritis and hepatorenal syndrome If >1% but <2% = indeterminate If >2% = more likely intrinsic renal cause (ie, ATN) or severe obstruction
FeUr (more reliable if patient has received diuretics, but still unreliable if underlying CKD)	$FeUr = [(Ur_{Urea} \times S_{Cr})/(S_{Urea} \times Ur_{Cr})] \times 100$ If <35% = likely prerenal source If >35% = more likely intrinsic renal cause (ie, ATN/other)
Creatinine clearance	Creatinine clearance $= [(Ur_{Cr} \times Ur_{Vol})/(S_{Cr} \times T_{min})] \times (1.73/BSA^a)$
Fluid overload (%)	Fluid overload (%) $= [(\Sigma$ Fluid$_{Input} - \Sigma$ Fluid$_{Output})/$admit Wt$_{kg}] \times 100$

Abbreviations: Σ, Sum; ATN, acute tubular necrosis; eGFR, estimated GFR; S$_{cr}$, serum creatinine; S$_{Na}$, serum sodium; T$_{min}$, time over which urine collected (min); UrCr, urine creatinine; Ur$_{Na}$, urine sodium; Ur$_{Vol}$, total volume of urine collected; Wt$_{kg}$, weight in kilograms.
^{a} BSA (m^2) $= 0.007184 \times$ height (cm)$^{0.725} \times$ weight (kg)$^{0.425}$.
Data from Patel HP. The abnormal urinalysis. Pediatr Clin North Am 2006;53:325–37; and Ringsrud KM. Cells in the urine sediment. Lab Med 2001;32:153–5.

underlying diagnosis. If possible, review by a pediatric nephrologist provides the best evaluation, because this has been proved superior to hospital laboratory reporting.[17] **Table 10** gives a list of sediment found in urine and the implications of their presence. Although **Table 10** gives a list of many possible causes for cells or sediment present, the following patterns and observations may point to more specific causes:

- BUN/Cr ratio of >20, although not particularly sensitive, suggests a prerenal cause, whereas a value of <10 points toward an intrinsic renal injury.
- Low specific gravity (given abnormal function and no evidence of diabetes insipidus) may indicate acute interstitial nephritis or other intrinsic renal dysfunction, because the kidney has lost its ability to concentrate the urine, especially with characteristic sediments present.
- High specific gravity may indicate relative intravascular volume depletion, or prerenal causes, and adrenal dysfunction.
- Red cell casts with red cells and proteinuria are highly suggestive of acute glomerulonephritis or vasculitis.
- White cells and white cell casts, especially with little or no proteinuria, suggests acute interstitial nephritis. Glomerulonephritis (especially postinfectious glomerulonephritis) can also present with white cell casts, but other cells or casts will likely be present (see above).

Table 10
Urine sediments and their significance

Urine Sediment	Interpretation and Significance
Hematologic origin	
Erythrocytes (RBCs)	A few (<5) present may be normal May be a result of bleeding (any location) In isolation (no casts present), may point toward lower urinary tract bleeding (ie, Foley catheter trauma, stones), but other diagnoses must be excluded
RBC casts	Glomerulonephritis, ATN (less common), or tubulointerstitial nephritis (rarely)
Leukocytes (WBCs)	A few present (<5) may be normal
Neutrophils	Most commonly seen WBCs in urine Often indicate inflammation along urogenital tract Associated with bacterial infection Concurrent low protein = more likely lower UTI Concurrent high protein = more likely renal involvement Neutrophils with no bacteria may reflect uncommon bacteria (or inflammatory response)
Eosinophils	Improved detection with Hansel or Wright stain Associated with drug-induced interstitial nephritis
Lymphocytes	Very few present may be normal Can be early indicator of rejection after transplant Leukocyte esterase test may be (-) with (+) lymphocytes
WBC casts	Pyelonephritis, tubulointerstitial nephritis, or glomerulonephritis (with other cells present)
Epithelial origin	
Renal epithelial cells	Few present may be normal Multiple etiologies possible including ATN, viral infections (inclusion bodies in CMV), renal transplant rejection, chemical toxins, drug toxicity, heavy metals, inflammation, and neoplasms
Squamous cells	Significant amount = likely contamination
Transitional cells	Few present may be normal Increased numbers with infection Large clumps/sheets may indicate transitional cell carcinoma
Other casts	
Fat bodies/fatty casts	Nephrotic syndrome (usually massive proteinuria)
Hyaline casts	Can be seen in normal health or after exercise Diuretic therapy Intrinsic renal disease
Granular casts	Glomerular disease Tubular injury Pyelonephritis/viral infections
"Dirty brown casts"	Granular casts with pigment, often caused by hemoglobin Context important as multifactorial Often seen in ATN, can suggest intravascular hemolysis
Waxy casts	Advanced renal failure/injury
Crystals	
Calcium oxalate crystals	Ethylene glycol ingestion

(continued on next page)

Table 10 *(continued)*	
Urine Sediment	**Interpretation and Significance**
Uric acid crystals	Tumor lysis syndrome
Cystine crystals	Cystinuria
Magnesium ammonium phosphate crystals	Struvite stones Increased ammonia production with increased pH Can be seen with urease-producing infections (eg, *Proteus* or *Klebsiella*)

Abbreviations: ATN, acute tubular necrosis; CMV, cytomegalovirus; RBC, red blood cell; UTI, urinary tract infection; WBC, white blood cell.

From Patel HP. The abnormal urinalysis. Pediatr Clin North Am 2006;53:325–37, with permission; and Ringsrud KM. Cells in the Urine Sediment. Lab Med 2001;32:153–5, with permission.

- Eosinophilia in the urine suggests drug-induced acute interstitial nephritis.
- Positive nitrite suggests infection.

Renal ultrasound can give additional data regarding the onset of AKI and the presence or absence of hydronephrosis and other abnormalities. Relatively large kidneys suggest an acute process, whereas kidneys that are smaller than expected may suggest CKD or other long-term injury. In addition, renal ultrasound can identify renal vascular anomalies, as can Doppler studies.

Although there is no current method for predicting AKI, high clinical suspicion based on risk and diligence in the prompt identification and treatment of AKI gives the greatest chance for the best outcomes. To that end, biomarkers are now being introduced and studied that may be able to improve the prompt identification of AKI and begin to move clinicians closer to establishing predictions for AKI. Although there are many biomarkers being evaluated, the most common and the most widely available for clinical use are cystatin c, neutrophil gelatinase-associated lipocalin, kidney injury molecule-1, and interleukin-18. Most are measured in serum and urine, but of those listed, all but cystatin c seem to have superior ability for early identification of AKI using the urinary measurement. In a recent study of urinary biomarkers in the pediatric emergency department, urinary neutrophil gelatinase-associated lipocalin, kidney injury molecule-1, and β_2 microglobulin all demonstrated accuracy in predicting pRIFLE injury versus those with pRIFLE risk or those without AKI.[18] Urinary neutrophil gelatinase-associated lipocalin has been shown in more than one study to show promise as an early marker for AKI and its severity in critically ill children and in children after cardiac surgery.[19] In addition, new methods are being developed to identify biomarkers. In one study, microarray data taken from children with septic shock–associated AKI identified two specific genes that showed a high sensitivity for predicting septic shock–associated AKI (matrix metalloproteinase-8 and elastase-2).[20] The ability to use biomarkers in the early identification of AKI is limited to the measurements available in any given center, but widespread use is likely in the near future.

The best overall management of pAKI involves prevention when possible; early identification, including the use of biomarkers where available; adequate fluid resuscitation with appropriate fluid management, including RRT if needed; avoidance or minimization of nephrotoxic exposures; optimal nutritional support and blood glucose management; and prompt identification of the underlying disorder with appropriate therapeutic intervention. **Fig. 1** presents an algorithm for suggested evaluation and points of intervention for patients at risk for or who are developing AKI. Although the algorithm is a guideline, continued discussion must be maintained with the pediatric

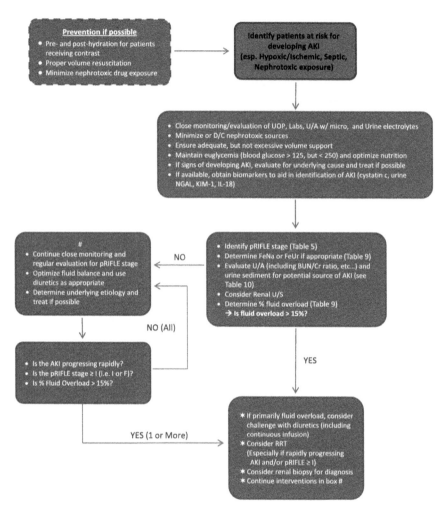

Fig. 1. Algorithm for evaluating AKI.

nephrologist regarding proper timing for the initiation of RRT if needed, and the need for renal biopsy to identify the underlying disorder. Because the care of these children is often complex, an organized team approach that includes the intensivist, nephrologist, bedside nurse, and other supportive staff is most optimal.

Finally, even with the best available data, biomarkers, and tools currently available, clinicians are still only reacting to injury that has already taken place. The greatest impact on pAKI in the future will come when clinicians begin to develop tools to predict pAKI. Although biomarkers may help clinicians move toward developing models for prediction, it is unlikely that these markers alone will provide the key. As a result, the concept of "renal angina" is being pursued, which serves to meld clinical, laboratory, and other data together to develop prediction models similar to the predictive capabilities of clinical and laboratory data that are used to identify cardiac ischemia in the setting of cardiac angina.[20] It is hoped that in the future these predictive models will be available, enabling one to intervene before significant injury occurs, improving the outcomes for children with pAKI.

RRT FOR AKI

RRT can be used for AKI, inborn error of metabolism, or intoxication. Specifically, the use of RRT for AKI is discussed in this section.[21] Options for RRT include hemodialysis (HD), peritoneal dialysis (PD), or continuous RRT (CRRT). Data have yet to show that the modality choice affects outcome in AKI. Most institutions pick modalities based on experience and clinical situations.

RRT is used for fluid removal (ultrafiltration) or solute clearance. If one compares the three forms of RRT, solute clearance is superior in HD, then CRRT, and then finally PD. This is directly related to the dialysate exposure during that period of time. Alternatively, ultrafiltration can be achieved by all modes yet hemodynamic instability is more stable with CRRT, then PD, then HD. This is typically because HD is used for a 3- to 4-hour period of time and CRRT and PD are used over a 24-hour period. Specific discussions around each modality follow.

Hemodialysis

HD requires a water source, often a reverse-osmosis system, and a machine. The machine has an acid and a base solution that allows for physiologic solution. Classically, the components of the dialysate are 0 to 2 potassium mEq/L, and 0 phosphorus. Otherwise, there are normal physiologic levels of bicarbonate, calcium, and sodium. Dialysate flow rates run between 30 and 50 L per hour, maximizing solute clearance. Ultrafiltration is determined by changes in transmembrane pressure. One can dialyze without ultrafiltrating and one can ultrafiltrate without dialyzing, or one can do both on HD.[22]

The extracorporeal therapy of HD is determined often by the intravascular blood volume of the child. Knowing that, the smaller the child the smaller the extracorporeal circuit should be to avoid hemodynamic instability. HD machines also have in-line heaters to avoid thermic abnormalities.[23]

Vascular access for HD in AKI is the same vascular access used in CRRT. Data by Hackbarth and colleagues[24] suggest that preferentially a catheter that is placed in the internal jugular vein and proportional to the size of the patient gives optimum of flow and minimizes recirculation. Choice optimal catheters can be found at www.pcrrt.com.

The benefit of HD is that it allows rapid clearance of solute and does not require ICU nursing staff; rather, dialysis nursing staff can take care of the system while the ICU nursing staff takes care of the child. The risk of HD may be from hemodynamic instability, although that can be controlled, but more importantly an excess of solute clearance. Patients with very high BUN (>100 mg/dL), high glucose, or high sodium have high osmolality. HD osmolality is roughly 280 mOsm/L. Therefore, if the patient is hyperosmolar and one dialyzes on HD, one may drop the osmolar quickly and develop what is referred to as "dialysis disequilibrium," which results in neurologic changes including seizures. This can be prevented by using an alternative form or RRT or making HD less efficient.[25]

Anticoagulation for HD can be none or heparin. Heparin is used to have a targeted activated clotting in the 150 to 200 range, similar to that of extracorporeal membrane oxygenation and CRRT.

Peritoneal Dialysis

PD is an alternative and is used more commonly in postcardiac and infant populations.[26] PD requires the placement of a catheter, either cuffed or acute, in the peritoneum as an inflow and an outflow system.[27,28] PD solutions in North America are lactate based. This is quite different than the bicarbonate-based solutions used for CRRT and for HD.

Lactate-based solutions deliver lactate to the patient with resulting rising plasma lactate levels. This may lead to confusion at bedside knowing whether rising lactate level is that of the patient or that of the solution.

At the initiation of PD, often a manual system is used with an inflow of roughly 10 mL/kg per pass, and that solution is placed in the peritoneum for roughly 45 minutes and drained over 15 minutes, resulting in a 1-hour cycle. Often the volume is not increased for a few weeks because of the risk for early leakage, which results in loss of ability to use PD as an option for RRT. PD has an advantage at bedside of rapid onset and ease of use with simplicity. PD has a disadvantage because it changes intra-abdominal pressure and thoracic pressure with impedance on respiratory effect including the risk of leakage of the peritoneal solution into the pulmonary space.[29] PD additionally has a low risk of developing peritonitis or infection in the peritoneum, which usually can be treated very easily with instillation of intraperitoneal antibiotics targeted at plasma concentrations. An example of this is the use of vancomycin intraperitoneally at 20 mg/L and tobramycin at 4 mg/L, which results in minimum inhibitory concentration of 20 μg/mL of vancomycin and 4 μg/mL of tobramycin.

Intraperitoneal heparin is often used at 250 to 500 units per liter to minimize activation of fibrin, avoiding clotting in the peritoneum. The use of intraperitoneal heparin does not give systemic affects; therefore, it can be used even in patients at risk for having systemic bleeding.

If one needs significant ultrafiltration, then one either goes up on the volume per pass, the frequency of cycles, or the glucose concentration of the dialysate to have a higher osmolar pole for ultrafiltration. If one needs higher solute clearance on PD, one need to either go up on the volume per pass or to lessen the cycle numbers and prolong the time in the peritoneum for better solute clearance.[30]

CRRT

CRRT can be as continuous venoveno-hemofiltration, venoveno-hemodiafiltration, or venovenohemo-diafiltration with dialysis. Data to date identify that the use of convective clearance (CVVH) or diffusive clearance (CVVHD) results in equal solute clearance with small-molecular-weight substances approaching, such as urea.[31] Larger molecular weight substances are highly protein-bound substances (eg, vancomycin) and have a preferential clearance on CVVH versus CVVHD.

Nonpublished studies by our group have identified a preferential clearance of inflammatory mediators and cytokines in patients with CVVH. Furthermore, work by Flores and colleagues[32] identified that in the stem cell population survival may be better in the convective mode.

Machinery to date used in North America allows for either a CVVH or a CVVHD or a CVVHDF combination. There is no additive benefit of doing convective and diffusive techniques in patients over purely convective or purely diffusive. Solutions in North America now are bicarbonate-based, often calcium free or calcium rich. The choice of calcium free is often used in patients using citrate anticoagulation. Calcium rich are often used in patients using heparin-based anticoagulation.

The federal government has identified that fluids given as a CVVH are referred to as drugs, yet fluids used for dialysate clearance are called devices. Based on Food and Drug Administration requirements, only fluids sold for the use of CVVH should be used for convection and dialysate fluids should not be used in a convective mode.

Anticoagulation in CRRT can be none or heparin as in HD or citrate anticoagulation. Classically, heparin-based protocols include a bolus of 10 to 20 units per kilogram and in a continuous infusion at 10 to 20 units/kg/h of heparin with target activated clotting between 150 and 200.

Work by our group over a decade ago identified the use of citrate anticoagulation as an alternative to heparin.[33] Comparison data by Brophy and coworkers[34] has identified similar outcome in circuit life between the two anticoagulation protocols. They also demonstrated that anticoagulation-free circuits do not last as long when compared with heparin- or citrate-based circuits. Citrate anticoagulation offers a benefit to the patient because it does not affect patient anticoagulation risk.

Citrate works by binding calcium in the plasma, thus chelating calcium from the coagulation's cascade, minimizing the risk of a clotted circuit. Calcium must be repleted back to the patient, preferably in the form of calcium chloride, to offset any risk of hypocalcemia to the patient.

A typical prescription for CVVH or CVVHD includes a blood flow rate of 5 to 10 mL/kg/h based on excess pressures, replacement or a diffusive rate of 2 to 3000 mL/1.73 m^2/h, and a net ultrafiltration rate based on hemodynamic stability between 0.5 and 2 mL/kg/h.[31] Anticoagulation could be done by heparin or by citrate. Vascular access in CRRT is identical to that for vascular access for AKI therapy by HD.

Comparison data of HD versus PD versus CRRT have identified no benefit in modality affecting outcome. Work by Fleming and coworkers[35] and Maxvold and coworkers[36] has identified equal outcome. Fleming's data suggest a better delivery of nutrition in patients on CVVH as opposed to patients on PD. Maxvold's paper identified that those patients who are at risk for hemodynamic compromise seem to be more stable on CRRT and there is a preference of CRRT in this population. Further work by our group identified similar outcomes in patients on PD and CRRT, with an improved outcome in patients on HD.[37] This retrospective database is biased for patients on HD, were less hemodynamically compromised, with less pressure use at the initiation of RRT.

To summarize, there are no data to date that the choice of RRT affects outcome. The choice of RRT modality is best decided on local expertise. In most cases of AKI, RRT modality may not have an effect on outcome. In certain populations (eg, postoperative infant cardiac surgical patients) PD may be preferable because of ease of use of PD and avoiding the use of veins that may need to be used with future cardiac catheterization.[38] In clinical events of intoxications the use of HD may be preferable because of the high clearance of solute.[39] In cases of inborn error of metabolism, the sequential use of HD followed by CRRT may be optimal.[40] Drug and nutritional clearance are affected by all forms of RRT and need to be attended.

REFERENCES

1. Din-Dzietham R, Liu Y, Bielo MV, et al. High blood pressure trends in children and adolescents in national surveys, 1963 to 2002. Circulation 2007;116(13):1488–96.
2. Jones DW, Hall JE. Seventh report of the joint national committee on prevention, detection, evaluation, and treatment of high blood pressure and evidence from new hypertension trials. Hypertension 2004;43(1):1–3.
3. Peacock FW, Hilleman DE, Levy PD, et al. A systematic review of nicardipine vs labetalol for the management of hypertensive crises. Am J Emerg Med 2012;30: 981–93.
4. Harambat J, va Stralen KJ, Kim JJ, et al. Epidemiology of chronic kidney disease in children. Pediatr Nephrol 2012;27:363–73.
5. Furth SL, Abraham AG, Jerry-Fluer J, et al. Metabolic abnormalities, cardiovascular disease risk factors, and GFR decline in children with chronic kidney disease. Clin J Am Soc Nephrol 2011;6:2132–40.

6. Lerner G, Kale AS, Warady BA, et al. Pharmacokinetics of darbepoetin alfa in pediatric patients with chronic kidney disease. Pediatr Nephrol 2002;17:933–9.

7. Schneider J, Khemani R, Grushkin C, et al. Serum creatinine as stratified in the RIFLE score for acute kidney injury is associated with mortality and length of stay for children in the pediatric intensive care unit. Crit Care Med 2010;38:933–9.

8. Akcan-Arikan A, Zappitelli M, Loftis LL, et al. Modified RIFLE criteria in critically ill children with acute kidney injury. Kidney Int 2007;71:1028–35.

9. Zappitelli M, Bernier PL, Saczkowski RS, et al. A small post-operative rise in serum creatinine predicts acute kidney injury in children undergoing cardiac surgery. Kidney Int 2009;76:885–92.

10. Himmelfarb J, Joannidis M, Molitoris B, et al. Evaluation and initial management of acute kidney injury. Clin J Am Soc Nephrol 2008;3:962–7.

11. Bunchman TE. Treatment of acute kidney injury in children: from conservative management to renal replacement therapy. Nat Clin Pract Nephrol 2008;4:510–4.

12. Payden D, de Pont AC, Sakr Y, et al. A positive fluid balance is associated with a worse outcome in patients with acute renal failure. Crit Care 2008;12:R74.

13. Goldstein SL, Somers MJ, Baum MA, et al. Pediatric patients with multi-organ dysfunction syndrome receiving continuous renal replacement therapy. Kidney Int 2005;67:653–8.

14. Foland JA, Fortenberry JD, Warshaw BL, et al. Fluid overload before continuous hemofiltration and survival in critically ill children: a retrospective analysis. Crit Care Med 2004;32:1771–6.

15. Venkataram R, Kellum JA. The role of diuretic agents in the management of acute renal failure. Contrib Nephrol 2001;132:158–70.

16. Van der Voort PH, Boerma EC, Koopmans M, et al. Furosemide does not improve renal recovery after hemofiltration for acute renal failure in critically ill patients: a double blind randomized controlled trial. Crit Care Med 2009;37:533–8.

17. Tsai JJ, Yeun JY, Kumar VA, et al. Comparison and interpretation of urinalysis performed by a nephrologist versus a hospital based clinical laboratory. Am J Kidney Dis 2005;46:820–9.

18. Du Y, Zappitelli M, Mian A, et al. Urinary biomarkers to detect acute kidney injury in the pediatric emergency center. Pediatr Nephrol 2011;26:267–74.

19. Basu R, Standage S, Cvijanovich NZ, et al. Identification of candidate serum biomarkers for severe septic shock-associated kidney injury via microarray. Crit Care 2011;15:R273.

20. Basu R, Chawla L, Wheeler DS, et al. Renal angina: an emerging paradigm to identify children at risk for acute kidney injury. Pediatr Nephrol 2012;27:1067–78.

21. Parekh RS, Bunchman TE. Dialysis support in the pediatric intensive care unit. Adv Ren Replace Ther 1996;3:326–36.

22. Donckerwolcke RA, Bunchman TE. Hemodialysis in infants and small children [review]. Pediatr Nephrol 1994;8:103–6.

23. Bunchman TE. Pediatric hemodialysis: lessons from the past, ideas for the future. Kidney Int 1996;53:S64–7.

24. Hackbarth R, Bunchman TE, Chua AN, et al. The effect of vascular access location and size on circuit survival in pediatric continuous renal replacement therapy: a report from the PCRRT registry. Int J Artif Organs 2007;30(12):1116–21.

25. Bunchman TE, Hackbarth RM, Maxvold NJ, et al. Prevention of dialysis disequilibrium by use of CVVH. Int J Artif Organs 2007;30:441–4.

26. Flynn JT, Kershaw DB, Smoyer WE, et al. Peritoneal dialysis for management of pediatric acute renal failure. Perit Dial Int 2001;21:390–4.

27. Chadha V, Warady BA, Blowey DL, et al. Tenckhoff catheters prove superior to cook catheters in pediatric acute peritoneal dialysis. Am J Kidney Dis 2000;35:1111–6.

28. Bunchman TE. Acute peritoneal dialysis in infant renal failure. Perit Dial Int 1996; 16(Suppl 1):S509–11.

29. Bunchman TE, Wood EG, Lynch RE. Hydrothorax as a complication of pediatric peritoneal dialysis. Perit Dial Bull 1987;7:237–9.

30. Smoyer WE, Maxvold NJ, Remenapp R, et al. Renal replacement therapy in pediatric critical care. In: Farhman BP, Zimmerman JJ, editors. Pediatric Critical Care - 2nd edition. St Louis (MO): Mosby; 1998:Chapter 64; p. 764–78.

31. Maxvold NJ, Smoyer WE, Custer JR, et al. Amino acid loss and nitrogen balance in critically ill children with acute renal failure: a prospective comparison between classic hemofiltration and hemofiltration with dialysis. Crit Care Med 2000;28: 1161–5.

32. Flores FX, Brophy PD, Symons JM, et al. CRRT after stem cell transplantation: a report from the Prospective Pediatric CRRT Registry Group. Pediatr Nephrol 2008;23:625–30.

33. Bunchman TE, Maxvold NJ, Brophy PD. Pediatric convective hemofiltration (CVVH): normocarb replacement fluid and citrate anticoagulation. Am J Kidney Dis 2003;42:1248–52.

34. Brophy PD, Somers MJ, Baum MA, et al. Multi-centre evaluation of anticoagulation in patients receiving continuous renal replacement therapy (CRRT). Nephrol Dial Transplant 2005;20:1416–21.

35. Fleming F, Bohn D, Edwards H, et al. Renal replacement therapy after repair of congenital heart disease in children: a comparison of hemofiltration and peritoneal dialysis. J Thorac Cardiovasc Surg 1995;109:322–31.

36. Maxvold NJ, Smoyer WE, Gardner JJ, et al. Management of acute renal failure in the pediatric patient: hemofiltration versus hemodialysis. Am J Kidney Dis 1997; 30(Suppl 4):S84–8.

37. Bunchman TE, McBryde KD, Mottes TE, et al. Pediatric acute renal failure: outcome by modality and disease. Pediatr Nephrol 2001;16:1067–71.

38. Bonilla-Felix M. Peritoneal dialysis in the pediatric intensive care unit setting. Perit Dial Int 2009;29(Suppl 2):S183–5.

39. Bunchman TE, Ferris ME. Management of toxic ingestions with the use of renal replacement. Pediatr Nephrol 2011;26:535–41.

40. Bunchman TE, Barletta GM, Winters JW, et al. Phenylacetate and benzoate clearance in a hyperammonemic infant on sequential hemodialysis and hemofiltration. Pediatr Nephrol 2007;22:1062–5.

Anemia and Transfusion in Critically Ill Pediatric Patients
A Review of Etiology, Management, and Outcomes

Daniel Sloniewsky, MD

KEYWORDS

- Anemia • Transfusion • Transfusion trigger • Transfusion-related acute lung injury
- Immunomodulation • Storage lesion • Child

KEY POINTS

- Anemia is commonly seen in critically ill pediatric patients.
- This anemia is caused by decreased erythropoiesis and increased blood loss.
- Anemia can worsen outcomes in critically ill patients.
- Transfusion of red blood cells may not improve outcomes in anemic critically ill children because of problems related to its storage and some inherent properties of the red blood cells.
- There are some therapeutic options available to critical care practitioners that may minimize the risks associated with transfusion.

INTRODUCTION

Anemia in critically ill pediatric patients is common. The etiology is multifactorial and includes diminished erythropoietin activity, poor iron use by the body, and blood loss (both iatrogenic and noniatrogenic). In addition, anemia has been shown in a variety of studies to worsen patient outcomes, presumably because of diminished oxygen delivery. For these reasons, transfusion of blood products, and in particular packed red blood cells (pRBCs), has become a significant therapeutic intervention. However, over the last 20 years it has become evident that transfused blood does not necessarily demonstrate the same characteristics as autologous blood. In fact, transfused blood products demonstrate metabolic, physiologic, and immunomodulatory effects that may worsen patient outcomes, possibly because of problems associated with the storage process. Subsequently multiple clinical studies have demonstrated that although critically ill patients with significant anemia have

Disclosures: The author has no financial relationships to disclose.
Division of Pediatric Critical Care Medicine, Department of Pediatrics, Stony Brook Long Island Children's Hospital, 100 Nicolls Road Stony Brook, NY 11794, USA
E-mail address: daniel.sloniewsky@sbumed.org

Crit Care Clin 29 (2013) 301–317
http://dx.doi.org/10.1016/j.ccc.2012.11.005   criticalcare.theclinics.com

increased morbidity and mortality, transfusion of blood products may not improve outcomes. The complications associated with transfusion are the stimulus for the research and development of new blood transfusion strategies and blood substitutes.

ANEMIA IN CRITICALLY ILL PATIENTS
Incidence of Anemia in Critically Ill Patients

Anemia is a common finding in critically ill adults and children, and its course in critically ill patients is predictable. In both populations, a substantial portion of the patients who present to an intensive care unit (ICU) are anemic as a baseline, although this percentage appears to be higher in adults than in children.[1-3] Bateman and colleagues[3,4] reported anemia in 33% of children on admission to the pediatric intensive care unit (PICU) compared with the 60% to 70% reported in adult studies. The incidence of anemia increases after admission to the ICU in critically ill children and adults, although the time frame differs between the groups. The majority of critically ill adults will eventually become anemic and they tend to reach the nadir of their hemoglobin concentration after the second week of hospitalization.[4] In the study by Bateman and colleagues,[3] an additional 41% of the critically ill pediatric patients enrolled became anemic during their course in the PICU. However, the appearance of anemia occurred soon after admission to the PICU (within 1–3 days) and 74% of the pRBCs administered were given within 48 hours of admission.[3] The etiology of anemia in the critically ill can help explain this time difference.

Etiology of Anemia

There are multiple reasons for anemia in critically ill patients. Although hemodilution seen with fluid resuscitation may play some role, the more important causes include inadequate production and blood loss.

Normal erythropoiesis

To better understand the pathology behind diminished erythrocyte production in critical illness, it is important to understand erythropoiesis. At birth, the marrow of all long bones produces red blood cells (RBCs) until the age of 5 years when the majority of erythropoiesis takes place in the vertebral bodies, ribs, sternum, and pelvis. There are several growth factors involved in RBC production, the primary one being erythropoietin (Epo), which is responsible for the maturation and proliferation of the erythroid cell line. In the fetus and newborn, this glycoprotein hormone is made by the Kupffer cells in the liver until around 4 to 6 weeks of age, when its production gradually shifts to the renal peritubular cells.[5] Its production is stimulated by both hypoxemia and anemia, although the fetal liver requires significantly lower levels of oxygen and RBCs before production of Epo is simulated. This lack of responsiveness to the usual stimuli can diminish erythropoiesis in critically ill premature fetuses and term newborns.[6] In addition to Epo, the normal production of new RBCs also requires iron as well as other substrates such as folic acid. Iron availability, in particular, can be affected in critically ill patients. Once released into the circulation, the normal RBC life span is approximately 120 days. When RBCs become senescent or damaged they are then removed from the circulation, primarily by the reticuloendothelial system, and their components are recycled.

Effect of critical illness on erythropoietin

The development of multiorgan dysfunction syndrome (MODS) is common in critically ill children, and involves a host of inflammatory mediators that are released in response to a physiologic stress, such as infection or trauma. These mediators as well as renal injury from MODS have been shown to affect Epo levels. Compared with healthy pediatric subjects, Epo levels in critically ill children are elevated, possibly secondary to increased interleukin (IL)-6 levels, which has been shown to stimulate hypoxia-induced erythropoiesis in in vitro models.[7] However, when comparing chronically anemic pediatric patients with acutely critically ill hypoxemic as well as acutely critically ill anemic patients, the levels of Epo are not elevated to the same degree. In their work in *Critical Care Medicine*, Krafte-Jacobs and colleagues[8] demonstrated that acutely anemic critically ill children did not have the same Epo levels as chronically anemic children with the same hemoglobin levels, even though the levels were checked hours after an increase in Epo should have occurred (Epo mRNA has been shown to increase 200-fold within 4–8 hours after a hemorrhagic insult). The Epo levels were also diminished in the acutely hypoxemic critically ill children in comparison with the chronically anemic subjects. The levels of Epo in both the anemic and hypoxemic groups were similar to levels in critically ill children who were not hypoxemic or anemic. The study was not designed to explain this blunted response to anemia and hypoxemia, although other studies have demonstrated the inhibitory effects some proinflammatory mediators, such as tumor necrosis factor (TNF)-α, IL-1α, IL-1β, and transforming growth factor β, have on Epo gene transcription.[6,9] Not only do these mediators suppress the levels of Epo and its receptors, thereby decreasing the bone marrow's response to hypoxemia or anemia, they have been shown to induce apoptosis of medullar progenitors in critically ill patients.[10] In addition, responsiveness to Epo becomes blunted, as its receptors have also been shown to be downregulated during critical illness.[9]

Effect of critical illness on iron use

More than two-thirds of the iron content in the human body is incorporated into hemoglobin (Hgb). Because there is minimal dietary intake of iron compared with consumption, the majority of the body's iron stores comes from the recycling of Hgb in senescent RBCs by macrophages.[10] The iron that is subsequently contained within these macrophages, as well as hepatocytes, binds to ferroportin, an iron exporter. However, under normal conditions ferroportin is degraded by hepcidin, a small peptide mainly produced by the liver. This peptide, when stimulated, can also decrease duodenal absorption of iron. Hepcidin, therefore, acts to limit iron availability for heme biosynthesis. Hepcidin synthesis is closely regulated and increases or decreases under different circumstances, such as inflammation or hypoxia and anemia, respectively.[10] The proinflammatory cytokine IL-6, for example, has been shown to upregulate hepcidin levels and diminish iron stores.[9] In addition, other proinflammatory cytokines such as IL-1 and TNF have been linked to increased synthesis of ferritin, the major protein associated with iron storage, by macrophages and hepatocytes.[11] It is thought that this "anemia of inflammation," which can occur within less than a week of the onset of inflammation, is an evolutionary response to sequester iron away from invading microorganisms.[9,12]

Iron-deficiency anemia caused by increased blood loss or inadequate dietary intake can also occur in critically ill patients. The diagnosis of total body iron depletion, however, can be complicated by the presence of anemia of inflammation, because the usual markers of iron deficiency are themselves affected by inflammation. Novel indicators such as Erythrocyte Zinc Protoporphyrin and Transferrin Receptor levels have been proposed as potentially useful in the diagnosis of iron deficiency.[10]

Phlebotomy-induced anemia in critical illness

As mentioned earlier, in comparison with adult patients, the onset of anemia in critically ill pediatric patients occurs early in the course of illness. One possible explanation for this may be related to the amount of blood loss associated with phlebotomy. There have been studies in neonatal ICUs that demonstrate the association between transfusion and unnecessary blood loss from phlebotomy overdraw.[13] In 2008, Bateman and colleagues[3] demonstrated that phlebotomy draws accounted for 73% of daily blood loss in critically ill children and that phlebotomy-related blood loss within the first 2 days of hospitalization was independently associated with transfusion. Pediatric patients with central venous catheters tend to exhibit greater overdraw volumes.[14]

Effects of Anemia in Critically Ill Patients

Delivery of oxygen

The most important consequence related to anemia involves the reduction of delivered oxygen (Do_2). The relationship between Hgb levels and Do_2 can be seen in the following equation:

$$Do_2 = CO \times CaCo_2, \text{ where}$$

$$CaCo_2 = (Sao_2 \times Hgb \times 1.36) + (0.003 \times Pao_2)$$

(CO = cardiac output; $CaCo_2$ = oxygen-carrying capacity; Sao_2 = oxygen saturation; Pao_2 = partial pressure of oxygen in the blood).

Based on these equations, the delivery of oxygen to the tissue depends heavily on the amount of hemoglobin available and little on dissolved oxygen in the blood.

However, more important than the actual delivery of oxygen to the tissue in critically ill children may be the relationship between delivery of oxygen and the consumption of oxygen by the tissues. Under normal circumstances, Do_2 exceeds the consumption of oxygen (Vo_2) by the body's organs by a factor of 3 to 5, thus allowing for an increase in extraction percentage under conditions of elevated Vo_2, which is true in both adults and children.[15] However, there is a critical level of Do_2 below which the body cannot meet its metabolic demands. Weiskopf and colleagues[16] studied healthy adult subjects who underwent isovolemic hemodilution, and found no evidence of tissue hypoxemia until they reached an Hgb level of 4 to 5 g/dL. Lieberman and colleagues[15,17] also examined resting healthy adult subjects who underwent isovolemic hemodilution as well as β-blockade to limit cardiac output, and found the critical Do_2 level to be less than 7.3 mL O_2/kg/min.

It must be mentioned that other hemodynamic measures also become altered under conditions of anemia and decreased Do_2. Increased cardiac output and changes in microcirculatory blood flow (due to such variables as changes in blood-vessel radius or decreased blood viscosity) can improve the delivery of oxygen and other metabolites to the tissues under anemic conditions.[6]

Tolerance of Anemia in Critical Ill Patients

Although significant anemia with a subsequent decrease in oxygen delivery is well tolerated by healthy subjects, the same cannot be said of critically ill patients. In the adult population, multiple studies have demonstrated a strong association between anemia and poor patient outcomes, such as the failure to liberate from mechanical ventilation after cardiac surgery and an increased risk of death.[1,18–20] Carson and colleagues[20] performed a retrospective cohort study involving surgical patients who refused blood transfusion for religious reasons, and concluded that morbidity increased as Hgb levels dropped below 8 g/dL and that the risk of mortality and/or morbidity became very high at Hgb levels below 6 g/dL. In addition, a study by Hebert and colleagues[21] concluded that anemia increased the risk of death in critically ill adult patients with acute cardiac disease.

The association between anemia and critically ill children, however, has not been studied as extensively. The largest studies of the effects of anemia in critically ill children involve pediatric patients with malaria, who have been shown to have increased mortality with severe anemia (Hgb <5 g/dL).[22,23]

BLOOD TRANSFUSION IN CRITICALLY ILL PATIENTS
History of Transfusion

The origins of transfusion medicine can be found in the 1600s when an English physician named Richard Lower successfully transfused the blood from one dog to another. In 1667, Jean-Baptiste Denis performed the first animal to human transfusion, a practice that was soon thereafter outlawed because of the number of reactions. Subsequently, many other physicians attempted to transfuse blood as well as other fluids (such as milk) from humans to improve patient outcomes. However, it was not until the early 1900s when Karl Landsteiner discovered the first blood groups that important strides were subsequently made in the storage and transfusion of blood products such that, nowadays, allogeneic pRBC transfusions are currently mainstays of therapy for several conditions.

Along with this revolution of blood banking, however, emerged new issues concerning the safety of the blood supply. Initial concerns about the transmission of infections, particularly viral infections, led to an avoidance of transfusions by many practitioners. However, now that these risks have been substantially reduced, other concerns related to the deleterious effects of pRBC transfusion, such as the metabolic, physiologic, and immunomodulatory effects, have arisen.

Transfusion Triggers in Critically Ill Adults

Before the 1990s, critically ill patients were typically transfused with pRBCs when Hgb levels dropped below 10 g/dL. This "trigger" for transfusion has its origins in an opinion piece by Adams and Lundy,[24] who claimed that

> Anemia...is present often when the patient is debilitated and when the risk of operation and anesthesia is great...interferes with adequate transportation of oxygen to the tissue. When the concentration of hemoglobin is less than 8–10 g per 100 cc of whole blood it is wise to give a blood transfusion before operation.[24]

This trigger was supported by work done by Crowell and Smith,[25] who examined the problem of increasing viscosity in the microvasculature with increasing hematocrit. Using a mathematical model, they suggested that the optimal Do_2 could be reached using a hematocrit of 30% as a trigger. This trigger was additionally supported by work done by Shoemaker and Czer[26] in the 1970s to 1980s. Later, Rivers and colleagues[27,28] used an Hgb trigger of 10 g/dL in the landmark Early Goal Directed Therapy Study for the treatment of severe sepsis and septic shock, which was also supported by the Surviving Sepsis Campaign in their guidelines for the treatment of pediatric sepsis.

At the same time that these studies demonstrated the ill-effects of anemia and proposed a transfusion trigger of 10 g/dL of Hgb, other studies were also done that showed potential problems related to transfused pRBCs, including the immunomodulatory effects.[29,30] Because of this increasing evidence of the deleterious effects of transfused pRBCs, a landmark study was undertaken by Hebert and the Canadian Critical Trials Group, comparing two different transfusion triggers to compare the risks of transfusion with the risks of anemia.[21] In this work, called the TRICC (Transfusion Requirements In Critical Care) study, the investigators enrolled 838 critically ill subjects and randomly assigned them to one of two groups: a liberal-strategy group who received pRBC transfusions at Hgb levels less than 10 g/dL, and a restrictive-strategy group who only received transfused pRBCs at Hgb levels less than 7 g/dL. Both groups were matched for demographics and severity of illness using Acute Physiology and Chronic Health Evaluation (APACHE II) scores. The investigators discovered that there were cumulatively no differences in outcomes for the two groups, including in patients with cardiac disease. However, there were statistically significant differences in outcomes concerning subjects with decreased severity of illness (APACHE scores <20) and subjects who were younger than 55 years. In both these populations, mortality was less in the restrictive-strategy groups than in the liberal-strategy groups.

Transfusion Triggers in Critically Ill Children

The TRICC study started the process of examining optimal Hgb levels in critically ill adults, but more needed to be done for critically ill children. In 2007, Lacroix and colleagues[31] took the first step in their study of transfusion triggers in critically ill children. In this work the investigators hypothesized that, just as in the TRICC study, critically ill children could tolerate a lower transfusion trigger than had been historically used, without any evidence of new or worsening MODS. A cohort of 637 stable, critically ill children were recruited from 19 tertiary-care PICUs in 4 countries, and were again divided into two groups: a liberal-strategy group whose Hgb level would be maintained to a threshold of 9.5 g/dL and a restrictive-strategy group whose Hgb level would be maintained to a threshold of 7 g/dL. Both groups of subjects again had similar demographics and degrees of illness. The restrictive group had a 96% reduction in the number of patients with a transfusion exposure without any increases in new or progressive MODS. There were no differences in any of the secondary outcomes, including mortality.

Some other studies have examined the effects transfused blood may have on clinically significant outcomes in critically ill children using even lower transfusion triggers. In 2 studies conducted in Africa consisting of hospitalized children with malaria, the investigators determined that pRBC transfusion could improve outcomes in such children with severe anemia (Hgb levels <5 g/dL) or respiratory symptoms such as dyspnea.[22,23] Taken together, it is clear from these studies that the benefits of transfusing critically ill children do not outweigh the risks at Hgb levels higher than 7 g/dL and perhaps even less.

Anemia and Transfusion in Critically Ill Premature Infants

In healthy term infants, improved oxygenation after birth leads to diminished Epo production, which then leads to diminished erythrocyte production. Over the course of the next several weeks, the infants will go from a relative polycythemic state to their physiologic nadir. Subsequently, the Hgb levels increase in response to increasing Epo levels until they reach "normal" levels by the fourth to sixth month of life.[32]

Premature infants suffer more readily than term infants from anemia. For example, 90% of infants with a birth weight of less than 1000 g are transfused.[33] This "anemia of prematurity" occurs because of both physiologic and iatrogenic factors. Premature infants require significant amounts of blood draws during the first few critical weeks of life. Shannon[34] reported in the early 1990s that a week's worth of blood samples could exceed 40 mL, which comprises more than half of a small infant's total blood volume. Neonatologists are more sensitive to this problem today, so these numbers may not currently be as high, although it is clear that iatrogenic blood loss remains a significant source of anemia of prematurity.[35] In addition to this blood loss, premature infants also have diminished Epo levels (because more hypoxia and anemia are needed to stimulate Epo production by the liver, as mentioned earlier), a reduced erythrocyte life span of only 35 to 50 days, and a relatively hyporegenerative bone marrow.[35,36]

Despite this high frequency of critically ill premature infants with anemia, the decision to transfuse such patients remains complex. Some have advocated the use of markers of poor oxygen delivery such as lactate or infrared spectroscopy to measure the extraction of fractional oxygen. These methods, however, have not proved to be conclusively helpful in making the decision to transfuse.[37] One of the reasons for this may lie in the decreased amount of fetal Hgb relative to that of adult Hgb present in transfused blood, which can alter Do_2.[38]

Along the same lines as the adult and pediatric studies, Bell and colleagues[39] attempted to discern a transfusion trigger in 100 preterm infants with birth weights between 500 and 1300 g in a randomized prospective trial. The investigators divided the infants into a liberal-transfusion group and a restrictive-transfusion group, using transfusion triggers based on hematocrits as well as the amount of respiratory support the subjects were receiving; that is, patients requiring mechanical ventilation had higher baseline hematocrits than those simply requiring supplemental oxygen only. No difference was found between the groups in survival, length of ventilation, retinopathy, development of bronchopulmonary dysplasia, or length of stay in hospital. However, the restrictive-transfusion group had a higher incidence of adverse neurologic events, specifically the development of grade 4 intraventricular hemorrhage or periventricular leukomalacia This finding has been called into question, because it had not been previously reported and there were significant questions about the methodology.[40] Of interest is that McCoy and colleagues[41] examined neurocognitive outcomes for 56 of the 100 subjects used in the Bell study[39] when the subjects were school age, and found that those children who had been in the liberal-transfusion group performed more poorly than the other group in various tests of intelligence, including verbal fluency and reading.

In 2006, Kirpalani and colleagues[42] looked for transfusion thresholds in extremely low-birth-weight babies (<1000 g). Again, the cohort of 451 infants was divided into two groups, low and high threshold, in regard of Hgb levels, amount of respiratory support, and age. Although these investigators found no benefit in maintaining higher hemoglobin levels in the initial study, a follow-up study was done on 430 of these subjects when they were 18 to 21 months corrected age, looking at their neurodevelopmental outcomes. In this report, the subjects with a low transfusion threshold showed a decreased Mental Development Index Score compared with the group with a high transfusion threshold.[43] More controlled studies are necessary to delineate the transfusion trigger for premature infants.

Anemia and Transfusion in Children with Congenital Heart Disease

Critically ill children with cyanotic heart disease are typically transfused to keep Hgb levels above 15 g/dL or hematocrit levels above 40%; this is done to ensure adequate Do_2 in patients who may only be able to maintain oxygen saturations as high as 70% to 75%. Transfusion may even benefit some children with noncyanotic congenital heart disease (CHD), as higher Hgb levels can increase blood viscosity, thereby maintaining a favorable shunt balance.[44,45] However, the true risk-to-benefit ratio of this practice is not known. In fact, Cholette and colleagues[46] demonstrated that children with single-ventricle physiology who have undergone cavopulmonary connection have no increased risks with a transfusion trigger of 9 g/dL in comparison with 13 g/dL. In addition, Szekely and colleagues[47] conducted a study on 657 children with CHD who underwent cardiac surgery, and found that blood transfusion was independently associated with infection, though not mortality. Patients undergoing repair of their CHD may have significant exposure to blood products during cardiopulmonary bypass, but further study is needed to elicit the ideal transfusion requirements in the perioperative period.

COMPLICATIONS OF BLOOD TRANSFUSION

Based on the aforementioned studies it is clear that, although anemia is potentially harmful to some critically ill patients, transfusion of pRBCs may not ameliorate the problem and may, in some cases, worsen outcomes. The reasons for this are certainly multifactorial, so a discussion about the complications of transfusion, while not providing definitive evidence, may lend some insight into the potential reasons for this discrepancy. There are several complications associated with transfusion. For the purposes of this review, the causes that can be seen in critically ill patients have been divided into infectious, immunologic, and physiologic.

Infectious Complications

Over the course of the past few decades, the amount of viral testing done on the blood supply has grown significantly. At present in the United States, a voluntary donor pool undergoes extensive interviewing before donating blood, which will then be tested for hepatitis B and C, human T-lymphotropic virus 1 and 2, human immunodeficiency virus (HIV) 1 and 2, West Nile virus, Chagas disease, and syphilis. This testing has greatly reduced the incidence of transmitted infectious diseases. The current rates of transmitted HIV, hepatitis B, and hepatitis C by blood product transfusion are 1 in 2,135,000, 1 in 205,000, and 1 in 1,935,000 transfusions, respectively.[48] Cytomegalovirus (CMV) positivity in transfused blood is very common (seen in 40% of donors) and can be devastating in immunocompromised hosts, although leukocyte reduction and γ-irradiation of the blood can obviate the risks of transmission.

In fact, the incidence of transfusion-related viral infections, now calculated using mathematical models, has been superseded by contamination by bacteria, particularly gram-negative bacteria such as *Yersinia enterocolitica* that replicate at cold temperatures. Septic transfusion reactions are now the leading cause of infectious transfusion–mediated morbidity and mortality, accounting for 12% of the transfusion-related mortalities reported to the Federal Food and Drug Administration (FDA) between 2005 and 2009.[49]

Immunologic Complications

Transfusion-related acute lung injury
Transfusion-related acute lung injury (TRALI) is one of the most frequent causes of transfusion-related mortality or severe morbidity, with a reported incidence of 1 per 5000 transfusions.[50,51] Although there are several definitions of this condition, they all remain consistent with the one developed by the National Heart, Lung, and Blood Institute (NHLBI) Working Group on TRALI in 2005.[51] According to this group, TRALI is defined as the development of acute lung injury in patients without any risk factors within 6 hours after the end of a transfusion of 1 or more plasma-containing blood products (although symptoms usually appear within 2 hours). The NHLBI Working Group definition of acute lung injury was as follows: (1) acute onset; (2) hypoxemia: Pao_2/Fio_2 less than 300 mm Hg regardless of positive end-expiration pressure level or oxygen saturation of 90% on room air; (3) bilateral infiltrates on frontal chest

radiograph; (4) pulmonary artery occlusion pressure less than 18 mm Hg when measured or lack of clinical evidence of left atrial hypertension. The trouble with this definition lies in the patients who may have a predisposing reason to develop acute lung injury, but whose new onset of hypoxia may be temporally related to a transfusion but not causally related. Because there are no laboratory tests available to confirm the diagnosis of TRALI in these patients, the Canadian Consensus Conference included a designation of "possible TRALI" in their definition, which emphasized the temporal relationship of the development of acute lung injury and transfusion.[52]

There are two proposed mechanisms by which TRALI develops. The first theory involves the presence of anti–human leukocyte antigen (HLA) I, anti–HLA II, and/or antineutrophil antibodies present in the transfused plasma that bind to their antigens and activate complement, which stimulates neutrophils that subsequently sequester in the lung to cause endothelial damage. This theory is supported by the observation that transfusion of fresh frozen plasma, which contains donor-derived antibodies, carries a higher risk of TRALI development. The second theory involves a 2-hit phenomenon whereby partially activated neutrophils, drawn to the lung because of an already activated pulmonary endothelium, become fully activated by either biological response modifiers contained within the stored blood and/or specific antibodies directed against antigens on the neutrophil surface. These immune mediators fully activate the neutrophils, causing endothelial damage, capillary leak, and acute lung injury.[53] Because both theories involve primed antibodies, the use of male-only plasma or plasma from nulliparous women has become more widespread, as there has been some epidemiologic evidence that parous women are higher-risk donors because of pregnancy-induced alloimmunization.[49] At present, there are only observational studies linking this shift in potential donors to a decrease in TRALI.

Patients with TRALI will typically present acutely with severe dyspnea (often requiring positive pressure ventilation), fever, and often hypotension. The findings on chest radiography can vary from infiltrates in dependent lung segments to complete white-out of the lungs, even with a paucity of adventitial sounds on lung examination.[50] The treatment is mainly supportive, as therapies such as diuretics and steroids have not been shown to be helpful. The natural course of this disease, although potentially fatal with a mortality rate of 6% to 10%, is short lived, typically lasting less than 24 hours.[50]

Transfusion-associated circulatory overload

Transfusion-associated circulatory overload (TACO), although not an immunologic phenomenon, is mentioned here because it can also present as pulmonary edema and, therefore, may be difficult to discern from TRALI. Its incidence has been quoted as from 1% to 10%, but is difficult to truly know because of the lack of an accepted definition. However, unlike TRALI, the etiology of TACO is thought to be related to an increase in hydrostatic pressure in the pulmonary vasculature, and patients with cardiopulmonary compromise and/or renal failure are at higher risk, as are infants.[54] Just as for TRALI there is no definitive test to diagnose TACO, although echocardiography, B-type natriuretic peptide level, and alveolar fluid protein content can be helpful. Because it can be somewhat prevented by using slow infusion rates in at-risk patients and does respond to diuretic therapy, there is a benefit in a diagnosis of TACO rather than TRALI.[49]

Transfusion-related immunomodulation

There are 2 plausible explanations for the seeming lack of benefit from transfusion in critically ill patients. The first relates to the consequences of prolonged RBC storage (ie, the "storage lesion") that can affect the metabolic state of the patient as well as the delivery of oxygen (see later discussion).

The other explanation relates to the effect of transfused blood on the native immune system. The notion that transfused blood can affect a patient's immunity first arose following the observation that cadaveric renal transplant patients who had received blood transfusions had a decreased incidence of rejection.[55] In addition, there have been other observations of immunosuppression related to transfusion in patients with malignancies and Crohn disease.[56,57] This immunomodulation has also been demonstrated in the increase in nosocomial infections in critically ill patients, although this last point has been argued in other works.[58,59]

The etiology of transfusion-related immunomodulation (TRIM) is poorly understood, although there is a suggestion that the immunosuppressive effect arises from contaminating leukocytes present in the transfused blood. These leukocytes become immunologically active and may directly downregulate the recipient's immune function.[60,61] Other possible mechanisms involve the release of biological response modifiers from leukocytes into the supernatant fluid of transfused pRBCs during storage,[62] or even the presence of soluble HLA peptides that are present in allogeneic plasma and result in immunosuppression.[59,62–64]

Immunomodulation has been described as a cause for the increased development of MODS and mortality in critically ill patients, including pediatric patients.[65] However, conflicting studies demonstrating an increase in nosocomial infections related to transfusion make the role of immunomodulation after transfusion difficult to discern.[1,4,59,66–68]

Transfusion-associated graft-versus-host disease and microchimerism

Still other immunologic phenomena that can occur involve the presence and activity of contaminating leukocytes that are transfused along with the pRBCs. Transfusion-associated graft-versus-host disease (GVHD) is a rare complication of transfusion that is characterized by viable donor leukocytes attacking recipient cells, primarily in severely immunocompromised hosts. This condition carries a significant mortality rate (84%) but can be prevented by irradiating pRBCs that are to be infused into at-risk patients.[49]

Along the same lines, the unwitting transfusion of leukocytes with pRBCs, even in leukocyte-reduced units, can result in transfusion-associated microchimerism (TA-MC). TA-MC occurs when a small percentage of donated lymphocytes persist in a recipient. These cells can proliferate and persist in the recipient for years after the transfusion. The clinical implication of this finding is unclear.[69]

Storage Lesions

The US FDA mandates that all RBC units have a maximum storage period of 42 days. However, during storage RBCs undergo several alterations including biochemical, biomechanical, and oxidative changes that progress over time. These alterations are collectively labeled the storage lesion. At 42 days, the assumption is that 75% of the transfused pRBCs will still maintain cellular integrity 24 hours after the transfusion, the rest being lost because of the storage lesion.[9]

Some of the changes that occur include increased lactate and potassium, and decreased cellular adenosine triphosphate, 2,3-diphosphoglycerate (2,3-DPG), calcium, and S-nitrosohemoglobin. The altered level of 2,3-DPG makes oxygen less available to the tissues, and the depletion of S-nitrosohemoglobin can result in depleted nitric oxide activity, causing vasoconstriction and compromising blood flow.[70] Some of the biomechanical changes seen in stored RBCs include decreased deformability and increased cell density and viscosity, which can also decrease Do_2. Oxidative changes include Hgb oxidation and denaturation as well as diminished oxidant defenses. The increase in phosphatidylserine exposure and the release of bioactive substances can also lead to immunomodulation.[54,71] These changes associated with the storage lesion are well documented and can lead to poor Do_2 and increased inflammation, thereby producing untoward clinical effects. Although there are some contradictory studies, the age of the blood has been correlated with morbidity and mortality in several studies, with "older" units (typically defined as storage for >14 days) leading to diminished Do_2 and worse outcomes than "fresher" (storage <14 days) units.[72,73] A recent randomized controlled study by Gauvin and colleagues[74] involving 455 stable but critically ill children demonstrated that the transfusion of RBC units older than 2 weeks was associated with a greater risk of developing new or progressive MODS. However, because the notion of deleterious clinical effects from the transfusion of older erythrocytes is still in dispute, a prospective, multicenter, randomized trial was designed examining the effects of storage age on 90-day all-cause mortality in adult patients requiring positive pressure in the ICU, and is currently expected to be completed in 2013.[49]

THERAPEUTIC INTERVENTIONS

Numerous interventions can be used to minimize both the risks of anemia and the risks associated with transfusions, some of which are outlined here.

Iron and Erythropoietin Supplementation

As mentioned earlier, iron homeostasis in critically ill patients shifts from a mobilizing form to a storage form. In addition, Epo levels in critically ill children, although elevated, do not reach appropriate levels based on the degree of anemia or hypoxemia. Multiple studies have been done to determine the efficacy of iron and Epo supplementation on outcomes in critically ill patients.

Iron supplementation can be administered via enteral or intravenous routes. The enteral route seems to be ineffective, as absorption may be downregulated in patients with increased iron stores.[75] Enteral iron also requires an acidic environment to be absorbed, which may be hindered by medications commonly given to critically ill patients to suppress secretion of gastric acid. Pieracci and Barie[12] demonstrated that enteral iron supplementation did not raise hematologic or iron markers in critically ill patients, although there was no increased risk of infection. Parenteral iron has also not been shown to improve erythropoiesis in critically ill patients. Van Iperen and colleagues[76] demonstrated that without adjunctive Epo, intravenous iron supplementation did not affect reticulocyte counts or serum transferrin levels.

The research detailing the use of erythropoietin in critically ill anemic patients has been conflicting. Multiple small studies have demonstrated an increase in reticulocyte counts with Epo supplementation, although with no increase in final hemoglobin levels or decrease in transfusion requirements.[76,77] However, 2 larger studies demonstrated that supplemental Epo could lead to reduced transfusion requirements in critically ill patients, although no other benefit was noted.[78,79] Finally, Corwin and colleagues[80] performed a third trial including 1460 critically ill patients, the largest to date, and demonstrated no difference between rates of transfusion or amount of pRBCs transfused in those receiving Epo supplements compared with those who did not, although at 29 days the Hgb levels increased more in the former than in the latter. Of note, those patients who received Epo also had an increased risk of thrombosis.

The use of Epo and iron in anemic premature infants has been more readily accepted, with the majority of studies demonstrating an increase in reticulocyte count and decreased transfusion requirement after Epo administration.[36] A recent Cochrane review demonstrated a decrease in the number of transfusions and amount of pRBCs transfused related to Epo administration early in the course of their hospital stays, although the investigators claimed that these numbers were of little clinical significance.[81] An association between Epo administration and the occurrence of retinopathy of prematurity was also reported, although some other studies have not found the same association.

Acute Normovolemic Hemodilution

Although not a procedure necessarily appropriate for medical patients, pediatric patients undergoing elective surgery may be candidates for acute normovolemic hemodilution (ANH). In this process, the patient's whole blood is removed while the circulating blood volume is maintained with (preferably) colloid solutions. Using this technique of blood preservation, the delivery of oxygen becomes less dependent on Hgb and more dependent on an increased cardiac output and increased oxygen extraction by the tissues when possible.[6] Cardiac output is increased because of increased preload, increased left ventricular ejection fraction, and decreased systemic vascular resistance.[82] If blood is necessary because of diminished Do_2, the patient's own blood can then be returned, without the risks associated with storage. The safe use of ANH in pediatric patients has been reported in orthopedic surgeries and liver transplantation, although there may only be a modest clinical benefit.[83–85]

Leukoreduction

Leukoreduction is the process whereby leukocytes in a blood product are decreased by filtration before storage or by a filter before infusion. There are specific, well-accepted reasons to decrease this leukocyte exposure in recipients, including the reduction of exposure to CMV, a decrease in the rates of febrile nonhemolytic transfusion reactions, and HLA alloimmunization.[86] However, other proposed benefits, such as the reduction in TRIM and a subsequent decrease in infection, have not been conclusively proved and are hotly debated.[49] Despite this lack of convincing evidence, several countries such as Canada and England and, although not mandated by the US FDA, major blood suppliers in the United States, including the American Red Cross, have elected to release only leukoreduced blood. Although potentially not beneficial, the complications from leukoreduction are few, and include increased costs, a reduction in the quantity of pRBC mass contained in each unit, and significant hypotension in transfused patients receiving angiotensin-converting enzyme inhibitors who had bedside filtration of their blood products.[86]

Blood Substitutes

Several synthetic alternatives to erythrocytes have been developed and tested. These blood substitutes can be divided into two categories: hemoglobin-based oxygen carriers (HBOCs) and perfluorocarbons (PFCs).

HBOCs are polymerized hemoglobin solutions that can deliver oxygen to the tissues while having the advantages of being universally compatible, requiring no refrigeration, being free of infectious risks, and having a very long shelf life of 1 to 2 years. To date, however, only one HBOC, Hemopure, remains a potential therapy, as others, notably Polyheme, have not been proved to be more effective than current standards[87] (though in the case of Polyheme, this may be reflective of the study protocol).[88] Because of the advantages noted there is still a push, primarily by the military, to continue research on this product.[87]

PFCs do not bind oxygen but instead are liquid fluorocarbons that deliver increased dissolved oxygen to the tissue at lower partial pressures in comparison with normal mechanisms. PFCs have the advantages of fast unloading of oxygen, improved delivery of oxygen through small capillaries owing to flow characteristics, and a long shelf life. Despite PFC having recently been shown to be able to sustain organ function during extreme anemia in an animal model, the only available formulation is in Russia.[89,90]

SUMMARY

Anemia is a common phenomenon in critically ill children. The causes of the anemia are multifactorial, but can be placed into the categories of decreased erythrocyte production because of certain effects of Epo and iron use, and increased blood loss. Although anemia has been linked to worse outcomes in these patients, the maximum amount of anemia that is tolerable and, subsequently, the lowest Do_2, has not been identified. The transfusion of pRBCs is considered an important supportive measure for anemic critically ill children, although there is variety of infectious, immunologic, metabolic, and physiologic complications associated with this process. To reduce the rates of complications associated with transfusion, steps can be taken to decrease the need for transfusion (such as the lowering of transfusion triggers) as well as to decrease the risks associated with transfusion itself (such as the use of leukoreduction). Blood substitutes, though potentially advantageous in some circumstances, have not yet been shown to be helpful, and more research is needed in this sphere.

REFERENCES

1. Corwin HL. The CRIT study: anemia and blood transfusion in the critically ill—current clinical practice in the United States. Crit Care Med 2004;32(1):39–52.
2. Thomas J. Anemia and blood transfusion practices in the critically ill: a prospective cohort review. Heart Lung 2010;39(3):217–25.
3. Bateman ST. Anemia, blood loss, and blood transfusions in North American children in the intensive care unit. Am J Respir Crit Care Med 2008;178(1):26–33.
4. Vincent JL. Anemia and blood transfusion in critically ill patients. JAMA 2002; 288(12):1499–507.
5. Salsbury DC. Anemia of prematurity. Neonatal Netw 2001;20(5):13–20.
6. Shander A. Anemia in the critically ill. Crit Care Clin 2004;20(2):159–78.
7. Krafte-Jacobs B, Bock GH. Circulating erythropoietin and interleukin-6 concentrations increase in critically ill children with sepsis and septic shock. Crit Care Med 1996;24(9):1455–9.
8. Krafte-Jacobs B. Erythropoietin response to critical illness. Crit Care Med 1994; 22(5):821–6.
9. Hayden SJ. Anemia in critical illness: insights into etiology, consequences, and management. Am J Respir Crit Care Med 2012;185(10):1049–57.
10. Lasocki S. Hepcidin and anemia of the critically ill patient: bench to bedside. Anesthesiology 2011;114(3):688–94.
11. Weiss G, Goodnough LT. Anemia of chronic disease. N Engl J Med 2005;352(10): 1011–23.
12. Pieracci FM, Barie PS. Diagnosis and management of iron-related anemias in critical illness. Crit Care Med 2006;34(7):1898–905.

13. Lin JC. Phlebotomy overdraw in the neonatal intensive care nursery. Pediatrics 2000;106(2):E19.
14. Valentine SL, Bateman ST. Identifying factors to minimize phlebotomy-induced blood loss in the pediatric intensive care unit. Pediatr Crit Care Med 2012; 13(1):22–7.
15. Istaphanous GK. Red blood cell transfusion in critically ill children: a narrative review. Pediatr Crit Care Med 2011;12(2):174–83.
16. Weiskopf RB. Human cardiovascular and metabolic response to acute, severe isovolemic anemia. JAMA 1998;279(3):217–21.
17. Lieberman JA. Critical oxygen delivery in conscious humans is less than 7.3 ml O_2 x kg(-1) x min(-1). Anesthesiology 2000;92(2):407–13.
18. Rady MY, Ryan T. Perioperative predictors of extubation failure and the effect on clinical outcome after cardiac surgery. Crit Care Med 1999;27(2):340–7.
19. Rasmussen L. Anemia and 90-day mortality in COPD patients requiring invasive mechanical ventilation. Clin Epidemiol 2011;3:1–5.
20. Carson JL. Mortality and morbidity in patients with very low postoperative Hb levels who decline blood transfusion. Transfusion 2002;42(7):812–8.
21. Hebert PC. A multicenter, randomized, controlled clinical trial of transfusion requirements in critical care. Transfusion requirements in critical care investigators, Canadian Critical Care Trials Group. N Engl J Med 1999;340(6):409–17.
22. English M. Blood transfusion for severe anaemia in children in a Kenyan hospital. Lancet 2002;359(9305):494–5.
23. Lackritz EM. Effect of blood transfusion on survival among children in a Kenyan hospital. Lancet 1992;340(8818):524–8.
24. Adams RC, Lundy JS. Anesthesia in cases of poor surgical risk: some suggestions for decreasing the risk. Surg Gynecol Obstet 1942;74:1011–5.
25. Crowell JW, Smith EE. Determinant of the optimal hematocrit. J Appl Physiol 1967; 22(3):501–4.
26. Czer LS, Shoemaker WC. Optimal hematocrit value in critically ill postoperative patients. Surg Gynecol Obstet 1978;147(3):363–8.
27. Rivers E. Early goal-directed therapy in the treatment of severe sepsis and septic shock. N Engl J Med 2001;345(19):1368–77.
28. Parker MM, Hazelzet JA, Carcillo JA. Pediatric considerations. Crit Care Med 2004;32(Suppl 11):S591–4.
29. van de Watering LM. Beneficial effects of leukocyte depletion of transfused blood on postoperative complications in patients undergoing cardiac surgery: a randomized clinical trial. Circulation 1998;97(6):562–8.
30. Bordin JO, Heddle NM, Blajchman MA. Biologic effects of leukocytes present in transfused cellular blood products. Blood 1994;84(6):1703–21.
31. Lacroix J. Transfusion strategies for patients in pediatric intensive care units. N Engl J Med 2007;356(16):1609–19.
32. Ohls RK. Erythropoietin to prevent and treat the anemia of prematurity. Curr Opin Pediatr 1999;11(2):108–14.
33. Maier RF. Changing practices of red blood cell transfusions in infants with birth weights less than 1000 g. J Pediatr 2000;136(2):220–4.
34. Shannon KM. Anemia of prematurity: progress and prospects. Am J Pediatr Hematol Oncol 1990;12(1):14–20.
35. Crowley M, Kirpalani H. A rational approach to red blood cell transfusion in the neonatal ICU. Curr Opin Pediatr 2010;22(2):151–7.
36. Attias D. Pathophysiology and treatment of the anemia of prematurity. J Pediatr Hematol Oncol 1995;17(1):13–8.

37. Murray NA, Roberts IA. Neonatal transfusion practice. Arch Dis Child Fetal Neonatal Ed 2004;89(2):F101–7.

38. Desmet L, Lacroix J. Transfusion in pediatrics. Crit Care Clin 2004;20(2):299–311.

39. Bell EF. Randomized trial of liberal versus restrictive guidelines for red blood cell transfusion in preterm infants. Pediatrics 2005;115(6):1685–91.

40. Boedy RF, Mathew OP. Randomized trial of liberal versus restrictive guidelines for red blood cell transfusion in preterm infants. Pediatrics 2005;116(4):1048–9 [author reply: 1049–50].

41. McCoy TE. Neurocognitive profiles of preterm infants randomly assigned to lower or higher hematocrit thresholds for transfusion. Child Neuropsychol 2011;17(4): 347–67.

42. Kirpalani H. The Premature Infants in Need of Transfusion (PINT) study: a randomized, controlled trial of a restrictive (low) versus liberal (high) transfusion threshold for extremely low birth weight infants. J Pediatr 2006;149(3):301–7.

43. Whyte RK. Neurodevelopmental outcome of extremely low birth weight infants randomly assigned to restrictive or liberal hemoglobin thresholds for blood transfusion. Pediatrics 2009;123(1):207–13.

44. Istaphanous GK. Comparison of the neuroapoptotic properties of equipotent anesthetic concentrations of desflurane, isoflurane, or sevoflurane in neonatal mice. Anesthesiology 2011;114(3):578–87.

45. Lister G. Physiologic effects of increasing hemoglobin concentration in left-to-right shunting in infants with ventricular septal defects. N Engl J Med 1982; 306(9):502–6.

46. Cholette JM. Children with single-ventricle physiology do not benefit from higher hemoglobin levels post cavopulmonary connection: results of a prospective, randomized, controlled trial of a restrictive versus liberal red-cell transfusion strategy. Pediatr Crit Care Med 2011;12(1):39–45.

47. Szekely A. Risks and predictors of blood transfusion in pediatric patients undergoing open heart operations. Ann Thorac Surg 2009;87(1):187–97.

48. Dodd RY, Notari EP, Stramer SL. Current prevalence and incidence of infectious disease markers and estimated window-period risk in the American Red Cross blood donor population. Transfusion 2002;42(8):975–9.

49. Gilliss BM, Looney MR, Gropper MA. Reducing noninfectious risks of blood transfusion. Anesthesiology 2011;115(3):635–49.

50. Moore SB. Transfusion-related acute lung injury (TRALI): clinical presentation, treatment, and prognosis. Crit Care Med 2006;34(Suppl 5):S114–7.

51. Toy P. Transfusion-related acute lung injury: definition and review. Crit Care Med 2005;33(4):721–6.

52. Kleinman S. Toward an understanding of transfusion-related acute lung injury: statement of a consensus panel. Transfusion 2004;44(12):1774–89.

53. Silliman CC. The two-event model of transfusion-related acute lung injury. Crit Care Med 2006;34(Suppl 5):S124–31.

54. Hendrickson JE, Hillyer CD. Noninfectious serious hazards of transfusion. Anesth Analg 2009;108(3):759–69.

55. Opelz G. Effect of blood transfusions on subsequent kidney transplants. Transplant Proc 1973;5(1):253–9.

56. Heiss MM. Blood transfusion-modulated tumor recurrence: first results of a randomized study of autologous versus allogeneic blood transfusion in colorectal cancer surgery. J Clin Oncol 1994;12(9):1859–67.

57. Peters WR. Multiple blood transfusions reduce the recurrence rate of Crohn's disease. Dis Colon Rectum 1989;32(9):749–53.

58. Taylor RW. Impact of allogenic packed red blood cell transfusion on nosocomial infection rates in the critically ill patient. Crit Care Med 2002;30(10):2249–54.
59. Vamvakas EC. Pneumonia as a complication of blood product transfusion in the critically ill: transfusion-related immunomodulation (TRIM). Crit Care Med 2006; 34(Suppl 5):S151–9.
60. Gafter U, Kalechman Y, Sredni B. Induction of a subpopulation of suppressor cells by a single blood transfusion. Kidney Int 1992;41(1):143–8.
61. Kirkley SA. Blood transfusion and total joint replacement surgery: T helper 2 (TH2) cytokine secretion and clinical outcome. Transfus Med 1998;8(3):195–204.
62. Nielsen HJ. Time-dependent, spontaneous release of white cell- and platelet-derived bioactive substances from stored human blood. Transfusion 1996; 36(11–12):960–5.
63. Magee CC, Sayegh MH. Peptide-mediated immunosuppression. Curr Opin Immunol 1997;9(5):669–75.
64. Puppo F. Soluble human MHC class I molecules induce soluble Fas ligand secretion and trigger apoptosis in activated CD8(+) Fas (CD95)(+) T lymphocytes. Int Immunol 2000;12(2):195–203.
65. Kneyber MC. Red blood cell transfusion in critically ill children is independently associated with increased mortality. Intensive Care Med 2007;33(8):1414–22.
66. Bilgin YM. Effects of allogeneic leukocytes in blood transfusions during cardiac surgery on inflammatory mediators and postoperative complications. Crit Care Med 2010;38(2):546–52.
67. Vamvakas EC, Blajchman MA. Universal WBC reduction: the case for and against. Transfusion 2001;41(5):691–712.
68. Hebert PC, Tinmouth A, Corwin HL. Controversies in RBC transfusion in the critically ill. Chest 2007;131(5):1583–90.
69. Lee TH. High-level long-term white blood cell microchimerism after transfusion of leukoreduced blood components to patients resuscitated after severe traumatic injury. Transfusion 2005;45(8):1280–90.
70. Reynolds JD. S-nitrosohemoglobin deficiency: a mechanism for loss of physiological activity in banked blood. Proc Natl Acad Sci U S A 2007;104(43): 17058–62.
71. Hovav T. Alteration of red cell aggregability and shape during blood storage. Transfusion 1999;39(3):277–81.
72. Kiraly LN. Transfusion of aged packed red blood cells results in decreased tissue oxygenation in critically injured trauma patients. J Trauma 2009;67(1):29–32.
73. Purdy FR, Tweeddale MG, Merrick PM. Association of mortality with age of blood transfused in septic ICU patients. Can J Anaesth 1997;44(12):1256–61.
74. Gauvin F. Association between length of storage of transfused red blood cells and multiple organ dysfunction syndrome in pediatric intensive care patients. Transfusion 2010;50(9):1902–13.
75. Andrews NC. Disorders of iron metabolism. N Engl J Med 1999;341(26):1986–95.
76. van Iperen CE. Response of erythropoiesis and iron metabolism to recombinant human erythropoietin in intensive care unit patients. Crit Care Med 2000;28(8): 2773–8.
77. Gabriel A. High-dose recombinant human erythropoietin stimulates reticulocyte production in patients with multiple organ dysfunction syndrome. J Trauma 1998;44(2):361–7.
78. Corwin HL. Efficacy of recombinant human erythropoietin in the critically ill patient: a randomized, double-blind, placebo-controlled trial. Crit Care Med 1999;27(11):2346–50.

79. Corwin HL. Efficacy of recombinant human erythropoietin in critically ill patients: a randomized controlled trial. JAMA 2002;288(22):2827–35.

80. Corwin HL. Efficacy and safety of epoetin alfa in critically ill patients. N Engl J Med 2007;357(10):965–76.

81. Ohlsson A, Aher SM. Early erythropoietin for preventing red blood cell transfusion in preterm and/or low birth weight infants. Cochrane Database Syst Rev 2012;(9):CD004863.

82. Bak Z. Transesophageal echocardiographic hemodynamic monitoring during preoperative acute normovolemic hemodilution. Anesthesiology 2000;92(5): 1250–6.

83. Copley LA. Hemodilution as a method to reduce transfusion requirements in adolescent spine fusion surgery. Spine (Phila Pa 1976) 1999;24(3):219–22 [discussion: 223–4].

84. Jawan B. Perioperative normovolemic anemia is safe in pediatric living-donor liver transplantation. Transplantation 2004;77(9):1394–8.

85. Segal JB. Preoperative acute normovolemic hemodilution: a meta-analysis. Transfusion 2004;44(5):632–44.

86. Dzik WH. Leukoreduction of blood components. Curr Opin Hematol 2002;9(6): 521–6.

87. Santry HP, Alam HB. Fluid resuscitation: past, present, and the future. Shock 2010;33(3):229–41.

88. Bernard AC. Postinjury resuscitation with human polymerized hemoglobin prolongs early survival: a post hoc analysis. J Trauma 2011;70(Suppl 5):S34–7.

89. Cabrales P, Carlos Briceno J. Delaying blood transfusion in experimental acute anemia with a perfluorocarbon emulsion. Anesthesiology 2011;114(4):901–11.

90. Jahr JS, Walker V, Manoochehri K. Blood substitutes as pharmacotherapies in clinical practice. Curr Opin Anaesthesiol 2007;20(4):325–30.

Coagulopathies in the PICU
DIC and Liver Disease

Robert I. Parker, MD

KEYWORDS

- Coagulopathy • Disseminated intravascular coagulation
- Pediatric intensive care unit • Liver disease

KEY POINTS

- Bleeding in pediatric-intensive-care-unit patients is associated with an increased risk of mortality. Fortunately, however, most patients with an abnormal coagulation profile do not bleed because this is generally secondary to liver disease or dietary-induced vitamin K deficiency.
- When the laboratory markers of coagulopathy are the result of disseminated intravascular coagulation (DIC), bleeding is common and the risk of mortality extreme.
- Although interventions directed toward correcting the abnormal coagulation test results are generally initiated, they are also generally either not warranted (in the case of liver disease) or not fully successful (in the case of DIC).
- Newer more biologically based therapies to reestablish normal hemostasis in patients with a consumptive coagulopathy have not been shown to be effective.
- Consequently, the treatment of choice for DIC (and related conditions) remains treating the underlying process that initiated the coagulopathic state along with supporting the hemostatic components by transfusion as best we can.

Bleeding is a common occurrence in intensive-care-unit (ICU) patients. Although it may be the primary reason for ICU admission, it more often occurs as a component of a systemic process. Even in patients who are not actively bleeding, concern for an increased risk of bleeding often affects how the intensivist cares for his or her patients. In surgical patients, one must always consider that although there may have been adequate surgical hemostasis at the completion of surgery, this situation may no longer exist and the cause for the bleeding is anatomic rather than medical (ie, caused by the surgical procedure itself). The list for causes of medical bleeding is long and includes inherited and acquired deficiencies of clotting factors, abnormalities of platelet number and function, abnormalities in the regulation of fibrinolysis, and vascular structural abnormalities (eg, collagen defects). (**Box 1**) This list also

Pediatric Hematology/Oncology, Stony Brook Long Island Children's Hospital, Stony Brook University School of Medicine, 100 Nicolls Road, Stony Brook, NY 11794, USA
E-mail address: rparker@notes.cc.sunysb.edu

Crit Care Clin 29 (2013) 319–333
http://dx.doi.org/10.1016/j.ccc.2012.12.003
0749-0704/13/$ – see front matter © 2013 Published by Elsevier Inc.

criticalcare.theclinics.com

Box 1
Conditions associated with serious bleeding or a high probability of bleeding

Disseminated intravascular coagulation

Liver disease/hepatic insufficiency

Vitamin K deficiency/depletion

Massive transfusion syndrome

Anticoagulant overdose (heparin, warfarin)

Congenital coagulopathies (eg, factor VIII deficiency) [hemophilia A], factor IX deficiency [hemophilia B])

Thrombocytopenia (drug induced, immunologic)

Acquired platelet defects (drug induced, uremia)

Laboratory abnormalities not associated with clinical bleeding

Lupus anticoagulant

Reactive hyperfibrinogenemia

Depressed clotting factor levels (newborns)

Specific factor deficiencies associated with specific diseases

Amyloidosis: factor X deficiency

Gaucher disease: factor IX deficiency

Nephrotic syndrome: factor IX deficiency, antithrombin-III deficiency

Cyanotic congenital heart disease (polycythemia, qualitative platelet defect, acquired von Willebrand disease)

---

includes drug effects on each of these components. Of the strictly medical causes of bleeding, consumptive coagulopathies (embodied in disseminated intravascular coagulation [DIC]) and liver disease are some of the more serious (DIC) or common (liver disease) encountered. Consequently, the focus of this review is to discuss current concepts on the pathophysiology and management of each. Additionally, the data regarding the use and efficacy of recombinant human activated factor VII (rhFVIIa) are reviewed.

DIC
Pathophysiology

DIC is one of the most serious hemostatic abnormalities seen in the pediatric ICU (PICU) but is generally noted in conjunction with other life-threatening conditions that warrant PICU admission. The clinical syndrome itself results from the activation of blood coagulation leading to excessive thrombin generation. The final result of this process is the widespread formation of fibrin thrombi in the microcirculation, with resultant consumption of certain clotting factors and platelets. Once the rate of consumption of clotting factors and platelets is greater than the ability to increase production, bleeding ensues.[1] Several specific conditions associated with the development of DIC are presented in **Table 1**. In general, the conditions associated with DIC are the same in adults and children and include a wide variety of disorders, the common feature of which is their ability to initiate coagulation to varying degrees. The mechanisms involved generally can be considered in 2 categories: (1) those intrinsic processes that enzymatically activate procoagulant proteins and (2) those

Table 1 Underlying diseases associated with DIC	
Sepsis	Retained placenta
Liver disease	Hypertonic saline abortion
Shock	Amniotic fluid embolus
Penetrating brain injury	Retention of a dead fetus
Necrotizing pneumonitis	Eclampsia
Tissue necrosis/crush injury	Localized endothelial injury
Intravascular hemolysis	(aortic aneurysm,
Acute promyelocytic leukemia	giant hemangiomata,
Thermal injury	angiography)
Freshwater drowning	Disseminated malignancy
Fat embolism syndrome	(prostate, pancreatic)

that cause the release of tissue factor (TF), which then triggers coagulation. These events are complex and can lead to significant bleeding and often complicate the management of an already critically ill child.

Fibrinolysis invariably accompanies thrombin formation in DIC,[1] and thrombin generation or release of tissue plasminogen activator usually initiates this process. Plasmin is generated and then digests fibrinogen and fibrin clots as they form. Plasmin also inactivates several activated coagulation factors and impairs platelet aggregation. As such, DIC represents an imbalance between the activity of thrombin, which leads to microvascular thrombi with coagulation factor and platelet consumption, and plasmin, which degrades these fibrin-based clots as they form. Therefore, thrombin-induced coagulation factor consumption, thrombocytopenia, and plasmin generation contribute to the presence of bleeding. Globally, DIC represents an imbalance between clot formation (coagulation) and clot breakdown (fibrinolysis). Initially, DIC is a thrombotic disorder characterized by microvascular thrombosis with bleeding occurring only when the consumption of platelets and clotting factors out paces the ability to replace these critical elements.

In addition to bleeding complications, the presence of fibrin thrombi in the microcirculation can lead to ischemic tissue injury. Pathologic data indicate that renal failure, acrocyanosis, multifocal pulmonary emboli, and transient cerebral ischemia may be related clinically to the presence of such thrombi. The presence of fibrinopeptides A and B (resulting from enzymatic cleavage of fibrinogen) leads to pulmonary and systemic vasoconstriction, which can potentiate an existing ischemic injury. In a given patient with DIC, either bleeding or thrombotic tendencies may predominate; in most patients, bleeding is usually the predominant problem. However, in up to 10% of patients with DIC, the presentation is exclusively thrombotic (eg, pulmonary emboli with pulmonary hypertension, renal insufficiency, altered mental status, acrocyanosis) without hemorrhage. Whether the presentation of DIC is thrombotic, hemorrhagic, or compensated (ie, laboratory results consistent with DIC without overt bleeding), microvascular thrombosis likely contributes to the development and progression of multiorgan failure.

Clinical Presentation and Diagnosis

The suspicion that DIC is present usually stems from one of two conditions: (1) unexplained, generalized oozing or bleeding or (2) unexplained, abnormal laboratory parameters of hemostasis. Consideration of DIC usually occurs in the context of a suggestive clinical scenario or associated disease (see **Table 1**). Although infection and multiple trauma are the most common underlying conditions associated with the development of DIC, certain other organ system dysfunctions predispose to DIC, including hepatic insufficiency and splenectomy.[2,3] Both of these conditions are associated with impaired reticuloendothelial system function and consequent impaired clearance of activated coagulation proteins and fibrin/fibrinogen degradation fragments, which may inhibit fibrin polymerization and clot formation.

The clinical severity of DIC frequently has traditionally been assessed by the severity of bleeding and coagulation abnormalities. Scoring tools that use a panel of laboratory tests along with severity-of-illness scores to assess the likelihood and severity of DIC have been proposed in an attempt to determine the prognosis at the time of diagnosis to better direct initial therapy. The tests most commonly used in many of these scoring systems for the diagnosis of DIC are listed in **Table 2**. Although no data exist for pediatric patients, this approach does have prognostic value, particularly in patients with sepsis.[4–6] The more commonly used scoring systems may serve as a template for the diagnosis of DIC; one[7] involves a qualitative score (3 out of 5 tests positive), whereas others[8] involve a quantitative score. Although each has been shown to be useful in identifying patients with suspected or confirmed DIC, they have not been fully validated for critically ill children. Limited studies have shown that early identification of DIC, before the onset of a gross hemorrhagic diathesis, improves survival in critically ill children.[8,9]

The combination of a prolonged PT, hypofibrinogenemia, and thrombocytopenia in the appropriate clinical setting is sufficient to suspect the diagnosis of DIC in most instances. Severe hepatic insufficiency (with splenomegaly and splenic sequestration of platelets) can yield a similar laboratory profile and must be ruled out. In addition to liver disease, several other conditions have presentations similar to DIC and must be considered in the differential diagnosis; they include massive transfusion, primary fibrinolysis, thrombotic thrombocytopenic purpura (TTP)/hemolytic uremic syndrome (HUS), heparin therapy, and dysfibrinogenemia. With the exception of massive transfusion syndrome, these disorders generally have only two of the three characteristic laboratory findings of DIC; a comparison of the laboratory findings in these disorders is noted in **Table 3**.

To confirm a diagnosis of suspected DIC, tests that indicate increased fibrinogen turnover (ie, elevated fibrin degradation products [FDPs] or D-dimer assay) may be necessary. The D-dimer assay for the D-dimer fragment of polymerized fibrin has been shown to be both highly sensitive and specific for proteolytic degradation of polymerized fibrin (fibrin clot that has been produced in the presence of thrombin). Consequently, this test is used with increasing frequency in patients with suspected DIC and is often stated to be the preferred test of fibrin/fibrinogen consumption. However, remembering that thrombin is produced whenever coagulation is activated in the presence of bleeding, the clinician must interpret a modest elevation

Table 2	
Laboratory tests for the diagnosis of DIC	
Test	**Discriminator Value**
Platelet count	<80–100,000 or a decrease of >50% from baseline
Fibrinogen	<100 mg/dL or a decrease of >50% from baseline
Prothrombin time	>3-s prolongation more than upper limit of normal
Fibrin degradation products	>80 mg/dL
D dimer	Moderate increase

Table 3
Hemorrhagic syndromes and associated laboratory findings

Clinical Syndrome	Screening Tests	Supportive Tests
DIC	Prolonged PT, aPTT, TT; decreased fibrinogen, platelets; microangiopathy	(+) FDPs, D-dimer; decreased factors V, VIII, and II (late)
Massive transfusion	Prolonged PT, aPTT; decreased fibrinogen, platelets ± prolonged TT	All factors decreased; (−) FDPs, D dimer (unless DIC develops); (+) transfusion history
Anticoagulant overdose		
Heparin	Prolonged aPTT, TT; ± prolonged PT	Toluidine blue/protamine corrects TT; reptilase time normal
Warfarin (same as vitamin K deficiency)	Prolonged PT; ± prolonged aPTT (severe); normal TT, fibrinogen, platelets	Vitamin K–dependent factors decreased; factors V, VIII normal
Liver disease		
Early	Prolonged PT	Decreased factor VII
Late	Prolonged PT, aPTT; decreased fibrinogen (terminal liver failure); normal platelet count (if splenomegaly absent)	Decreased factors II, V, VII, IX, and X; decreased plasminogen; ± FDPs unless DIC develops
Primary fibrinolysis	Prolonged PT, aPTT, TT; decreased fibrinogen ± platelets decreased	(+) FDPs, (−) D dimer; short euglobulin clot lysis time
TTP	Thrombocytopenia, microangiopathy with mild anemia; PT, aPTT, fibrinogen generally within normal limits/mildly abnormal	ADAMTS-13 deficiency/inhibitor, unusually large von Willebrand factor multimers between episodes; mild increase in FDPs or D dimer
HUS	Microangiopathic hemolytic anemia, ± thrombocytopenia; PT, aPTT generally within normal limits	Renal insufficiency; FDPs and D dimer generally (−)

Abbreviations: aPTT, activated partial thromboplastin time; FDPs, fibrin degradation products; PT, prothrombin time; TT, thrombin time.

of D dimer in postoperative or trauma patients with some degree of caution. The presence of a marked elevation of D dimer in nonbleeding patients essentially excludes primary fibrinogenolysis as the sole cause of measurable FDPs in the serum. The thrombin time (TT) is a less sensitive test for DIC, but may be useful in cases of suspected heparin overdose, because it corrects in the test tube with the addition of protamine sulfate or toluidine blue. Similarly, the euglobulin clot lysis time may not be sensitive to fibrinolysis associated with DIC but is significantly shortened in most cases of primary fibrinolysis. Other tests of purported value, such as soluble fibrin monomer or thrombin-antithrombin complex formation, either have problems with sensitivity or are impractical for widespread use outside of a research setting.

MENINGOCOCCAL PURPURA FULMINANS

Purpura fulminans is a systemic coagulopathy similar, if not identical, to DIC that classically accompanies meningococcal sepsis and is sporadically noted with other similarly severe infections. The hallmark of this syndrome is tissue ischemia and necrosis caused by marked microvascular thrombosis. Patients are generally noted to have severely depressed levels of protein C (PC), with a degree of suppression that correlates with mortality. The presence of the plasminogen activator inhibitor type 1 (PAI-1) 4G/4G genotype producing the highest plasma levels of PAI-1 have been described in patients with meningococcal sepsis and has been shown to be associated with increased sepsis and mortality but not with meningococcal meningitis.[10] Activated PC (APC) can stimulate fibrinolysis by forming a tight 1:1 complex with PAI-1, which leads to inactivation of this fibrinolysis inhibitor. Thus, because APC complexes to PAI-1, these findings of increased PAI-1 and decreased PC are probably interrelated. High levels of thrombin lead to high levels of APC, APC complexes to PAI-1, and finally, PC is depleted.[11] This mechanism is possibly the explanation for the extremely low levels of PC found in meningococcal disease. The purpura seen in this disease is similar to that seen in congenital PC deficiency. From a therapeutic point of view, meningococcal sepsis has been considered as a model for sepsis-associated PC deficiency; many open-label studies of PC-concentrate therapy have been published in this patient population. The suggestion of one study that a disturbed activation process of PC by semiquantitative analysis of expression of thrombomodulin and the endothelial PC receptor in the dermal microvasculature of children with severe meningococcemia and purpuric or petechial lesions[12] calls into question the therapeutic benefit of PC concentrates. A randomized, placebo-controlled, dose-finding study of PC concentrate in the same patient population demonstrated adequate activation of PC to APC, even in the most severely ill patients, with a dose-dependent improvement in coagulation parameters.[13]

Recently, patients with sepsis with thrombocytopenia-associated multiple organ failure (TAMOF) have been described; in many of these patients, a decrease in the von Willebrand factor (vWf) cleaving protease ADAMST-13 has been documented. Intensive plasma exchange by apheresis has been shown to reverse the course of disease and multiorgan failure in many of these children.[14] In some patients, prolongation of the PT suggested activation of coagulation and fibrin consumption; on autopsy, patients were noted to have fibrin- and vWf-rich thrombi similar to those seen in classic DIC.

Management

The primary treatment of DIC is correction of the underlying problem that led to its development. Specific therapy for DIC should not be undertaken unless patients have significant bleeding or organ dysfunction secondary to DIC, significant thrombosis has occurred, or treatment of the underlying disorder (eg, acute promyelocytic leukemia) is likely to increase the severity of DIC.

Supportive therapy for DIC includes the use of several component blood products.[15,16] Packed red blood cells are given according to accepted guidelines in the face of active bleeding. Fresh whole blood (ie, <24–48 hours old) may be given to replete both volume and oxygen-carrying capacity, with the potential additional benefit of providing coagulation proteins, including fibrinogen and platelets. Cryoprecipitate is the component of choice if critical hypofibrinogenemia (eg, <75 mg/dL) is present because cryoprecipitate contains a much higher concentration of fibrinogen than does whole blood or fresh frozen plasma (FFP). Fibrinogen concentrates available in Europe are not yet available in the United States. FFP is of limited value for the treatment of significant hypofibrinogenemia because of the large volumes required to produce any meaningful increase in plasma fibrinogen concentration. FFP infusions may effectively replete other coagulation factors consumed with DIC, such as PC, although the increase in these proteins may be quite small unless large volumes of FFP are infused. The use of cryoprecipitate or FFP in the treatment of DIC has been open to debate in the past because of the concern that these products merely provide further substrate for ongoing DIC and, thus, increase the amount of fibrin thrombi formed. However, clinical (autopsy) studies have failed to confirm this concern.

The goal of blood component therapy is not to produce normal numbers but rather to produce clinical stability. If the serum fibrinogen level is less than 75 to 50 mg/dL, repletion with cryoprecipitate to increase plasma levels to 100 mg/dL or more is the goal. A reasonable starting dose is 1 bag of cryoprecipitate for every 10 kg of body weight every 8 to 12 hours. Because cryoprecipitate is not a standardized component (ie, its content varies from bag to bag), the fibrinogen level should be rechecked after an infusion to assess the increase. The amount and timing of the next infusion is then adjusted according to the results. Platelet transfusions may also be used when thrombocytopenia is thought to contribute to ongoing bleeding. Many of the fibrin/fibrinogen fragments produced in DIC have the potential to impair platelet function by inhibiting fibrinogen binding to platelets, an effect that may be clinically significant at the concentration of FDPs achieved with DIC. Platelet transfusions in patients with DIC should be considered to maintain platelet counts up to 40,000 to 80,000/mcL depending on the clinical status of the patient. In the case of children with sepsis-associated TAMOF and low ADAMST-13, plasma exchange may represent an intervention that is simultaneously supportive and therapeutic.

Pharmacologic therapy for DIC has 2 primary aims: to turn off ongoing coagulation so that repletion of coagulation factors may begin and to impede thrombus formation and ensuing ischemic injury. Recombinant activated factor VII (rhFVIIa), a recombinant hemostatic factor, has been used to treat bleeding in DIC refractory to other therapies as well as in trauma and in other medical and surgical causes of severe, life-threatening bleeding.[17–22] Improved outcome with rhFVIIa infusions in comparison with standard treatment with FFP and/or plasma concentrates has not been shown. A brief discussion of the use of rhFVIIa to treat refractory bleeding can be found later.

Various synthetic and natural modulators of hemostasis have shown some efficacy in moderating multiorgan dysfunction in animal models of sepsis. These modulators include anticoagulant molecules (eg, heparin, antithrombin-III [AT-III], tissue factor pathway inhibitor, APC) and thrombolytic modulators (eg, tissue plasminogen activator, thrombin-activatable fibrinolysis inhibitor). Although initial reports of the use of recombinant human APC in sepsis demonstrated a benefit on survival in adults with sepsis, there was increased bleeding in the elderly; the pediatric trial was stopped because of futility and increased bleeding in infants. Subsequent reanalysis of data demonstrated no benefit of this agent in the treatment of sepsis and it was withdrawn from the US market. Except in the setting of meningococcal purpura fulminans, clinical trials addressing the use of natural modulators of thrombosis and fibrinolysis have not consistently demonstrated a benefit in patients with sepsis.[13,23–27]

LIVER DISEASE AND HEPATIC INSUFFICIENCY
Pathophysiology of Abnormal Hemostasis in Liver Disease

Liver disease is a common cause of abnormal hemostasis in patients in the ICU, with abnormal coagulation studies or overt bleeding occurring in approximately 15% of patients who have either clinical or laboratory evidence of hepatic dysfunction. It is a common cause of a prolonged prothrombin time (PT) and/or activated partial thromboplastin time (aPTT), often without any clinical manifestations. The hemostatic defect associated with liver disease is multifactorial, with essentially all phases of hemostasis being affected.[28,29] In liver disease, synthesis of many plasma coagulation proteins, including factors II, V, VII, IX, and X, is impaired. Fibrinogen synthesis by the liver is usually maintained at levels that prevent bleeding until terminal liver failure is present. Factor VIII and vWf levels are generally normal to increased in acute and chronic liver disease; neither factors are synthesized in the liver and both are acute phase reactants.

In addition to decreased levels of plasma coagulation proteins, many patients with liver disease, particularly cirrhosis, exhibit increased fibrinolytic activity. An increase in fibrinolytic potential is a frequent occurrence in patients who have undergone portacaval shunt procedures. The mechanism for this heightened fibrinolytic state is not clear, although increased amounts of plasminogen activator can often be demonstrated. It may be difficult to discern whether fibrinolysis occurs solely because of underlying severe liver disease or as a result of concurrent, compensated, DIC because patients with cirrhosis are at an increased risk for the development of DIC. The clinical distinction can be virtually impossible to make if active bleeding is present. In liver disease, levels of FDPs may be increased as a result of increased fibrinolysis and by decreased hepatic clearance of the fibrinogen fragments.

A variable degree of thrombocytopenia may be present in patients with hepatic dysfunction; this is usually ascribed to splenic sequestration. It is rarely profound; although it generally does not produce clinically significant bleeding in and of itself, it may exacerbate bleeding from other causes. In vitro platelet aggregation and adhesion may be affected.[30,31] Increased plasma concentrations of FDPs are a possible cause of these abnormalities. The thrombocytopenia of liver disease in conjunction with other coagulation/hemostatic defects secondary to liver disease may result in bleeding that is difficult to manage, particularly if all aspects of the problem are not addressed.

Patients with synthetic liver disease may also exhibit decreased synthesis of the vitamin K–dependent anticoagulant proteins PC and protein S as well as AT-III.[29] Decreased levels of these natural anticoagulants may increase the risk of thrombosis, a risk that is further increased if fibrinolysis is impaired. The usual tests used to measure coagulation, PT, aPTT, and TT, are insensitive to conditions of increased risk for thrombosis and will not be affected by variations in the levels of any of these naturally occurring anticoagulants.

LIVER DISEASE AND THE INTERNATIONAL NORMALIZED RATIO

Many clinicians use the international normalized ratio (INR) as a surrogate measure of the PT. The INR was developed to compare the intensity of vitamin K antagonist (VKA) anticoagulant therapy between clinical laboratories using reagents of differing sensitivities; although it is calculated from the PT, it is not a surrogate for the PT. It has only been standardized and validated for the purpose of quantifying the intensity of VKA anticoagulation. Because INR is calculated from the PT, any condition that produces a prolonged PT will give an increased INR. Many clinicians have assumed that the presence of an elevated INR indicates an increased risk for bleeding, as in patients on VKA therapy. However, no data exist to confirm this assumption. Multiple studies on patients with liver disease and prolonged PT have demonstrated a rebalanced hemostasis system with maintenance of thrombin generation and decreased fibrinolytic potential with a resulting increased risk for thrombosis rather than an increased risk of bleeding.[32–35] However, other investigators have shown an increase in global fibrinolytic potential in patients with liver disease; but these studies have not linked this finding to an increase in bleeding.[36] The lack of correlation of PT (and consequently INR) in patients with liver disease may be explained by the fact that, in contrast to VKA therapy in which only one pathway involved in hemostasis is affected, liver disease effects essentially all phases of hemostasis: primary (platelet-dependent) hemostasis, fibrin clot initiation, coagulation inhibition, and fibrinolysis. Of these phases, only fibrin clot production is measured by the PT and (coincidentally) the INR. Although a prolonged PT in these patients reflects decreased in vitro fibrin clot formation, the net result of these multiple effects is a rebalancing of in vivo hemostasis in patients with liver disease in which the decreased fibrin clot production is counterbalanced by a decrease in natural inhibitors of coagulation. As a consequence, adequate hemostasis is maintained and neither the PT nor the INR accurately reflects the risk of bleeding in these patients.[37–40] However, patients with liver disease may still experience clinically significant bleeding as a consequence of severe thrombocytopenia, a rebalanced hemostatic system that does not adequately compensate for a decrease in procoagulant clotting factors and/or increased fibrinolysis. Anatomic lesions, such as esophageal varices caused by portal hypertension, also represent a significant risk for upper gastrointestinal hemorrhage in these patients. Consequently, the intensive care clinician must carefully and thoroughly assess his or her patients for these risks. However, the role traditional measures of coagulation (ie, PT, aPTT) play in this assessment are limited at best.

Presentation

The hemostatic defect in liver disease is multifactorial, and each patient should be approached accordingly. The most common scenario is a patient with liver disease and a prolonged PT without overt bleeding in whom the potential for bleeding is a concern. In patients with liver disease and impaired synthetic capabilities, particularly those who are critically ill, rhFVIIa activity levels are usually the first to decrease because of its short half-life (4–6 hours) and increased turnover. This results in a prolonged PT and can be noted even when usual markers of hepatocellular injury/hepatic insufficiency remain relatively normal.[28,29] As the severity of liver disease increases, the aPTT may also be affected, reflecting more severely impaired synthetic. In this setting, plasma concentrations of the vitamin K–dependent coagulation factors (II, VII, IX, X) decrease, as do those of FV (which is synthesized in the liver but not vitamin K dependent). A prolonged TT in the setting of liver disease may indicate the presence of dysfibrinogenemia as a result of altered hepatic fibrinogen synthesis. Although fibrinogen synthesis occurs in the liver, its plasma level is maintained until the disease approaches the end stage. When fibrinogen levels are severely depressed as a consequence of decreased synthesis and not increased degradation (fibrinolysis) or consumption (conversion to fibrin), liver failure has typically reached the terminal phase.

In more severe forms of liver disease, fibrinolysis may complicate clinical management. The differentiation between concomitant DIC and fibrinolysis attributable to liver disease alone may be difficult. The D-dimer assay result should be negative in patients who have liver disease, elevated FDPs, and fibrinolysis but no active bleeding because thrombin is not being generated. Further clinical distinction is usually not possible; in practice, it is very difficult to distinguish between a patient with fibrinolysis alone without activation of coagulation and one who has a DIC-like process.

Therapy

If patients are not actively bleeding, no specific therapy is required, with certain provisos. In patients with a prolonged PT who are in a postoperative state or are scheduled for an invasive procedure, correction of the PT may be considered; FFP is the component of choice for this purpose. However, studies have shown inconsistent and incomplete correction of the PT in liver disease and also call into question the need to correct this parameter at all. Multiple studies have shown that invasive procedures can be performed safely without correction of a prolonged PT.[37,41,42] When a correction of the PT is desired, a decrease of the PT to a value of 3 or less seconds more than the upper limit of normal for the testing laboratory is considered adequate.[42–44]

Cryoprecipitate is required only if fibrinogen levels are less than 50 to 100 mg/dL or if significant dysfibrinogenemia is documented. Vitamin K deficiency is also relatively common in this patient population, and replacement may be necessary. In contrast to children with dietary vitamin K deficiency and normal liver function, correction of the PT in vitamin K–responsive critically ill patients typically requires longer than 12 to 24 hours and repeated dosing of parenteral vitamin K. Patients with significant hepatic impairment may manifest a partial response or may not respond at all. The immediate use of FFP is, therefore, appropriate when rapid correction is necessary. rhFVIIa infusions have been shown to control bleeding in severe liver disease, although reduced mortality does not necessarily result.[45,46] To date, no studies have conclusively shown rhFVIIa concentrate to be superior to prothrombin complex concentrates (PCC) for the management of bleeding.[21]

When the synthetic capability of the liver becomes more profoundly impaired and the aPTT is prolonged, greater volumes of FFP or more specific therapy may be necessary. The use of FIX concentrates (PCC) or rhFVIIa has been advocated, particularly if bleeding is present. However, their use remains controversial. The products produced from plasma pooled from multiple donors carry a relatively low but still measurable risk of hepatitis (both types B and C) and human immunodeficiency virus. In addition, PCCs or rhFVIIa may initiate thromboembolic events, provoke DIC, and worsen hemostasis.[47] The use of PCCs or rhFVIIa should be reserved for patients with poorly controlled bleeding that is unresponsive to other more established therapeutic modalities, such as infusion of FFP.

A comprehensive therapeutic approach is required in patients with active bleeding as a result of liver disease. Initially, FFP, 10 to 15 mL/kg body weight, may be given every 6 to 8 hours until bleeding slows significantly; it should then be continued at maintenance levels as dictated by clinical status and coagulation studies. Continuous infusions of FFP (starting dose 2–4 mL/kg/h) have also been used with success to control bleeding following a bolus infusion.[48] Recombinant FVIIa or prothrombin complex concentrates may be used in those patients who are unresponsive to FFP infusions.[46,49] Cryoprecipitate should be infused for fibrinogen levels less than 50 to 100 mg/dL. Platelet transfusions may also be required if the platelet count is less than 40,000 to 80,000/μL, depending on the clinical situation. Vitamin K should be empirically administered on the presumption that part of the synthetic defect may result from a lack of this cofactor. However, a poor response to vitamin K in the presence of severe liver disease should be anticipated. Transfusions of packed cells are administered as deemed appropriate by the clinician. In the future, 4-factor prothrombin complex concentrates (PCCs containing factors II, VII, IX, and X) and fibrinogen concentrates in development may be available to treat refractory bleeding and hypofibrinogenemia not effectively managed with current blood products.

RHFVIIA

rhFVIIa is a novel clotting factor that enhances fibrin clot formation by enhancing the generation of activated factor X (F.Xa). This enhancement occurs by forming a complex with TF at sites of vascular injury, which then catalyzes the conversion of FX to its activated form Xa. The increase in VIIa/TF complex formation occurs in part by the increase in plasma F.VIIa concentrations following infusion and in part by the binding of F.VIIa to the platelet surface, which results in the concentration of F.VIIa at sites of vascular injury. Infusion of rhFVIIa has been reported to control bleeding refractory to therapy with FFP and platelet infusions. Most of the reports are of single cases or case series with only a limited number of randomized controlled trials. Owing to the positive reports in the literature, and to the difficulty of controlling severe bleeding with standard therapies, the use of rhFVIIa has increased dramatically over the past decade in both adults and children.[50,51] Although most randomized studies have demonstrated efficacy in the control of hemorrhage, most have not demonstrated a reduction in mortality.[17–21] Most of the randomized controlled trials reported have compared the effect of rhFVIIa with placebo rather than with FFP or PCCs.[52–55] With the exception of those patients with acquired inhibitors to FVIII, no controlled trials have been conducted in children. Recombinant activated factor rhFVIIa has also been shown to correct the hemostatic defect caused by the antiplatelet agents aspirin and clopidogrel, to be beneficial in the treatment of bleeding secondary to congenital platelet defects, and to effectively reverse the anticoagulation produced by the anti-Xa agent fondaparinux.[56–58] Reports have noted that the use of rhFVIIa may result in an increase in thrombosis and thromboembolic events in adults; although the incidence seems to be small, there is a suggestion of increased incidence with an increased dose of rhFVIIa.[59,60] However, limited studies suggest an increase in thromboembolic events in neonates, although the rate may be similar to that noted with FFP infusions.[51,61,62] A reasonable conclusion to be drawn from these data is that although rhFVIIa may be effective in controlling bleeding in selected clinical settings, there are insufficient data to conclude that it is superior to other available sources of clotting factors (eg, FFP, PCCs) or to conclude that use of rhFVIIa has a beneficial effect on mortality in bleeding patients. Better-designed randomized controlled trials in which FVIIa is tested against FFP or PCCs are warranted.

SUMMARY

Bleeding in PICU patients is associated with an increased risk of mortality. Fortunately, however, most patients with an abnormal coagulation profile do not bleed because this is generally secondary to liver disease or dietary-induced vitamin K deficiency. When the laboratory markers of coagulopathy are the result of DIC, bleeding is common and the risk of mortality extreme. Although interventions directed toward correcting the abnormal coagulation test results are generally initiated, they are also generally either not warranted (in the case of liver disease) or not fully successful (in the case of DIC). Newer more biologically based therapies to reestablish normal hemostasis in patients with a consumptive coagulopathy have not been shown to be effective. Consequently, the treatment of choice for DIC (and related conditions) remains treating the underlying process that initiated the coagulopathic state along with supporting the hemostatic components by transfusion as best we can. Our enthusiasm for new products coupled with frustration with the limited usefulness of standard therapeutic measures should not move us in the direction of using unproven therapies outside the context of clinical trials.

REFERENCES

1. Bick RL, Arun B, Frenkel EP. Disseminated intravascular coagulation. Clinical and pathophysiological mechanisms and manifestations. Haemostasis 1999;29(2–3): 111–34.
2. Chuansumrit A, Hotrakitya S, Sirinavin S, et al. Disseminated intravascular coagulation findings in 100 patients. J Med Assoc Thai 1999;82(Suppl 1):S63–8.
3. Oren H, Cingoz I, Duman M, et al. Disseminated intravascular coagulation in pediatric patients: clinical and laboratory features and prognostic factors influencing survival. Pediatr Hematol Oncol 2005;22(8):679–88.
4. Cauchie P, Cauchie CH, Boudjeltia KZ, et al. Diagnosis and prognosis of overt disseminated intravascular coagulation in a general hospital—meaning of the ISTH score system, fibrin monomers, and lipoprotein-C-reactive protein complex formation. Am J Hematol 2006;81(6):414–9.
5. Gando S, Iba T, Eguchi Y, et al. A multicenter, prospective validation of disseminated intravascular coagulation diagnostic criteria for critically ill patients: comparing current criteria. Crit Care Med 2006;34(3):625–31.
6. Voves C, Wuillemin WA, Zeerleder S. International Society on Thrombosis and Haemostasis score for overt disseminated intravascular coagulation predicts organ dysfunction and fatality in sepsis patients. Blood Coagul Fibrinolysis 2006;17(6):445–51.
7. Leclerc F, Hazelzet J, Jude B, et al. Protein C and S deficiency in severe infectious purpura of children: a collaborative study of 40 cases. Intensive Care Med 1992;18(4):202–5.
8. Gando S. The utility of a diagnostic scoring system for disseminated intravascular coagulation. Crit Care Clin 2012;28:373–88.
9. El-Nawawy A, Abbassy AA, El-Bordiny M, et al. Evaluation of early detection and management of disseminated intravascular coagulation among Alexandria University pediatric intensive care patients. J Trop Pediatr 2004;50(6):339–47.
10. Geishofer G, Binder A, Muller M, et al. 4G/5G promoter polymorphism in the plasminogen-activator-inhibitor-1 gene in children with systemic meningococcaemia. Eur J Pediatr 2005;164:486–90.
11. Hermans PW, Hibberd ML, Booy R, et al. 4G/5G promoter polymorphism in the plasminogen-activator-inhibitor-1 gene and outcome in meningococcal disease. Meningococcal Research Group. Lancet 1999;354(9178):556–60.
12. Faust SN, Levin M, Harrison OB, et al. Dysfunction of endothelial protein C activation in severe meningococcal sepsis. N Engl J Med 2001;345(6):408–16.
13. De Kleijn ED, De Groot R, Hack CE, et al. Activation of protein C following infusion of protein C concentrate in children with severe meningococcal sepsis and purpura fulminans: a randomized, double-blinded, placebo-controlled, dose-finding study. Crit Care Med 2003;31(6):1839–47.
14. Nguyen TC, Han YY, Kiss JE, et al. Intensive plasma exchange increases a disintegrin and metalloprotease with thrombospondin motifs-13 activity and reverses organ dysfunction in children with thrombocytopenia–associated multiple organ failure. Crit Care Med 2008;36:2878–87.
15. Erber WN. Plasma and plasma products in the treatment of massive haemorrhage. Best Pract Res Clin Haematol 2005;19(1):97–112.
16. Goldenberg NA, Manco-Johnson MJ. Pediatric hemostasis and use of plasma components. Best Pract Res Clin Haematol 2005;19(1):143–55.
17. Boffard KD, Riou B, Warren B, et al. Recombinant factor VIIa as adjunctive therapy for bleeding control in severely injured trauma patients: two parallel

randomized, placebo-controlled, double blind clinical trials. J Trauma 2005;59(1): 8–15 [discussion: 15–8].
18. Mathew P, Young G. Recombinant factor VIIa in paediatric bleeding disorders— a 2006 review. Haemophilia 2006;12(5):457–72.
19. Sallah S, Husain A, Nguyen NP. Recombinant activated factor VII in patients with cancer and hemorrhagic disseminated intravascular coagulation. Blood Coagul Fibrinolysis 2004;15(7):577–82.
20. Scarpelini S, Rizoli S. Recombinant factor VIIa and the surgical patient. Curr Opin Crit Care 2006;12(4):351–6.
21. Yank V, Tuohy CV, Logan AC, et al. Systematic review: benefits and harms of in-hospital use of recombinant factor VIIa administration. Ann Intern Med 2011;154: 529–40.
22. Franchini M, Manzato F, Salvagno GL, et al. Potential role of recombinant acti-vated factor VII for the treatment of severe bleeding associated with dissemi-nated intravascular coagulation: a systemic review. Blood Coagul Fibrinolysis 2007;18:589–93.
23. Afshari A. Evidence based evaluation of immune-coagulatory interventions in crit-ical care. Dan Med Bull 2011;58:B4316.
24. Davis-Jackson R, Correa H, Horswell R, et al. Antithrombin III (AT) and recombi-nant tissue plasminogen activator (R-TPA) used singly and in combination versus supportive care as treatment of endotoxin-induced disseminated intravascular coagulation (DIC) in the neonatal pig. Thromb J 2006;4:7.
25. Jaimes F, de la Rosa G, Arango C, et al. A randomized clinical trial of unfractio-nated heparin for treatment of sepsis (the HETRASE study): design and rationale. Trials 2006;7:19.
26. Munteanu C, Bloodworth LL, Korn TH. Antithrombin concentrate with plasma exchange in purpura fulminans. Pediatr Crit Care Med 2000;1:84–7.
27. Zenz W, Zoehrer B, Levin M, et al. Use of recombinant tissue plasminogen acti-vator in children with meningococcal purpura fulminans: a retrospective study. Crit Care Med 2004;32:1777–80.
28. Al Ghumias AK, Gader A, Faleh FZ. Haemostatic abnormalities in liver disease: could some haemostatic tests be useful as liver function tests? Blood Coagul Fibrinolysis 2005;16(5):329–35.
29. Lisman T, Caldwell SH, Leebeck FW, et al. Hemostasis in chronic liver disease. J Thromb Haemost 2006;4:2059.
30. Ordinas A, Escolar G, Cirera I, et al. Existence of a platelet-adhesion defect in patients with cirrhosis independent of hematocrit: studies under flow conditions. Hepatology 1996;24:1137–42.
31. Escolar G, Cases A, Vinas M, et al. Evaluation of acquired platelet dysfunctions in uremic and cirrhotic patients using the platelet function analyzer (PFA-100): influ-ence of hematocrit elevation. Haematologica 1999;84:614–9.
32. Sogaard KK, Horvath-Puho E, Gronbaek H, et al. Risk of venous thromboembo-lism in patients with liver disease: a nationwide population-based case-control study. Am J Gastroenterol 2009;104:96–101.
33. Roberts LN, Patel RK, Arya R. Haemostasis and thrombosis in liver disease. Br J Haematol 2009;148:507–12.
34. Lisman T, Potre RJ. Rebalanced hemostasis in patients with liver disease: evidence and clinical consequences. Blood 2010;116:878–85.
35. Lisman T, Bakhtiari K, Adelmeijer J, et al. Intact thrombin generation and decreased fibrinolytic capacity in patients with acute liver injury or acute liver failure. J Thromb Haemost 2012;10:1312–9.

36. Rijken DC, Kock EL, Guimaraes AH, et al. Evidence for an enhanced fibrinolytic capacity in cirrhosis as measured with two different global fibrinolysis tests. J Thromb Haemost 2012;10:2116–22.

37. Townsend JC, Heard R, Powers ER, et al. Usefulness of international normalized ratio to predict bleeding complications in patients with end-stage liver disease who undergo cardiac catheterization. Am J Cardiol 2012;110:1062–5.

38. Tripodi A, Caldwell SH, Hoffman M, et al. Review article: the prothrombin time test as a measure of bleeding risk and prognosis in liver disease. Aliment Pharmacol Ther 2007;26:141–8.

39. Tripodi A, Baglin T, Robert A, et al. Reporting prothrombin time results as international normalized ratios for patients with chronic liver disease. J Thromb Haemost 2010;8:1410–2.

40. Wei YX, Li J, Zhang LW, et al. Assessment of validity of INR system for patients with liver disease associated with viral hepatitis. J Thromb Thrombolysis 2010; 30:84–9.

41. Fisher NC, Mutimer DJ. Central venous cannulation in patients with liver disease and coagulopathy – a prospective audit. Intensive Care Med 1999;25:481–5.

42. Segal JB, Dzik WH. Paucity of studies to support that abnormal coagulation test results predict bleeding in the setting of invasive procedures: an evidence-based review. Transfusion 2005;45:1413–25.

43. Dasher K, Trotter JF. Intensive care unit management of liver-related coagulation disorders. Crit Care Clin 2012;28:389–98.

44. Youssef WI, Salazar F, Dasarathy S, et al. Role of fresh frozen plasma infusion in correction of coagulopathy of chronic liver disease: a dual phase study. Am J Gastroenterol 2003;98:1391–4.

45. Ganguly S, Spengel K, Tilzer LL, et al. Recombinant factor VIIa: unregulated continuous use in patients with bleeding and coagulopathy does not alter mortality and outcome. Clin Lab Haematol 2006;28(5):309–12.

46. Ramsey G. Treating coagulopathy in liver disease with plasma transfusions or recombinant factor VIIa: an evidence based review. Best Pract Res Clin Haematol 2005;19(1):113–26.

47. Goodnough LT. A reappraisal of plasma, prothrombin complex concentrates, and recombinant factor VIIa in patient blood management. Crit Care Clin 2012;28: 413–26.

48. Bonduel MM. Oral anticoagulation therapy in children. Thromb Res 2006;118(1): 85–94.

49. Brady KM, Easley RB, Tobias JD. Recombinant activated factor VII (rFVIIa) treatment in infants with hemorrhage. Paediatr Anaesth 2006;16(10):1042–6.

50. Logan AC, Yank V, Stafford RS. Off-label use of recombinant factor VIIa in U.S. hospitals: analysis of hospital records. Ann Intern Med 2011;154:516–22.

51. Witmer CM, Huang YS, Lynch K, et al. Off-label recombinant factor VIIa use and thrombosis in children: a multi-center cohort study. J Pediatr 2011;158:820–5.

52. Yuan ZH, Jiang JK, Huang WD, et al. A meta-analysis of the efficacy and safety of recombinant activated factor VII for patients with acute intracerebral hemorrhage without hemophilia. J Clin Neurosci 2010;17:685–93.

53. Chavez-Tapia NC, Alfaro-Lara R, Tellez-Avila F, et al. Prophylactic activated recombinant factor VII in liver resection and liver transplantation: systemic review and meta-analysis. PLoS One 2011;6:e22581.

54. Simpson E, Lin Y, Stanworth S, et al. Recombinant factor VIIa for the prevention and treatment of bleeding in patients without haemophilia. Cochrane Database Syst Rev 2012;(3):CD005011.

55. Marti-Carvajal AJ, Karakitsiou DE, Salanti G. Human recombinant activated factor VII for upper gastrointestinal bleeding in patients with liver diseases. Cochrane Database Syst Rev 2012;(3):CD004887.

56. Altman R, Scazziota A, De Lourdes Herrera M, et al. Recombinant factor VIIa reverses the inhibitory effect of aspirin or aspirin plus clopidogrel on in vivo thrombin generation. J Thromb Haemost 2006;4(9):2022–7.

57. White GC. Congenital and acquired platelet disorders: current dilemmas and treatment strategies. Semin Hematol 2006;43(Suppl 1):S37–41.

58. Elmer J, Wittels KA. Emergency reversal of pentasaccharide anticoagulants: a systemic review of the literature. Transfus Med 2012;22:108–15.

59. O'Connell KA, Wood JJ, Wise RP, et al. Thromboembolic adverse events after use of recombinant human coagulation factor VIIa. JAMA 2006;295(3):293–8.

60. Diringer MN, Skolnick BE, Mayer SA, et al. Risk of thromboembolic events in controlled trials of rFVIIa in spontaneous intracerebral hemorrhage. Stroke 2008;39:850–6.

61. Young G, Wicklund B, Neff P, et al. Off-label use of rFVIIa in children with excessive bleeding: a consecutive study of 153 off-label uses in 139 children. Pediatr Blood Cancer 2009;53:179–83.

62. Puetz J, Darling G, Brabec P, et al. Thrombotic events in neonates receiving recombinant factor VIIa or fresh frozen plasma. Pediatr Blood Cancer 2009;53:1074–8.

Common Endocrine Issues in the Pediatric Intensive Care Unit

Amelie von Saint Andre-von Arnim, MD[a], Reid Farris, MD[a],
Joan S. Roberts, MD[b], Ofer Yanay, MD[a], Thomas V. Brogan, MD[a],
Jerry J. Zimmerman, MD, PhD, FCCM[c],*

KEYWORDS

- Stress response • Renin-angiotensin-aldosterone axis • Euthyroid sick syndrome
- Diabetic ketoacidosis • Strict glycemic control • Diabetes insipidus
- Syndrome of inappropriate antidiuretic hormone • Cerebral salt wasting
- Critical illness-related corticosteroid insufficiency

KEY POINTS

- Critical illness pathogen-associated molecular patterns (PAMPS) and damage-associated molecular patterns (DAMPS) activate the neurogenic-endocrine-inflammatory stress response.
- Antidiuretic hormone (ADH), the renin-angiotensin-aldosterone axis, and natriuretic peptide signaling normally govern sodium and water homeostasis, all of which can be disrupted in critical illness.
- Stress-mediated protein catabolism provides amino acid substrate for gluconeogenesis, the antecedent to hyperglycemia commonly associated with critical illness; however, it remains unclear if strict glycemic control is beneficial in improving outcomes among critically ill children.
- Diabetic ketoacidosis (DKA) continues to represent a common admission diagnosis among pediatric intensive care patients, and cerebral edema (ischemia-reperfusion injury, impaired cerebral blood flow regulation, altered blood-brain barrier, effective osmolality imbalance) remains a potentially fatal complication encountered during DKA management.
- Critical illness related corticosteroid insufficiency (CIRCI) is commonly encountered in pediatric intensive care, but practitioners prescribing replacement corticosteroid, should be aware of not only the anti-inflammatory and hemodynamic stabilizing properties of the class of agents, but also the potential for enhanced muscle catabolism, hyperglycemia, hypernatremia, and acquired immunodeficiency adverse drug effects.
- Both insufficient and excess thyroid hormone can produce life-threatening illness. Critical non-thyroidal illness (also known as euthyroid sick syndrome) is common among critically ill patients, but it remains controversial if normalizing total and free tri-iodothyronine in this setting is beneficial.

[a] Seattle Children's Hospital, University of Washington School of Medicine, 4800 Sand Point Way NE, Seattle, WA 98105, USA; [b] Department of Pediatrics, Critical Care Division, Seattle Children's Hospital, University of Washington School of Medicine, 4800 Sand Point Way NE, Seattle, WA 98105, USA; [c] Seattle Children's Hospital, University of Washington School of Medicine, Room MB.10.625, 4800 Sand Point Way NE, Seattle, WA 98105, USA
* Corresponding author.
E-mail address: jerry.zimmerman@seattlechildrens.org

Crit Care Clin 29 (2013) 335–358
http://dx.doi.org/10.1016/j.ccc.2012.11.006
0749-0704/13/$ – see front matter © 2013 Elsevier Inc. All rights reserved.

ACTIVATION OF THE STRESS RESPONSE IN CRITICAL ILLNESS

Multiple stimuli encountered in critical illness activate an acute stress response.[1,2] Such afferent stimuli include pain, visual, auditory, and olfactory stimuli, baroreceptor, chemoreceptor and stretch receptor activation as well as inflammation. With regards to these stimuli, various surveillance aspects of innate immunity recognize pathogen-associated molecular patterns (PAMPS).[3] Perhaps less well appreciated are recognition systems for damage-associated molecular patterns (DAMPS), which arise after critical illness tissue injury.[4] For example, mitochondrial damage may lead to release of N-formyl proteins as well as bacterial DNA, both perceived as foreign antigens. Accordingly, both infection and tissue injury can activate the stress response through inflammation signaling via recognition of PAMPS and DAMPS.

Various mediators that provide afferent signaling for the stress response are transported to the brain and cross the blood-brain barrier via fenestrated capillaries and activated cytokine transport. In addition, afferent signaling is also provided by the vagus and other nerve input.[1] Afferent stress signals are integrated at the level of the hypothalamus, where a neurogenic-endocrine-inflammation stress response ensues.[1,5,6] Forward and reverse servo signaling occurs between each major biochemical element of the stress response. Four primary efferent events are activated and summarize the activity of the acute stress response:

Synthesis of Proinflammatory and Antiinflammatory Mediators

The former has evolved to contain and eliminate foreign antigens, particularly infectious.[7] This system is mediated through toll-like receptor signaling and augmentation of proinflammatory nuclear transcription factor pathways. Complement, lectin-binding proteins, and activation of macrophages, endothelial cells, neutrophils, and natural killer cells represent additional elements of the innate immune system. Increased production of interleukin 6 (IL-6) stimulates synthesis of acute phase proteins, including C-reactive protein, fibrinogen, and α_2-macroglobulin. Simultaneously, antiinflammatory mediator production is also upregulated in part via signaling via the vagus nerve, with nerve endings terminating on splenic and hepatic macrophages that activate the α-7 subunit of the acetylcholine receptor, resulting in decreased production of proinflammatory mediators with tumor necrosis factor α (TNF-α) being most extensively investigated to date.[8,9]

Activation of the Sympathetic and Parasympathetic Nervous System

Discussion of the feedback role of the parasympathetic nervous system has already been mentioned in regard to development of a compensatory antiinflammatory response.[10] Increased sympathetic activity promotes catecholamine synthesis and release that serves several functions: cardiac output and blood pressure are sustained via increases in heart rate as well as systemic vascular resistance. Catecholamine release also inhibits insulin release and action, and stimulates both glucagon and adrenocorticotropic hormone (ACTH) production. Glucagon mediates acute glucose energy substrate availability and ACTH stimulates cortisol production, with effects on transcription and translation of hundreds of genes (discussed later under CIRCI).[11]

Enhanced Release of Various Counterregulatory Hormones

Glucocorticoids, glucagon, and growth hormone (GH) are upregulated with concurrent modulation of thyroid activity. Both cortisol and thyroid hormone contributions to the stress response are discussed in subsequent sections of this article.

Release of Antidiuretic Hormone and Activation of the Renin-Angiotensin-Aldosterone Axis

This cascade results in reclamation of water via upregulation of aquaporin channels and enhanced reabsorption of sodium via aldosterone signaling in the renal collecting tubules. Alterations in antidiuretic hormone (ADH) states in the pediatric intensive care unit (PICU) are also discussed in the next section of this article. Renal macula densa cells in concert with contractile mesangial cells of the glomerulus sense increased α-adrenergic activity, distal convoluted tubule chloride/sodium concentration changes, and decreased perfusion and subsequently signal modified fenestrated endothelial cells in the renal afferent arteriole to produce and release renin from the so-called juxtaglomerular apparatus. Brain-kidney nerve connections can also directly activate this cascade. Renin converts hepatic-synthesized angiotensinogen to angiotensin 1. Subsequently, angiotensin-converting enzyme located diffusely among endothelial cells, but particularly in the pulmonary endothelia, catalyzes the conversion on angiotensin 1 to angiotensin 2. Angiotensin 2 facilitates a variety of activities essential to the acute stress response, as summarized in **Box 1**.

SALT/WATER BALANCE PROBLEMS
Normal Water Homeostasis

ADH and thirst maintain plasma osmolality in a narrow range, between 275 and 295 mOsm/L. ADH is produced in the supraoptic and paraventricular nuclei of the hypothalamus, and transported through axonal processes to the capillary plexi in the posterior pituitary. ADH binds to V2 receptors located on principal cells in the renal collecting ducts. This binding leads to a cyclic adenosine monophosphate–mediated increase in permeability of the luminal cell membrane, allowing back diffusion of water from the tubules to the plasma, and concentrating the urine via aquaporin-2 water channels. ADH is primarily regulated by osmoreceptors in the anterior hypothalamus. Nonosmotic regulatory factors include volume depletion and cardiac failure, as well as pain, nausea, and medications.

Syndrome of Inappropriate ADH

Syndrome of inappropriate ADH (SIADH) is a common disorder in the intensive care unit (ICU) characterized by the inability to suppress the secretion of ADH, resulting in partially impaired water excretion and hyponatremia. Criteria for the diagnosis of

---

Box 1
Activities of angiotensin 2

- Increases systemic vascular resistance and blood pressure
- Mediates aldosterone production by adrenal cortex
- Augments plasminogen activator inhibitor 1 release
- Stimulates thirst and salt craving
- Enhances release of vasopressin, ACTH, and norepinephrine
- Increases sodium reabsorption directly
- Promotes afferent and efferent renal vasoconstriction
- Induces cardiomyocyte hypertrophy
- Facilitates nuclear transcription factor NFkB activity

SIADH include hyponatremia, plasma hypotonicity, inappropriate urine concentration for the degree of plasma hypotonicity, natriuresis despite hyponatremia, euvolemia, and exclusion of other causes of euvolemic hypo-osmolality (hepatic, renal, thyroid, and adrenal dysfunction).[12]

Pathophysiology
Hyponatremia is initially mediated by inappropriate ADH-induced water retention. The ensuing volume expansion activates secondary natriuretic mechanisms. Renin and aldosterone activities downregulate, resulting in sodium and water loss and restoration of near euvolemia. The net effect is that, with chronic SIADH, sodium loss is more prominent than water retention.[13] Hence, urine osmolality is inappropriately high compared with plasma osmolality, and urine sodium levels are generally greater than 20 mEq/L. Conditions associated with SIADH are multiple and are summarized in **Box 2**.

Signs and symptoms
The severity of clinical manifestations depends on the rate of decrease in serum sodium, which determines the risk for cellular swelling, and cerebral edema. Hyponatremia developing over days to weeks may be symptom-free as a result of adaptation of brain cells. Rapid changes in serum sodium levels can result in nausea, vomiting, muscle cramps, decreased deep tendon reflexes, lethargy, coma, focal deficits, and seizures. There is marked individual variability regarding the degree of hyponatremia at which symptoms become apparent. Most patients develop seizures and coma with acute hyponatremia of less than 120 mEq/L.[14]

Treatment
Fluid restriction is the mainstay of therapy for SIADH. The total intake must be less than insensible losses and urinary output combined, which is generally around 0.75 L/m^2 body surface area or less. Further therapies depend on the presence or absence of CNS symptoms or imaging suggestive of cerebral edema, and the rate of hyponatremia development. For hyponatremia that has been present for less than 4 hours and is not associated with CNS symptoms, serum sodium correction can be safely corrected at rates of 0.7 to 1.0 mEq/L/h.[14] If hyponatremia has developed over a longer time interval or if CNS symptoms are present, the goal is to increase serum sodium levels slowly at a rate of 0.5 mEq/L/h to avoid osmotic demyelination syndrome.[14] Symptoms of osmotic demyelination may include obtundation, tremor, amnesia, quadriplegia, coma, and seizures.[15] In hyponatremic patients with signs of acute CNS cellular swelling, an initial rapid bolus of 5 to 6 mL/kg of 3% saline increases the serum sodium

---

Box 2
Conditions associated with SIADH

- Central nervous system (CNS) disease (infections, head trauma, brain tumors, cerebral thrombosis or hemorrhage, Guillain-Barré syndrome, postneurosurgical procedures)

- Pulmonary conditions (pneumonia, asthma, pneumothorax, positive pressure ventilation)

- Malignancies (lymphoma, Ewing sarcoma, mesothelioma, bronchogenic carcinomas)

- Multiple drugs (eg, vincristine, cyclophosphamide, carbamazepine, barbiturates, opiates, tricyclic antidepressants, salicylates)

From Fuhrman BP, Zimmerman JJ. Pediatric critical care. 4th edition. Philadelphia: Elsevier; 2011; with permission.

by approximately 5 mEq/L and can help stabilize cerebral swelling and avoid impending herniation. Further sodium needs in symptomatic patients can be replaced using 3% saline infusion according to the calculated sodium deficit: sodium deficit [mEq] = 0.6 × body weight [kg] × (125-measured [Na]). Frequently, a regimen of 3% saline at 1 to 2 mL/kg/h with periodic administration of loop diuretic to promote water excretion is an effective and safe regimen for patients with acute hyponatremia. Sodium levels should be monitored every 2 hours, initially. Further fluid restriction may be necessary if sodium levels do not normalize. In adults, use of the ADH V1 and V2 receptor antagonist conivaptan has been reported to increase urine volume and reduce urine osmolality in hyponatremia and fluid-retaining states.[16–18] Although pediatric usage has been reported, further data are necessary to evaluate its role in children.[19]

Cerebral Salt Wasting

Cerebral salt wasting (CSW) is characterized by hyponatremia and extracellular volume depletion caused by inappropriate sodium wasting in the urine in the setting of CNS disease.[20] The mechanism by which cerebral disease leads to renal salt wasting is poorly understood, and some believe that CSW does not really exist.[21,22]

Pathophysiology

There are 2 theories for the pathophysiologic mechanisms for CSW: (1) central function of a circulating natriuretic factor and (2) disruption of neural input to the kidney.[23,24] The first theory is that a circulating factor impairs renal tubular sodium reabsorption.[21,25,26] The primary candidate is brain natriuretic peptide (BNP), which decreases sodium reabsorption and inhibits renin release.[25,27] BNP may also decrease autonomic outflow at the level of the brainstem.[28] The second theory is that the sympathetic nervous system facilitates sodium, uric acid, and water reabsorption in the proximal tubule, as well as renin release. Impaired sympathetic output could therefore explain the decreased proximal sodium and uric acid reabsorption, and the impaired release of renin and aldosterone. Renal salt wasting leads to volume depletion, which provides a baroreceptor stimulus for the release of ADH with water retention, which further exacerbates hyponatremia.

Among patients with CNS disease and hyponatremia, CSW is less common than SIADH.[29–31] CSW has frequently been described in adults with subarachnoid hemorrhage, but can be associated with meningitis, encephalitis, poliomyelitis, CNS tumors, and after CNS surgery (and after trauma).[20,32]

Signs and symptoms

The typical onset of CSW is within the first 10 days after a neurosurgical procedure or event. Without volume replacement, it is associated with extracellular fluid depletion and signs of dehydration, such as orthostatic hypotension, dry mucous membranes, decreased skin turgor, and tachycardia. SIADH, on the other hand, is associated with a slightly increased or normal extracellular volume status.

Diagnosis

CSW should be considered in patients with CNS disease and hyponatremia (<135 mEq/L) with a low plasma osmolality; an increased urine osmolality caused by renal sodium wasting and ADH secretion in response to volume depletion; an increased urine sodium concentration caused by salt wasting; and a low serum uric acid concentration caused by uric acid wasting in the urine. Urine output is typically brisk. Clinical evidence of hypovolemia (or isotonic volume replacement to avoid it) is crucial, because these laboratory findings may overlap with SIADH, and the 2 disorders are managed differently.[20,33]

Treatment

Maintaining a positive water and salt balance is the key element of therapy. Volume repletion should be achieved with isotonic saline. Severe hyponatremia may require hypertonic saline administration or oral salt supplementation. It is essential to frequently monitor therapy and adjust treatment accordingly. Administration of a mineralocorticoid, such as fludrocortisone, can also be used.[31,34,35] Long-term therapy is not necessary, because CSW tends to resolve within 3 to 4 weeks.[24]

Diabetes Insipidus

Diabetes insipidus (DI) is characterized by excretion of large amounts of dilute, tasteless (insipid) urine, leading to hypernatremia.

Pathophysiology

The 2 most important pathophysiologic mechanisms are vasopressin (ADH) deficiency in central DI and renal vasopressin insensitivity in nephrogenic DI. Central DI is caused by a defect in secretion or synthesis of vasopressin by the neurohypophyseal system. Acquired forms of central DI are more commonly seen in the PICU. Causes of DI are summarized in **Box 3**.

There exist rare genetic forms of DI with autosomal-dominant and autosomal-recessive inheritance involving the ADP-neurophysin gene, as well as an X-linked recessive form of central DI. DI can be associated with congenital CNS malformations such as holoprosencephaly, agenesis of the pituitary, and midline craniofacial abnormalities.

Severe damage to the neurohypophysial system by neurosurgery or trauma often results in a typical triphasic response with an initial polyuric phase (hours to days), reflecting inhibition of ADH release caused by hypothalamic dysfunction.[32] This response is followed by unregulated release of vasopressin from the degenerating posterior pituitary, clinically inducing SIADH (days 6–12). DI may ensue in a third phase after the posterior pituitary ADP stores are depleted. This last phase may be permanent or transient.[13,36]

Nephrogenic DI results from partial or complete resistance of the kidney to ADH and is caused by acquired or genetic concentrating defects of the kidneys. Genetic forms may be caused by X-linked recessive alteration of the vasopressin V2 receptor or

---

Box 3
Causes of DI

- Head trauma
- Tumors (craniopharyngioma, meningioma, leukemia, lymphoma)
- Postneurosurgical procedures
- Cerebral vascular anomalies
- Infections (meningitis, encephalitis)
- Rheumatic disease (Wegener granulomatosis, systemic lupus erythematosus, scleroderma)
- Guillain-Barré syndrome
- CNS malformation
- Brain death

Data from Fuhrman BP, Zimmerman JJ. Pediatric critical care. 4th edition. Philadelphia: Elsevier; 2011.

mutations of the aquaporin-2 gene, with either autosomal-dominant or autosomal-recessive inheritance. Causes for acquired nephrogenic DI are more common and include chronic renal failure, renal tubulointerstitial diseases, medications (eg, lithium, diuretics, amphotericin B, cisplatin, rifampin), metabolic derangements (hypercalcemia, hypokalemia), sickle cell disease, or dietary abnormalities (primary polydipsia, decreased sodium intake, severe protein restriction).[32]

Signs and symptoms

Untreated central DI typically presents with polyuria and polydipsia if thirst is not impaired. Moderate to severe hypernatremia can develop, especially in infants and young children who cannot independently access free water and in postoperative patients with unrecognized DI. Irritability, high-pitched cry, and hyperpyrexia can be signs of hypernatremia in infants. Symptoms can progress to lethargy, increased muscle tone, and seizures. Hyperosmolar states can be complicated by shrinkage of brain cells, leading to tearing of cerebral vessels, subarachnoid hemorrhage, and venous sinus thrombosis.[32] Urine specific gravity is less than 1.005, and urine osmolality typically low (50–200 mOsm/L). Serum sodium concentration and serum osmolality depend on hydration status of the patient.

Treatment

Isotonic 0.9% saline boluses should be administered to a child presenting in shock. After reversal of shock, careful replacement of water deficits is conducted with hypotonic fluids, in conjunction with vasopressin replacement. The water deficit is calculated by the following equation: water deficit = $0.6 \times$ body weight $\times$ ([Na]−140)/140. To reduce the risk for cerebral edema, the water deficit is corrected slowly over 48 to 72 hours, with a goal decrease in serum sodium of 10 to 12 mEq/L/d using hypotonic fluid (0.2–0.45% normal saline) or enteral water. Vasopressin replacement should be initiated for central DI. A continuous infusion of vasopressin should be started at 0.5 mU/kg/h and titrated up to achieve antidiuresis. Alert patients who can regulate their thirst may be treated with intranasal or subcutaneous 1-demino-8-D-arginine vasopressin (DDAVP). It is crucial to follow patients' intake and output closely, and replace ongoing urine output and insensible losses in addition to the calculated water deficit to avoid iatrogenic hyponatremia. Serum sodium levels require frequent monitoring (every 2–6 hours), initially.

GLYCEMIC CONTROL IN PEDIATRIC PATIENTS

Hyperglycemia was first recognized during episodes of stress by Thomas Willis in the seventeenth century.[37] With data collected in the last 2 decades, it is clear that hyperglycemia is common in nondiabetic critically ill children, with peak blood glucose and duration directly associated with worse outcome.[38] Hyperglycemia is found frequently in subsets of critically ill children with specific disease process (traumatic brain injury, burns, sepsis, congenital heart disease [CHD], necrotizing enterocolitis).[39–43] In addition, 2 other dimensions of glycemic control, namely hypoglycemia and glucose variability, may independently contribute to morbidity and mortality.[44]

Control of blood glucose is complex, involving interactions between the pituitary, liver, pancreas, and adrenals. Insulin acts to lower blood glucose level, enhancing glucose uptake and glycogenesis and suppressing gluconeogenesis. Glucagon, catecholamines, GH, and cortisol increase blood glucose concentrations through upregulation of glycogenolysis and gluconeogenesis. As noted earlier, this finding represents an essential endogenous response to a stressful situation such as injury or infection, mobilizing glucose to meet increased cellular metabolic demand. Secretion of these hormones results from stimulation of the sympathetic nervous system or direct activation by proinflammatory mediators. Cytokines such as TNF-α and IL-1 can stimulate the hypothalamic-pituitary axis, releasing ACTH, whereas IL-1 and IL-2 can stimulate the adrenal cortex to directly enhance glucocorticoid synthesis.[37,45,46] High glucose loads from feeds and intravenous infusions accentuate serum glucose concentrations.

Hyperglycemia exacerbates the cytokine, inflammatory, and oxidative stress response, potentially setting up a vicious cycle whereby hyperglycemia leads to further hyperglycemia.[45] There are several mechanisms by which hyperglycemia is postulated to cause damage at a cellular level. These mechanisms include oxidative stress, advance glycation, and mitochondrial pathways.[38,47] Acute, short-term hyperglycemia affects all major components of innate immunity and impairs the ability of the host to combat infection, even although certain distinctive proinflammatory alterations of the immune response can be observed under these conditions.[9] It is unclear whether hyperglycemia contributes to the pathophysiology as a direct risk factor or serves as a surrogate marker for severity of illness,[43] representing a transient alteration of carbohydrate metabolism in response to stress.[48]

In 2001, a seminal study by Van den Berghe and colleagues[49] reported that tight glycemic control in critically ill adults lowered hospital mortality by more than 30%. It is perhaps not surprising that such a simple intervention with a significant impact prompted a change in practice, new guidelines for glycemic control development,[50,51] and a lot of hope. However, in following years, multiple prospective randomized adult studies failed to replicate this success. For example, the NICE-SUGAR (Normoglycemia in Intensive Care Evaluation—Survival Using Glucose Algorithm Regulation Study, ClinicalTrials.gov #NCT00220987) multicenter international study, which involved more than 6100 adult patients, showed that tight glycemic control increased mortality.[52] In a systematic review of adult prospective randomized controlled trials (RCTs) of tight glycemic control, Marik and Preiser concluded that "The NICE-SUGAR study, as well as 4 additional RCTs, were unable to replicate the findings of the 2 Leuven Intensive Insulin Therapy Trials and, indeed, raised the possibility that tight glycemic control may increase organ failure and death in patients fed according to current guidelines."[53]

Pediatric intensivists have been reluctant to embrace tight glycemic control. A survey involving 30 PICUs in the United States reported considerable disparity between physicians' beliefs that some pediatrics subsets should receive glycemic control, but few used a standard approach to treat hyperglycemia.[54] The population in the PICU is diverse both in terms of diagnosis and age. Extrapolating data from adult studies should therefore be limited. Two large prospective randomized studies examining glycemic control in children have been published. In 2009, Vlasselaers and colleagues[55] published a large single-center study (NCT00214916) involving 700 critically ill children (317 of whom were infants <1 year of age). Tight glycemic control targeted age-adjusted blood glucose concentration (2.8–4.4 mmol/L [50–80 mg/dL] for infants and 3.9–5.6 mmol/L [70–100 mg/dL] for children). In the conventional arm, patients received insulin only to prevent blood glucose from exceeding 11.9 mmol/L or 214 mg/dL. Intensive insulin therapy shortened ICU length of stay (LOS) and decreased extended LOS, attenuated inflammatory response (per C-reactive protein concentrations), and decreased mortality from 6% in the conventional arm to 3% in the intervention arm.

Hypoglycemia occurred in 25% of patients in the intensive insulin arm, and in only 1% in the conventional group. More importantly, hypoglycemia occurred on more than 2 occasions in 5% of patients in the intense insulin arm (and none on the conventional arm). Decreased mortality with intensive insulin therapy occurred with 2 categories of cause of death, namely neurologic and pulmonary. In 2010, the same group published a small study (14 neonates) focusing on patients with cardiac anomalies requiring surgery. These investigators reported reduction in myocardial injury and inflammatory response.[56] Although a small study, they again reported shorter PICU stay, especially in those who needed extended PICU stay, and decreased time to tracheal extubation in the tight glycemic control group.

Recently, Agus and colleagues[57] published a 2-center prospective randomized trial SPECS, Safe Pediatric Euglycemia after Cardiac Surgery, ClinicalTrials.gov #(00443599) that enrolled 980 children, 0 to 36 months of age, who underwent cardiac surgery using cardiopulmonary bypass. In this study, the targeted glucose level was higher (80–110 mg/dL, 4.4–6.1 mmol/L) than in the study by Vlasselaers and colleagues. Agus and colleagues' results indicated no change in infection rate, mortality, LOS, or measures of organ failure when compared with standard care.

Faced with 2 large trials with contradicting results, how does a clinician decide which recommendations to follow? Should the difference be attributed to the type of patients included in each study and should we treat only patients with pulmonary and neurologic disease? Should we target a lower glucose level[58]? There is no question that specific trial characteristics and study reproducibility should be considered before firm guidelines are published. At the time of this review, large-scale pediatric trials further examining tight glycemic control are under way. Emory Children's Center is conducting a large single-center prospective randomized clinical trial to evaluate the outcome, benefit, safety, and impact on resource use of maintaining strict glucose control among children with life-threatening conditions (http://clinicaltrials.gov/ct2/show/NCT01116752). A multicenter randomized open study is also being conducted in the United Kingdom: (http://www.chip-trial.org.uk/). The primary outcome for the Control of Hyperglycaemia in Pediatric Intensive Care (CHiP) trial is the number of days alive and free from mechanical ventilation within the 30 days after trial entry. The study is examining multiple secondary outcomes, including mortality, cost-effectiveness, and long-term outcomes (follow-up after 12 months). Data collection will be stratified data for patients with traumatic brain injury. The Heart And Lung Failure-Pediatric INsulin Titration (HALF-PINT) trial of strict glycemic control in critically ill children in the United States has also begun enrollment (NCT 01565941 ClinicalTrials.gov).

With the paucity of pediatric RCTs, conflicting results from existing studies, and loss of equipoise within the adult literature, pediatric intensivists are left with several unanswered questions. Glycemic control in critically ill children may be beneficial. However, tight glycemic control carries significant risk for hypoglycemia, and there is a lack of data regarding specific age groups and diagnoses, as well as absence of long-term outcomes among survivors. The ideal glycemic target and specific subpopulations that might benefit from glycemic control remain controversial. Large studies are under way and will probably help resolve some of these issues. Pediatric intensivists should also support research examining other potential therapies that can ameliorate hyperglycemia without the risks of hypoglycemia.

DIABETIC KETOACIDOSIS

Type 1 diabetes mellitus (T1DM) is an immune-mediated disease that results in total pancreatic β-cell loss and complete dependence on exogenous insulin.[59] The incidence of T1DM varies widely throughout the world and has been increasing globally over time.[59,60] Diabetic ketoacidosis (DKA) is seen in 15% to 70% of patients at the time of diagnosing T1DM. The risk of DKA in patients with known T1DM has been estimated from 1% to 10% per patient per year.[61] DKA represents the leading cause of morbidity and mortality in children with T1DM.[61,62]

The biochemical definition of DKA includes hyperglycemia (blood glucose >200 mg/dL), acidosis (venous pH <7.3 or bicarbonate <15 mmol/L), and ketonemia or ketonuria.[61–63] It is manifest as a consequence of relative or absolute insulin deficiency in the setting of increase of counterregulatory hormones, including glucagon, cortisol, catecholamines, and GH. This hormonal response, a specific example of the stress response, results in a catabolic state and impaired peripheral glucose use caused by lack of insulin and resultant endogenous glucose production via glycogenolysis and gluconeogenesis.

Ketoacidosis

The DKA catabolic state also leads to increased lipolysis and β-oxidation of fatty acids, with resultant ketone body production (β-hydroxybutyrate, acetoacetate, and acetone). Ketonemia results in an anion gap acidosis, which may be compounded by a lactic acidosis secondary to a hypoperfused state from significant dehydration. In addition, ketone bodies have centrally mediated emetogenic effects, potentially resulting in additional loss of hydrogen, chloride, and potassium ions. This situation may lead to a mixed picture, with a metabolic alkalosis overlying the anion gap acidosis.

Volume Depletion

Hyperglycemia and hyperketonemia lead to an osmotic diuresis once the blood glucose level exceeds the renal threshold for glucose reabsorption ($\approx$180 mg/dL). In addition, this hyperglycemic, hyperosmolar state results in a shift of intracellular fluid into the extracellular space, further contributing to electrolyte derangements. Total fluid deficit at the time of presentation to medical care is generally estimated to range from 5% to 10%, depending on the duration and severity of illness. Hypovolemic shock is possible although rare in pediatric DKA. Volume depletion further stimulates the cortisol and catecholamine response, resulting in increased endogenous glucose and ketone body production, exacerbating the metabolic derangements described.[63]

Electrolyte Derangements

The hyperosmolar state and resultant osmotic diuresis not only cause free water losses but significant electrolyte losses as well. Sodium, potassium, and phosphorus are all depleted from both the intracellular and extracellular compartments. Serum sodium concentration may be affected by dilution as a result of free water shifts related to hyperglycemia and physiologic ADH release as a result of intravascular volume depletion. Total body potassium losses are significant and result from vomiting, increased renal losses both from osmotic diuresis as well as increased levels of aldosterone in response to dehydration, and transcellular shifts into the extracellular space caused by both acidosis as well as increased plasma osmolality.[61–63] Serum potassium levels at the time of presentation can vary from low to high, depending on the relative contributions of the mechanisms described earlier and the duration of symptoms. Total body phosphate depletion is primarily a result of osmotic diuresis. However, like potassium, initiation of insulin therapy results in a transcellular shift of phosphate into the intracellular compartment.[61]

Cerebral Edema

Cerebral edema is a well-described and potentially fatal complication of DKA. Clinically significant cerebral edema has been reported to occur in about 1% of DKA cases. However, subtle or subclinical edema has been shown on imaging studies in a substantial proportion of patients with DKA.[64,65] Cerebral edema generally presents

4 to 12 hours after the start of rehydration and may present as late as 22 to 48 hours later, although it has also been reported before initiation of therapy.[61,63] The pathophysiology of cerebral edema in DKA remains unclear and is likely multifactorial. Possible contributory mechanisms include impaired cerebral blood flow caused by dehydration and hypocarbia, resulting in ischemia and tissue hypoxia, leading to vasogenic edema and prolonged serum hyperosmolarity, resulting in production of compensatory intracellular osmoles that persist while treatment with fluids and insulin decreases serum osmolarity, promoting an intracellular free water shift and cytotoxic edema.[64] Alteration of cerebral vascular regulation and of the blood brain barrier in children with DKA have also been suggested.[66] Many have evaluated risk factors for clinically significant cerebral edema in pediatric patients with DKA.[64,67–70] The results of many of these studies point to factors that are closely associated with severity of illness in this patient population.[63] Determining the relative contribution of underlying disease, individual variation, and treatment factors on progression to clinically significant cerebral edema is an as yet unrealized goal. Knowledge of described risk factors combined with pathophysiologic data informs the resuscitation and management of patients who present with potentially long-standing metabolic derangements in an effort to prevent the most severe of neurologic complications.

Treatment

The principal goals of therapy for DKA include correction of dehydration and electrolyte derangement, reversal of ketosis and acidosis, and the avoidance of cerebral edema. Recent international consensus guidelines provide a current standard approach to these patients, providing a baseline for iterative improvement.[61] Treatment of pediatric DKA should occur in a unit with nursing and physician expertise in inpatient DKA management, documented guidelines, access to laboratories to provide timely and frequent measurements, and the ability to access immediate treatment of cerebral edema.

The approach to fluid management is based on expert consensus because no treatment strategy has been definitively proved to treat DKA with a lower incidence of cerebral edema. The summarized features include: (1) estimated volume deficit is 5% to 7% in patients with moderate DKA and 7% to 10% in patients with severe DKA; (2) patients in shock or severe dehydration should receive 0.9% saline to restore peripheral circulation in 10 mL/kg/h boluses; (3) total rehydration fluid should be distributed over 48 hours, with frequent assessment of laboratory values; (4) calculation of effective osmolality (mosm/kg) = $[2 \times (Na + K) (mmol/L)] + [glucose (mg/dL)/18]$ and corrected sodium = $[measured\ Na\ (mmol/L)] + [0.016 \times (glucose\ (mg/dL) - 100)]$ provide additional information on the response to fluid replacement (eg, Ref.[71]); and (5) replacement fluids should be isotonic for the first 4 to 6 hours and at least 0.45% saline over the subsequent 36 hours, increasing tonicity as may be required to ensure that the measured serum sodium is increasing as serum glucose level is falling.

Insulin therapy should begin after the first hour of initial fluid replacement has occurred at 0.1 units/kg/h intravenously (IV) and continue until the resolution of DKA (pH >7.30, bicarbonate >15 mmol/L or closure of the anion gap). As plasma glucose decreases, 5% to 10% glucose should be added, aiming to keep blood glucose at ~200 mg/dL (11 mmol/L) to prevent hypoglycemia while continuing insulin infusion. Potassium replacement is also essential, and should continue throughout IV fluid therapy, as potassium chloride, potassium phosphate, or potassium acetate. Replacement of phosphate is indicated in cases with prolonged lack of food intake or clinical weakness and should be combined with careful monitoring of serum calcium to avoid hypocalcemia.

Treatment approaches linked with higher risk of cerebral edema and accordingly to be avoided include bicarbonate administration, diminished increase of corrected sodium during fluid replacement, insulin therapy in the first hour of fluid treatment, and high volume of fluid infusion in the first 4 hours. If cerebral edema is suspected, treatment responses include reduction of rehydration fluid infusion rate by one-third, administration of mannitol or hypertonic saline, elevation of the head of the bed, and avoidance of venous catheters in the large neck veins. Intubation and mechanical ventilation are required for impending respiratory failure or inability to protect the airway, but aggressive hyperventilation is not recommended.[72] After stabilizing therapies have been started, a cranial computed tomography scan should be obtained to rule out other potential contributing causes for neurologic impairment and to evaluate need for possible additional interventions, including neurosurgical evaluation.

CRITICAL ILLNESS-RELATED CORTICOSTEROID INSUFFICIENCY
Induction of the Cortisol Stress Response

Stimuli associated with critical illness facilitate the elaboration of proinflammatory cytokines such as IL-1, IL-2, IL-6, and interferon γ.[73] These cytokines signal the hypothalamus to release corticotropin-releasing hormone, which subsequently stimulates the anterior pituitary to release ACTH, which stimulates fasciculata cells of the adrenal cortex to produce hydrocortisone. Other mediators such as TNF-α, corticostatin, and macrophage inhibitory protein provide negative feedback for cortisol production. Cortisol exhibits a plasma half-life of approximately 80 to 115 minutes, although its duration of biologic action extends to approximately 8 hours. In an unstressed state, humans older than approximately 6 months generally show circulating total cortisol concentrations of 5 to 10 μg/dL. However, when stressed, total circulating cortisol levels are typically in the 25 μg/dL to 60 μg/dL range.[74] Although unstressed individuals characteristically show diurnal variation in terms of cortisol production, with a maximum value generally around 08:00 AM, critically ill patients lose this variability in cortisol production.

Corticosteroid (Glucocorticoid) Actions

Cortisol (hydrocortisone) is the major corticosteroid elicited in the stress response. Its chemical structure is unique, with a C4-C5 double bond and a C3 ketone group, which are required for adrenocorticoid activity. In addition, the hydroxyl moiety at C11 is essential for both antiinflammatory action as well as glucose homoeostasis functions. Cortisol shows approximately 1% the mineralocorticoid activity of aldosterone. Of primary interest to the intensivist, cortisol mediates broad antiinflammatory properties as well as augmentation of hemodynamics. The antiinflammatory activity of hydrocortisone occurs by 2 primary mechanisms[75]:

1. Glucocorticoids bind to a plasma glucocorticoid receptor comprised of heat shock proteins. This complex is subsequently transported to the nucleus, where it binds to glucocorticoid-responsive elements of the genome, generally enhancing transcription of antiinflammatory genes and inhibiting transcription of proinflammatory genes.
2. In addition, the glucocorticoid-glucocorticoid receptor complex binds to nuclear factor κ B (NFκB), that again would have the effect of inhibiting translation of proinflammatory genes generally stimulated by the NFκB nuclear transcription factor.[76]

Through these primary mechanisms, corticosteroids inhibit proinflammatory production and release of proinflammatory chemokines, adhesion molecules, inducible nitric oxide synthase, nicotinamide adenine dinucleotide phosphate oxidoreductase, as well as cyclooxygenase.[75] Glucocorticoids also augment antiinflammatory responses such as production of macrophage inhibitory protein, IL-10, IκB, IL-1 receptor antagonist as well as lipocortin, an inhibitor of phospholipase A and inhibitor of neutrophil adhesion and the respiratory burst.

Corticosteroids facilitate several positive hemodynamic actions, that include modulation of signal transduction; upregulation of catecholamine, angiotensin, endothelin, and mineralocorticoid receptor numbers and attenuation of their downregulation; inhibition of prostaglandin synthesis; alteration of sodium and calcium transport; modulation of microvascular permeability facilitated by vasocortin; and augmentation of erythrocyte 2, 3 diphosphoglycerate.[76]

Corticosteroids mediate multiple metabolic effects, but in the setting of acute stress, primarily mobilize substrate for energy production and protein synthesis through suppression of insulin action, resulting in augmentation of lipolysis, protein catabolism and subsequent gluconeogenesis, and expansion of synthesis of acute phase reactants as well as inflammation and immunity proteins.

Clinical Testing for Corticosteroid Sufficiency

Testing for adequacy of the cortisol stress response in critical illness has generally involved assessing random total cortisol concentration (in the setting of critical illness stress) or undertaking a corticotropin stimulation test. The latter involves either so-called standard-dose corticotropin (140 μg/kg for children or 250 μg maximum) or low-dose corticotropin (typically 1 μg). Best available adult data gleaned from metyrapone testing of critically ill adults suggest that a random cortisol less than 10 μg/dL or random free cortisol less than 2 μg/dL or a delta cortisol (corticotropin-stimulated minus baseline concentration) less than 9 μg/dL reflects an inadequate cortisol response to the stress of critical illness.[77,78] It has been suggested that monitoring free cortisol is probably more appropriate than monitoring total cortisol because it represents the biologically active fraction for the hormone.[79] This notion becomes particularly relevant for critically ill patients with low albumin, in whom total cortisol concentrations may be low (significant albumin binding) but adequate free cortisol concentrations maintained. Methodology is now available for real-time free cortisol assessment in critically ill children.[80] However, it has been reported that at least 30% of critically ill children may show free cortisol concentrations less than 2 μg/dL (generally considered a threshold for defining adrenal insufficiency) without any clinical evidence of adrenal insufficiency such as unstable hemodynamics, hypoglycemia, or hyponatremia.[81]

Multiple investigators have undertaken observational studies focused on the relationship between random serum total cortisol levels and outcomes among critically ill children.[82–86] These studies confirm loss of ACTH-cortisol circadian rhythm among children with sepsis. Generally, as illness severity increases, IL-6, TNF-α, and ACTH increase, whereas serum total cortisol decreases. Both cortisol and ACTH correlate with Pediatric Risk of Mortality (PRISM) illness severity score, organ dysfunction scores, lactate, C-reactive protein, and fibrinogen. Fewer observational studies have used standard-dose corticotropin stimulation testing.[87–89] These investigations confirm that, like adults, inadequate adrenal reserve is common among children with sepsis. Again, higher PRISM scores, requirement for vasoactive-inotropic support, vasoactive-inotropic resistant shock and multiple organ dysfunction syndrome were more common in children with inadequate adrenal reserve. Chronic illness and organ dysfunction as well as an inadequate adrenal reserve status in some studies were predictive of mortality. Using low-dose corticotropin stimulation, 30% of critically ill children were found to be adrenal insufficient using delta cortisol criteria (as described earlier) on PICU day 1 and were at risk for fluid resuscitation and need for vasoactive-inotropic infusions, but this condition was not associated with surgery, illness severity per PRISM score, or duration of mechanical ventilation.[90]

At least 3 investigations suggest that the methodology for testing adrenal sufficiency among critically ill patients is uninformative as currently practiced. One investigation examining adrenal insufficiency among adult trauma patients reported that 50% of a healthy adult cohort (averaging 35 years of age) showed inadequate adrenal response using corticotropin stimulation testing.[91] Similarly, the CORTICUS (Cortico-steroid Therapy of Septic Shock, ClinicalTrials.gov # NCT0014004) trial of hydrocorti-sone supplementation among adults with septic shock concluded that standard corticotropin stimulation testing assessing total cortisol concentrations does not adequately identify a critically ill sepsis population who might benefit from corticoste-roid replacement therapy.[92] In a third investigation of corticotropin stimulation testing of 522 adults receiving vasopressors for treatment of hemodynamic instability,[93] the investigators concluded that corticosteroid supplementation based on arbitrary base-line concentrations or increments of plasma cortisol was not associated with a survival benefit.

Adrenal Insufficiency Encountered in Pediatric Critical Care Medicine

Adrenal insufficiency may be categorized into 2 major categories. Primary adrenal insufficiency involves destruction or maldevelopment of the adrenal gland. Injury to the adrenal glands may occur by hemorrhage or thrombosis, particularly in the setting of a tenuous adrenal vasculature (Waterhouse-Friderichsen syndrome). Primary adrenal insufficiency is also seen in congenital adrenal hyperplasia[94] and Addison disease. Secondary adrenal insufficiency occurs secondary to loss of hypothalamic-pituitary-adrenal access integrity. Common clinical scenarios associ-ated with secondary adrenal insufficiency include acute and chronic steroid admin-istration and systemic inflammatory response syndrome, particularly associated with sepsis. In addition, medications such as etomidate and ketoconazole inhibit the 11β-hydroxylase cytochrome P450 involved in the rate-limiting step of hydrocor-tisone synthesis.

Even with seemingly adequate cortisol production in the setting of stress, patients may show relative adrenal insufficiency secondary to a variety of cortisol resistance syndromes.[95,96] Examples of such scenarios that may play out at the tissue level include depletion of corticosteroid-binding globulin, activation of the 11β-hydroxyste-roid dehydrogenase, depression of glucocorticoid receptors or diminution of receptor affinity for cortisol, alteration of secondary signaling, and increase of antiglucocorti-coid compounds and receptors. A recent investigation reported that glucocorticoid treatment of adults induced microRNA-124 levels 3-fold and that this finding was associated with T-lymphocyte downregulation of the α-glucocorticoid receptor and upregulation of the β-glucocorticoid receptor.[97]

Adverse Effects of Corticosteroid Administration

Although intensivists have focused on the favorable hemodynamic and antiinflamma-tory benefits of corticosteroids, perhaps the catabolic and immunodeficiency effects of corticosteroids have been inadequately considered.[98] Of particular relevance to critically ill patients are the adverse side effects of hyperglycemia (discussed earlier), reduced somatic growth, impaired wound healing, neuromuscular weakness (eg, Ref.[99]), hospital-acquired infection (eg, Ref.[100]), and altered neurodevelopment for neonates and infants (eg, Ref.[101]).

Best available evidence regarding corticosteroid supplementation

Although the debate continues regarding the use of corticosteroids as adjunctive therapy for unstable hemodynamics, particularly in sepsis, wide-based consensus suggests that corticosteroid replacement/supplementation should be provided in specific situations, as summarized in **Box 4**.[102]

When prescribed in setting of critical illness, corticosteroids should be used at the lowest dose appropriate for the shortest duration that is reasonable, and practitioners should appreciate the adverse side effects that can accompany corticosteroid dosing.[103] Clinicians should collectively support quality research that attempts to establish evidence-based medicine for the application of adjunctive corticosteroids for pediatric critical illness. Such research will involve identification of groups most likely to benefit from glucocorticoid supplementation with the lowest risk of adverse effects, maintenance of equipoise among the pediatric critical care community so that the research can occur with minimal bias; and use of clinically meaningful end points.[104]

THYROID METABOLISM IN CRITICAL ILLNESS

Thyroid hormone occupies a central role in metabolism in utero even before the thyroid gland develops; the fetus is dependent on maternal-derived thyroid hormone; and everyone requires thyroid hormones until the end of life.[105–107] Various activities of thyroid hormone are shown in **Box 5**.

Thyroid hormone enhances normal tissue development, especially normal neuronal maturation.[108] It helps to regulate metabolism, including stimulating oxygen consumption, amino acid and lipid metabolism, and thermogenesis by uncoupling adenosine triphosphate (ATP) production and oxidative phosphorylation. Thyroid hormone alters the activity of other hormones such as cortisol, insulin, GH, and parathyroid hormone activity. Beyond simple metabolic effects, thyroid hormone increases α-adrenergic receptor affinity and responsiveness to catecholamines as well as increasing the respiratory response to hypoxia and hypercarbia. The effect of thyroid hormone on hemodynamics is reviewed in detail in Ref.[109] Thyroid hormone deficiency can render life impossible and its excess can make it untenable.

Thyroid hormone production begins with the thyroid gland capturing iodide from the circulation by the sodium-iodide symporter, which requires energy in the form of ATP. Once in the follicular cell of the thyroid gland, thyroid peroxidase catalyzes the oxidation of iodide to iodine using hydrogen peroxide produced by thyroid oxidase. Thyroglobulin (TG), a large hormone precursor, is synthesized within the rough endoplasmic

---

Box 4
Corticosteroid supplementation in pediatric illness

- Acute or chronic cortical steroid dosing (eg, asthma, rheumatologic disease, cancer, hematopoietic stem cell or solid organ transplantation)
- Hypothalamic-pituitary-adrenal axis problem
- Congenital adrenal hyperplasia
- Multiple endocrinopathies
- Treatment with ketoconazole or etomidate
- Purpura fulminans
- Severe, true vasoactive-inotropic unresponsive septic shock

---

Box 5
Actions of thyroid hormone

- Facilitates fetal brain and skeletal development
- Aids postnatal growth and development
- Increases O_2 consumption and heat production
- Stimulates mitochondriogenesis
- Improves cardiac lusitropy
- Enhances systolic cardiac function
- Amplifies myocardial expression of α-adrenergic and β-adrenergic receptors
- Increases heart rate
- Lowers peripheral vascular resistance
- Increase β-adrenergic receptors in skeletal muscle adipose and lymphocytes
- Augments catecholamine action at the receptor
- Improves ventilatory responses to hypoxia and hypercarbia
- Increases erythropoietin synthesis
- Promotes gastrointestinal motility
- Stimulates bone turnover
- Increases hepatic gluconeogenesis and glycogenolysis
- Improves insulin sensitivity
- Facilitates multiple nonthyroidal collaborative endocrine effects

---

reticulum of the follicular cells. Iodine reacts with the tyrosine residues of TG to form monotyrosine and diiodotyrosine residues within the TG peptide. Thyroid peroxidase catalyzes the binding of adjacent iodotyrosines to form thyroxin (T4) and smaller quantities of triiodothyronine (T3). T4 is transported to distant tissue bound to the T4-binding globulin, transthyretin, and albumin, and as a result of this protein binding, T4 is not readily filtered by kidneys. Peripheral tissues contain isoforms of iodotyrosine deiodinases that cleave T4 to T3 and reverse T3 (rT3). Thyroid hormone production is tightly regulated by the hypothalamic-pituitary-thyroid axis. The hypothalamus produces thyroid-releasing hormone (TRH), which travels to the pituitary gland, stimulating it to produce thyroid-stimulating hormone (TSH), which in turn acts on the thyroid gland. TSH stimulates thyroid hormone production and release as well as growth of the follicular cells. In target organs, T3 binds to thyroid hormone receptors in the nucleus that interact with specific nucleotide sequences termed thyroid responsive elements within promoter regions of regulated genes. When T3 is bound to the thyroid responsive elements, it acts as a coactivator for appropriate gene sequences, and when T3 is not bound, the gene activity is repressed.

Critical Nonthyroidal Illness (Euthyroid Sick Syndrome)

The most common abnormality of thyroid function in patients in the ICU is critical nonthyroidal illness (also known as euthyroid sick syndrome), which arises in response to a wide variety of nonthyroidal diseases, both chronic or acute.[110,111] The changes are believed to be caused by cytokine activity such as TNF-α that inhibits 5'-deiodinase, decreasing peripheral conversion of T4 to T3. Thus, the initial decline in circulating total and free T3 levels is followed by an increase in rT3 levels. This situation seems to be attributable to diminished 5'-monoiododinase activity. Levels of free T4 are normal or slightly decreased, whereas TSH levels are normal or low normal. Certain medications, such as corticosteroids, amiodarone, iodinated cystographic dyes, propylthiouracil (PTU), and high-dose propranolol may also inhibit 5'-deiodinase, resulting in critical non-thyroidal illness. Prognostic usefulness of rT3 and T3/rT3 among critically ill patients has been reported,[112] including associations with illness severity and clinical outcomes.[110]

Ongoing debate about the benefit of treating critical nonthyroidal illness persists, particularly among children with CHD, in whom both congenital and acquired hypothy-roidism are common.[113] Infants younger than 3 months with CHD and with low T3 or high cortisol concentration on PICU admission had a more complicated PICU course in terms of duration of vasoactive-inotropic or mechanical ventilation support.[114] In an interventional trial involving 193 children with CHD (ClinicalTrials.gov NCT00027417), supplemental T3 provided no overall benefit in terms of decreasing the duration of mechanical ventilation (primary study end point), but post hoc analysis suggested a possible benefit for children younger than 5 months.[115] In a systematic review eval-uating risks and benefits of postoperative T3 therapy in adults undergoing cardiovas-cular surgery,[116] postoperative intravenous T3 therapy increased cardiac index but did not reduce mortality. As illness becomes more severe, total and free T4 levels also decrease. When T4 and TSH levels are low, critical nonthyroidal illness can be difficult to distinguish from hypothyroidism. However, low T4 with increased TSH levels signifies true hypothyroidism.

Hypothyroidism

Hypothyroidism may result from primary thyroid failure, may be secondary (caused by TSH deficiency) or tertiary (caused by inadequate TRH), or may be caused by periph-eral resistance to the action of thyroid hormone.[117] The most common precipitating factor for hypothyroidism worldwide is iodine deficiency.[118] Congenital hypothy-roidism arises as a result of thyroidal dysgenesis, thyroid dysfunction with abnormal hormone production, or abnormalities in the hypothalamic-pituitary axis.[119] In North American children older than 6 years, the most common cause of acquired hypothy-roidism is Hashimoto (or autoimmune) thyroiditis. This form of hypothyroidism is most common in girls, and 30% to 40% of patients have a family history of thyroid disease. Untreated infants with hypothyroidism develop short stature, mental retardation, char-acteristic puffy face and hands, and often deaf mutism, a constellation termed cretinism. In children, chronic hypothyroidism produces decreased growth, resulting in short stature. In addition, affected individuals may experience precocious puberty.

Acutely, patients with hypothyroidism may experience poor cardiac contractility, left ventricular dilatation, and decreased cardiac output with bradycardia, but despite these symptoms, congestive heart failure occurs uncommonly. Respiratory effort may be diminished, especially in patients with myxedema coma. Patients with hypo-thyroidism may experience hyponatremia as a result of decreased glomerular filtration rate and inability to excrete a water load. Anemia, muscle cramps, weakness and paresthesia, fatigue, and lethargy occur commonly. Patients also suffer constipation, fecal impaction, and ileus. Features of hypothyroidism are summarized in **Table 1**.

Myxedema Coma

This form of critical hypothyroidism remains uncommon in the pediatric age group. It usually presents in patients with long-standing hypothyroidism, but can be the initial presentation of hypothyroidism. It is often precipitated by other illnesses such as infection. Critical hypothyroidism is marked by progressive weakness stupor,

Table 1
Clinical features of hypothyroidism

Neurologic	General	Other
Fatigue	Decreased appetite	Constipation
Lethargy	Weight gain	Myalgias
Somnolence	Cold intolerance	Dry skin
Depression		Menstrual irregularities
Headache		Bradycardia
Dementia		

hypothermia, hypoventilation, hypoglycemia and hyponatremia progressing to coma, shock, and death. Usually, onset is gradual. Therapy for this medical emergency includes rapid institution of supportive measures and addition of thyroid hormone.

Hyperthyroidism

Although not commonly a critical illness, hyperthyroidism is usually manifest as Graves disease.[120,121] In Graves disease, an autoimmune process, autoantibodies bind the TSH receptor, producing hypertrophy and hyperplasia of the thyroid gland. Another cause of hyperthyroidism stems from TSH production by a pituitary adenoma. Hyperthyroidism in a teenager is most likely caused by Hashimoto thyroiditis. Amiodarone can produce hyperthyroidism, because its structure resembles that of thyroid hormone. Symptoms of hyperthyroidism, summarized in **Table 2**, can be varied but include, agitation, dysrhythmias, hyperreflexia, heat intolerance, and diarrhea.

Patients with critical hyperthyroidism or thyroid storm usually present with cardiac (supraventricular tachycardia or sinus tachycardia) or neurologic disease (confusion, delirium, or coma). Hyperthyroidism should be included in the differential diagnosis of pediatric pulmonary hypertension.[122] Other symptoms may include nausea, emesis, diarrhea, or weakness.[123] However, the most dire and dramatic presentation, thyroid storm, may progress to hyperthermia, cardiovascular collapse, coma, and potentially death, Treatment requires a deliberate broad-stroke approach, with:

1. Supportive care, including volume resuscitation, temperature control, and anxiolysis
2. Blockade of the peripheral activity of T3 with β-blockade (such as esmolol infusion) or thionamides
3. Limiting thyroid gland production of T4 with thionamides (such as PTU or methimazole), which block thyroid peroxidase iodination
4. Treat precipitating causes

Table 2
Clinical features of hyperthyroidism

Cardiac	Neurologic	General	Other
Palpitations	Nervousness	Increased appetite	Respiratory distress
Tachycardia	Hyperactivity	Weight loss	Diarrhea
Exercise intolerance	Anxiety	Fatigue	Abdominal pain
	Emotional lability	Muscle weakness	Proptosis
	Insomnia	Thirst	
	Personality change		

In summary thyroid hormone is central to normal development and metabolism. Abnormalities in thyroid function in North America often arise from autoimmune diseases, but they rarely present as critical illness. However, severe deficiency or excess of thyroid hormone both represent life-threatening disease, which must be treated expeditiously and thoroughly. Such deficiencies must be considered, because presentation may be nonspecific.

REFERENCES

1. Molina PE. Neurobiology of the stress response: contribution of the sympathetic nervous system to the neuroimmune axis in traumatic injury. Shock 2005;24:3–10.
2. Baumann H, Gauldie J. The acute phase response. Immunol Today 1994;15:74–80.
3. Abreu MT, Arditi M. Innate immunity and toll-like receptors: clinical implications of basic science research. J Pediatr 2004;144:421–9.
4. Zhang Q, Raoof M, Chen Y, et al. Circulating mitochondrial DAMPs cause inflammatory responses to injury. Nature 2010;464:104–7.
5. Besedovsky HO, del Rey A. Immune-neuro-endocrine interactions: facts and hypotheses. Endocr Rev 1996;17:64–102.
6. Turnbull AV, Rivier CL. Regulation of the hypothalamic-pituitary-adrenal axis by cytokines: actions and mechanisms of action. Physiol Rev 1999;79:1–71.
7. Franchi L, Nunez G. Immunology. Orchestrating inflammasomes. Science 2012; 337:1299–300.
8. Rosas-Ballina M, Olofsson PS, Ochani M, et al. Acetylcholine-synthesizing T cells relay neural signals in a vagus nerve circuit. Science 2011;334:98–101.
9. Tracey KJ. Cell biology. Ancient neurons regulate immunity. Science 2011;332: 673–4.
10. Bone RC. Sir Isaac Newton, sepsis, SIRS, and CARS. Crit Care Med 1996;24: 1125–8.
11. Galon J, Franchimont D, Hiroi N, et al. Gene profiling reveals unknown enhancing and suppressive actions of glucocorticoids on immune cells. FASEB J 2002;16:61–71.
12. Schrier RW, Bansal S. Diagnosis and management of hyponatremia in acute illness. Curr Opin Crit Care 2008;14:627–34.
13. Adrogue HJ, Madias NE. Hyponatremia. N Engl J Med 2000;342:1581–9.
14. Lynch RE, Wood EG. Fluid and electrolyte issues in pediatric critical illness. In: Fuhrman B, Zimmerman JJ, editors. Pediatric critical care. Philadelphia: Elsevier; 2011. p. 944–62.
15. Kumar S, Fowler M, Gonzalez-Toledo E, et al. Central pontine myelinolysis, an update. Neurol Res 2006;28:360–6.
16. Kumar S, Berl T. Vasopressin antagonists in the treatment of water-retaining disorders. Semin Nephrol 2008;28:279–88.
17. Wright WL, Asbury WH, Gilmore JL, et al. Conivaptan for hyponatremia in the neurocritical care unit. Neurocrit Care 2009;11:6–13.
18. Murphy T, Dhar R, Diringer M. Conivaptan bolus dosing for the correction of hyponatremia in the neurointensive care unit. Neurocrit Care 2009;11:14–9.
19. Rianthavorn P, Cain JP, Turman MA. Use of conivaptan to allow aggressive hydration to prevent tumor lysis syndrome in a pediatric patient with large-cell lymphoma and SIADH. Pediatr Nephrol 2008;23:1367–70.
20. Gutierrez OM, Lin HY. Refractory hyponatremia. Kidney Int 2007;71:79–82.
21. Singh S, Bohn D, Carlotti AP, et al. Cerebral salt wasting: truths, fallacies, theories, and challenges. Crit Care Med 2002;30:2575–9.

22. Carlotti AP, Bohn D, Rutka JT, et al. A method to estimate urinary electrolyte excretion in patients at risk for developing cerebral salt wasting. J Neurosurg 2001;95:420–4.

23. Palmer BF. Hyponatremia in patients with central nervous system disease: SIADH versus CSW. Trends Endocrinol Metab 2003;14:182–7.

24. Palmer BF. Hyponatraemia in a neurosurgical patient: syndrome of inappropriate antidiuretic hormone secretion versus cerebral salt wasting. Nephrol Dial Transplant 2000;15:262–8.

25. Berger TM, Kistler W, Berendes E, et al. Hyponatremia in a pediatric stroke patient: syndrome of inappropriate antidiuretic hormone secretion or cerebral salt wasting? Crit Care Med 2002;30:792–5.

26. Harrigan MR. Cerebral salt wasting syndrome: a review. Neurosurgery 1996;38: 152–60.

27. Berendes E, Walter M, Cullen P, et al. Secretion of brain natriuretic peptide in patients with aneurysmal subarachnoid haemorrhage. Lancet 1997;349: 245–9.

28. Levin ER, Gardner DG, Samson WK. Natriuretic peptides. N Engl J Med 1998; 339:321–8.

29. Ganong CA, Kappy MS. Cerebral salt wasting in children. The need for recognition and treatment. Am J Dis Child 1993;147:167–9.

30. Jimenez R, Casado-Flores J, Nieto M, et al. Cerebral salt wasting syndrome in children with acute central nervous system injury. Pediatr Neurol 2006;35: 261–3.

31. Taplin CE, Cowell CT, Silink M, et al. Fludrocortisone therapy in cerebral salt wasting. Pediatrics 2006;118:e1904–8.

32. Hannon MJ, Finucane FM, Sherlock M, et al. Disorders of water homeostasis in neurosurgical patients. J Clin Endocrinol Metab 2012;97:1423–33.

33. Maesaka JK, Imbriano LJ, Ali NM, et al. Is it cerebral or renal salt wasting? Kidney Int 2009;76:934–8.

34. Albanese A, Hindmarsh P, Stanhope R. Management of hyponatraemia in patients with acute cerebral insults. Arch Dis Child 2001;85:246–51.

35. Kinik ST, Kandemir N, Baykan A, et al. Fludrocortisone treatment in a child with severe cerebral salt wasting. Pediatr Neurosurg 2001;35:216–9.

36. Agha A, Sherlock M, Phillips J, et al. The natural history of post-traumatic neurohypophysial dysfunction. Eur J Endocrinol 2005;152:371–7.

37. Brealey D, Singer M. Hyperglycemia in critical illness: a review. J Diabetes Sci Technol 2009;3:1250–60.

38. Srinivasan V, Spinella PC, Drott HR, et al. Association of timing, duration, and intensity of hyperglycemia with intensive care unit mortality in critically ill children. Pediatr Crit Care Med 2004;5:329–36.

39. Cochran A, Scaife ER, Hansen KW, et al. Hyperglycemia and outcomes from pediatric traumatic brain injury. J Trauma 2003;55:1035–8.

40. Gore DC, Chinkes D, Heggers J, et al. Association of hyperglycemia with increased mortality after severe burn injury. J Trauma 2001;51:540–4.

41. Hall NJ, Peters M, Eaton S, et al. Hyperglycemia is associated with increased morbidity and mortality rates in neonates with necrotizing enterocolitis. J Pediatr Surg 2004;39:898–901 [discussion: 898–901].

42. Branco RG, Garcia PC, Piva JP, et al. Glucose level and risk of mortality in pediatric septic shock. Pediatr Crit Care Med 2005;6:470–2.

43. Klein GW, Hojsak JM, Schmeidler J, et al. Hyperglycemia and outcome in the pediatric intensive care unit. J Pediatr 2008;153:379–84.

44. Wintergerst KA, Buckingham B, Gandrud L, et al. Association of hypoglycemia, hyperglycemia, and glucose variability with morbidity and death in the pediatric intensive care unit. Pediatrics 2006;118:173–9.

45. Dungan KM, Braithwaite SS, Preiser JC. Stress hyperglycaemia. Lancet 2009; 373:1798–807.

46. Chrousos GP. The hypothalamic-pituitary-adrenal axis and immune-mediated inflammation. N Engl J Med 1995;332:1351–62.

47. Van den Berghe G. How does blood glucose control with insulin save lives in intensive care? J Clin Invest 2004;114:1187–95.

48. Mizock BA. Alterations in carbohydrate metabolism during stress: a review of the literature. Am J Med 1995;98:75–84.

49. van den Berghe G, Wouters P, Weekers F, et al. Intensive insulin therapy in critically ill patients. N Engl J Med 2001;345:1359–67.

50. Bates D, Clark NG, Cook RI, et al. American College of Endocrinology and American Association of Clinical Endocrinologists position statement on patient safety and medical system errors in diabetes and endocrinology. Endocr Pract 2005;11:197–202.

51. Dellinger RP. Steroid therapy of septic shock: the decision is in the eye of the beholder. Crit Care Med 2008;36:1987–9.

52. Finfer S, Chittock DR, Su SY, et al. Intensive versus conventional glucose control in critically ill patients. N Engl J Med 2009;360:1283–97.

53. Marik PE, Preiser JC. Toward understanding tight glycemic control in the ICU: a systematic review and metaanalysis. Chest 2010;137:544–51.

54. Preissig CM, Rigby MR. A disparity between physician attitudes and practice regarding hyperglycemia in pediatric intensive care units in the United States: a survey on actual practice habits. Crit Care 2010;14:R11.

55. Vlasselaers D, Milants I, Desmet L, et al. Intensive insulin therapy for patients in paediatric intensive care: a prospective, randomised controlled study. Lancet 2009;373:547–56.

56. Vlasselaers D, Mesotten D, Langouche L, et al. Tight glycemic control protects the myocardium and reduces inflammation in neonatal heart surgery. Ann Thorac Surg 2010;90:22–9.

57. Agus MS, Steil GM, Wypij D, et al. Tight glycemic control versus standard care after pediatric cardiac surgery. N Engl J Med 2012;367:1208–19.

58. Kavanagh BP. Glucose in the ICU–evidence, guidelines, and outcomes. N Engl J Med 2012;367:1259–60.

59. Knip M. Descriptive epidemiology of type 1 diabetes–is it still in? Diabetologia 2012;55:1227–30.

60. Onkamo P, Vaananen S, Karvonen M, et al. Worldwide increase in incidence of type I diabetes–the analysis of the data on published incidence trends. Diabetologia 1999;42:1395–403.

61. Wolfsdorf J, Craig ME, Daneman D, et al. Diabetic ketoacidosis in children and adolescents with diabetes. Pediatr Diabetes 2009;10(Suppl 12):118–33.

62. Dunger DB, Sperling MA, Acerini CL, et al. European Society for Paediatric Endocrinology/Lawson Wilkins Pediatric Endocrine Society consensus statement on diabetic ketoacidosis in children and adolescents. Pediatrics 2004; 113:e133–40.

63. Koul PB. Diabetic ketoacidosis: a current appraisal of pathophysiology and management. Clin Pediatr (Phila) 2009;48:135–44.

64. Levin DL. Cerebral edema in diabetic ketoacidosis. Pediatr Crit Care Med 2008; 9:320–9.

65. Glaser N. Cerebral injury and cerebral edema in children with diabetic ketoacidosis: could cerebral ischemia and reperfusion injury be involved? Pediatr Diabetes 2009;10:534–41.

66. Vavilala MS, Richards TL, Roberts JS, et al. Change in blood-brain barrier permeability during pediatric diabetic ketoacidosis treatment. Pediatr Crit Care Med 2010;11:332–8.

67. Marcin JP, Glaser N, Barnett P, et al. Factors associated with adverse outcomes in children with diabetic ketoacidosis-related cerebral edema. J Pediatr 2002; 141:793–7.

68. Glaser N, Barnett P, McCaslin I, et al. Risk factors for cerebral edema in children with diabetic ketoacidosis. The Pediatric Emergency Medicine Collaborative Research Committee of the American Academy of Pediatrics. N Engl J Med 2001;344:264–9.

69. Mahoney CP, Vlcek BW, DelAguila M. Risk factors for developing brain herniation during diabetic ketoacidosis. Pediatr Neurol 1999;21:721–7.

70. Edge JA, Jakes RW, Roy Y, et al. The UK case-control study of cerebral oedema complicating diabetic ketoacidosis in children. Diabetologia 2006;49:2002–9.

71. Hoorn EJ, Carlotti AP, Costa LA, et al. Preventing a drop in effective plasma osmolality to minimize the likelihood of cerebral edema during treatment of children with diabetic ketoacidosis. J Pediatr 2007;150:467–73.

72. Tasker RC, Lutman D, Peters MJ. Hyperventilation in severe diabetic ketoacidosis. Pediatr Crit Care Med 2005;6:405–11.

73. Sternberg EM, Chrousos GP, Wilder RL, et al. The stress response and the regulation of inflammatory disease. Ann Intern Med 1992;117:854–66.

74. Marik PE, Levitov A. The "koala stress syndrome" and adrenal responsiveness in the critically ill. Intensive Care Med 2010;36:1805–6.

75. Annane D, Cavaillon JM. Corticosteroids in sepsis: from bench to bedside? Shock 2003;20:197–207.

76. Rhen T, Cidlowski JA. Antiinflammatory action of glucocorticoids–new mechanisms for old drugs. N Engl J Med 2005;353:1711–23.

77. Annane D, Maxime V, Ibrahim F, et al. Diagnosis of adrenal insufficiency in severe sepsis and septic shock. Am J Respir Crit Care Med 2006;174:1319–26.

78. Marik PE, Pastores SM, Annane D, et al. Recommendations for the diagnosis and management of corticosteroid insufficiency in critically ill adult patients: consensus statements from an international task force by the American College of Critical Care Medicine. Crit Care Med 2008;36:1937–49.

79. Hamrahian AH, Oseni TS, Arafah BM. Measurements of serum free cortisol in critically ill patients. N Engl J Med 2004;350:1629–38.

80. Zimmerman JJ, Barker RM, Jack R. Initial observations regarding free cortisol quantification logistics among critically ill children. Intensive Care Med 2010; 36:1914–22.

81. Zimmerman JJ, Donaldson A, Barker RM, et al. Real-time free cortisol quantification among critically ill children. Pediatr Crit Care Med 2011;12:525–31.

82. Riordan FA, Thomson AP, Ratcliffe JM, et al. Admission cortisol and adrenocorticotrophic hormone levels in children with meningococcal disease: evidence of adrenal insufficiency? Crit Care Med 1999;27:2257–61.

83. Joosten KF, de Kleijn ED, Westerterp M, et al. Endocrine and metabolic responses in children with meningoccocal sepsis: striking differences between survivors and nonsurvivors. J Clin Endocrinol Metab 2000;85:3746–53.

84. De Kleijn ED, Joosten KF, Van Rijn B, et al. Low serum cortisol in combination with high adrenocorticotrophic hormone concentrations are associated with

poor outcome in children with severe meningococcal disease. Pediatr Infect Dis J 2002;21:330–6.

85. Onenli-Mungan N, Yildizdas D, Yapicioglu H, et al. Growth hormone and insulin-like growth factor 1 levels and their relation to survival in children with bacterial sepsis and septic shock. J Paediatr Child Health 2004;40:221–6.

86. den Brinker M, Joosten KF, Liem O, et al. Adrenal insufficiency in meningococcal sepsis: bioavailable cortisol levels and impact of interleukin-6 levels and intubation with etomidate on adrenal function and mortality. J Clin Endocrinol Metab 2005;90:5110–7.

87. Hatherill M, Tibby SM, Hilliard T, et al. Adrenal insufficiency in septic shock. Arch Dis Child 1999;80:51–5.

88. Pizarro CF, Troster EJ, Damiani D, et al. Absolute and relative adrenal insufficiency in children with septic shock. Crit Care Med 2005;33:855–9.

89. Casartelli CH, Garcia PC, Branco RG, et al. Adrenal response in children with septic shock. Intensive Care Med 2007;33:1609–13.

90. Menon K, Ward RE, Lawson ML, et al. A prospective multicenter study of adrenal function in critically ill children. Am J Respir Crit Care Med 2010;182: 246–51.

91. Dimopoulou I, Tsagarakis S, Kouyialis AT, et al. Hypothalamic-pituitary-adrenal axis dysfunction in critically ill patients with traumatic brain injury: Incidence, pathophysiology, and relationship to vasopressor dependence and peripheral interleukin-6 levels. Crit Care Med 2004;32:404–8.

92. Sprung CL, Annane D, Keh D, et al. Hydrocortisone therapy for patients with septic shock. N Engl J Med 2008;358:111–24.

93. Rady MY, Johnson DJ, Patel B, et al. Cortisol levels and corticosteroid administration fail to predict mortality in critical illness: the confounding effects of organ dysfunction and sex. Arch Surg 2005;140:661–8 [discussion: 669].

94. Hsieh S, White PC. Presentation of primary adrenal insufficiency in childhood. J Clin Endocrinol Metab 2011;96:E925–8.

95. Annane D. Time for a consensus definition of corticosteroid insufficiency in critically ill patients. Crit Care Med 2003;31:1868–9.

96. Adcock IM, Barnes PJ. Molecular mechanisms of corticosteroid resistance. Chest 2008;134:394–401.

97. Ledderose C, Mohnle P, Limbeck E, et al. Corticosteroid resistance in sepsis is influenced by microrna-124-induced downregulation of glucocorticoid receptor-alpha. Crit Care Med 2012;40:2745–53.

98. Britt RC, Devine A, Swallen KC, et al. Corticosteroid use in the intensive care unit: at what cost? Arch Surg 2006;141:145–9 [discussion: 149].

99. Puthucheary Z, Harridge S, Hart N. Skeletal muscle dysfunction in critical care: wasting, weakness, and rehabilitation strategies. Crit Care Med 2010;38: S676–82.

100. Costello JM, Graham DA, Morrow DF, et al. Risk factors for central line-associated bloodstream infection in a pediatric cardiac intensive care unit. Pediatr Crit Care Med 2009;10:453–9.

101. Yeh TF, Lin YJ, Lin HC, et al. Outcomes at school age after postnatal dexamethasone therapy for lung disease of prematurity. N Engl J Med 2004;350:1304–13.

102. Brierley J, Carcillo JA, Choong K, et al. Clinical practice parameters for hemodynamic support of pediatric and neonatal septic shock: 2007 update from the American College of Critical Care Medicine. Crit Care Med 2009;37:666–88.

103. Arafah BM. Hypothalamic pituitary adrenal function during critical illness: limitations of current assessment methods. J Clin Endocrinol Metab 2006;91:3725–45.

104. Zimmerman JJ. A history of adjunctive glucocorticoid treatment for pediatric sepsis: moving beyond steroid pulp fiction toward evidence-based medicine. Pediatr Crit Care Med 2007;8:530–9.

105. Cooper DS, Ladenson PW. The thyroid gland. In: Gardner DG, Shoback S, editors. Greenspan's basic and clinical endocrinology. 9th edition. San Francisco (CA): McGraw-Hill Medical; 2011. p. 162–226.

106. Ulate KP, Zimmerman JJ. Common endocrinopathies in the pediatric intensive care unit. In: Fuhrman B, Zimmerman JJ, editors. Pediatric critical care. 4th edition. Philadelphia: Elsevier; 2011. p. 1105–23.

107. Eyal O, Rose SR. Thyroid hormone. In: Nichols DG, editor. Roger's textbook of pediatric intensive care. 4th edition. Philadelphia: Wolters Kluwer Health, Lippincott Williams & Wilkins; 2011. p. 1649–60.

108. Bauer M, Silverman DH, Schlagenhauf F, et al. Brain glucose metabolism in hypothyroidism: a positron emission tomography study before and after thyroid hormone replacement therapy. J Clin Endocrinol Metab 2009;94:2922–9.

109. Klein I, Danzi S. Thyroid hormone treatment to mend a broken heart. J Clin Endocrinol Metab 2008;93:1172–4.

110. Marks SD, Haines C, Rebeyka IM, et al. Hypothalamic-pituitary-thyroid axis changes in children after cardiac surgery. J Clin Endocrinol Metab 2009;94:2781–6.

111. den Brinker M, Joosten KF, Visser TJ, et al. Euthyroid sick syndrome in meningococcal sepsis: the impact of peripheral thyroid hormone metabolism and binding proteins. J Clin Endocrinol Metab 2005;90:5613–20.

112. Peeters RP, Wouters PJ, van Toor H, et al. Serum 3,3',5'-triiodothyronine (rT3) and 3,5,3'-triiodothyronine/rT3 are prognostic markers in critically ill patients and are associated with postmortem tissue deiodinase activities. J Clin Endocrinol Metab 2005;90:4559–65.

113. Passeri E, Frigerio M, De Filippis T, et al. Increased risk for non-autoimmune hypothyroidism in young patients with congenital heart defects. J Clin Endocrinol Metab 2011;96:E1115–9.

114. Plumpton KR, Anderson BJ, Beca J. Thyroid hormone and cortisol concentrations after congenital heart surgery in infants younger than 3 months of age. Intensive Care Med 2010;36:321–8.

115. Portman MA, Slee A, Olson AK, et al. Triiodothyronine supplementation in infants and children undergoing cardiopulmonary bypass (TRICC): a multicenter placebo-controlled randomized trial: age analysis. Circulation 2010;122:S224–33.

116. Kaptein EM, Sanchez A, Beale E, et al. Clinical review: thyroid hormone therapy for postoperative nonthyroidal illnesses: a systematic review and synthesis. J Clin Endocrinol Metab 2010;95:4526–34.

117. Peter F, Muzsnai A. Congenital disorders of the thyroid: hypo/hyper. Pediatr Clin North Am 2011;58:1099–115, ix.

118. Eastman CJ. Screening for thyroid disease and iodine deficiency. Pathology 2012;44:153–9.

119. Abduljabbar MA, Afifi AM. Congenital hypothyroidism. J Pediatr Endocrinol Metab 2012;25:13–29.

120. Iraci GS, Fux-Otta C. Images in clinical medicine. Graves' hyperthyroidism. N Engl J Med 2009;360:e31.

121. Brent GA. Clinical practice. Graves' disease. N Engl J Med 2008;358:2594–605.

122. Trapp CM, Elder RW, Gerken AT, et al. Pediatric pulmonary arterial hypertension and hyperthyroidism: a potentially fatal combination. J Clin Endocrinol Metab 2012;97:2217–22.

123. Franklyn JA, Boelaert K. Thyrotoxicosis. Lancet 2012;379:1155–66.

Medical Ethics in Pediatric Critical Care

Alberto Orioles, MD[a,b], Wynne E. Morrison, MD, MBE[a,c],*

KEYWORDS

- Medical ethics • Pediatrics • Critical care • Multidisciplinary

KEY POINTS

- Medical ethics is a system of moral principles that apply values and judgments to the practice of medicine.
- Since the mid-twentieth century, concerns about human experimentation and the availability of new technologies have led to a larger role for ethical analysis in medicine, as witnessed by the increasing use of institutional review boards, hospital ethics committees, and the expansion of the role of clinical ethicists.
- In pediatric critical care, more children are surviving with chronic illnesses, and some of these children need ongoing or frequent intensive care and technological support.
- It is important to practice with a continuing awareness of areas in which controversies can develop and to be familiar with institutional resources.

MEDICAL ETHICS AND CRITICAL CARE

Medical ethics is a system of moral principles that apply values and judgments to the practice of medicine. Although the historical roots of Western medical ethics may be traced to early writings on the duties of physicians from Hippocrates to rabbinic and Christian teachings, the world's first official national code of medical ethics[1] was adopted by the American Medical Association in 1847, which served as a body of rules and regulations for the medical profession.

Since the mid-twentieth century, concerns about human experimentation[2–4] and the availability of new technologies have led to a larger role for ethical analysis in medicine, as witnessed by the increasing use of institutional review boards, hospital ethics committees, and the expansion of the role of clinical ethicists. At the same time that the complexity of medical decisions has been increasing, there has been growing respect for the autonomy of the patient and shared decision making. Medical ethics

a Departments of Anesthesiology and Critical Care, The Children's Hospital of Philadelphia, 3400 Civic Center Boulevard, Philadelphia, PA 19104, USA; b Division of Pediatric Critical Care, Children's Hospitals and Clinics of Minnesota, 2525 Chicago Avenue, Minneapolis, MN 55404, USA; c Perelman School of Medicine, University of Pennsylvania, Philadelphia, PA 19104, USA
* Corresponding author. Departments of Anesthesiology and Critical Care, The Children's Hospital of Philadelphia, 3400 Civic Center Boulevard, Philadelphia, PA 19104.
E-mail address: MORRISONW@email.chop.edu

Crit Care Clin 29 (2013) 359–375
http://dx.doi.org/10.1016/j.ccc.2012.12.002   criticalcare.theclinics.com
0749-0704/13/$ – see front matter © 2013 Elsevier Inc. All rights reserved.

has therefore of necessity evolved from a theoretic, philosophic justification of moral principles into a pragmatic approach to resolving everyday dilemmas in clinical care.[5]

Such dilemmas are particularly common in critical care, because of the wealth of issues surrounding imbalances of supply and demand between the resources of the health care system and the needs of the public, conflicts between the health care team and the patient/surrogate decision maker over whether life-sustaining technologies should be used, and appropriate use of experimental therapies in heroic attempts to save a life. Technological advances have enabled us to prolong life, but values play into the decisions about what quality or length of life is worth preserving at what costs of suffering on the part of the patient or of resources on the part of society. In pediatric critical care, more and more children are surviving with chronic illnesses,[6] and some of these children need ongoing or frequent intensive care and technological support. These questions are therefore likely to become even more common as time passes, and reaching shared goals among all parties involved is even more essential.[7]

MORAL THEORY AND MIDLEVEL PRINCIPLES

Theoretic biomedical ethics is grounded in philosophic traditions of moral theory, which underlie how individuals and society determine what is right. Deontology is a system of moral theory delineated by Immanuel Kant, in which certain actions are deemed intrinsically right or good based on whether they could logically and morally be universally applied[8(pp350-1)]. As an example, truth telling is held to be an intrinsically good action because society could not function if it could not be assumed that others were usually telling the truth. Kant also famously held that "the end does not justify the means," upholding the right of the individual to self-determination as more important than achieving a common good if doing so required sacrificing that individual. There are obvious implications in research ethics, in which it is inappropriate to knowingly harm 1 person even if the knowledge gained could benefit many others. An alternative moral theory is utilitarianism or consequentialism, which argues that an action is considered right that achieves the greatest good for the greatest number of people. Many policy and public health decisions by their nature rely on balancing such utilitarian concerns with the rights of individuals.

In their groundbreaking book *Principles of Biomedical Ethics*,[8] Tom Beauchamp and James Childress outline 4 midlevel principles that can be derived from either underlying moral theory to help guide clinical and policy decisions relating to health care. Most decisions require balancing the directives of these principles against one another. The 4 principles described by Beauchamp and Childress are:

- Respect for autonomy: a competent patient has the right to refuse or choose their treatment.
- Beneficence: a clinician should act in the best interest of the patient.
- Nonmaleficence: "first, do no harm" or avoid harming the patient
- Justice: making sure that those in similar circumstances are treated the same, whether concerning the distribution of scarce health resources or who receives which treatment (fairness and equality).

Other values that are sometimes discussed include:

- Respect for persons: the patient (and the person treating the patient) has the right to be treated with dignity. Autonomy derives from this underlying Kantian directive.
- Truthfulness and honesty: related to the concept of informed consent, emphasized since the historical events of the Nuremberg trials and Tuskegee syphilis experiments.[4,9]

Although ethical analysis using such principles is often helpful, it is important to avoid oversimplifying complex situations by setting up artificial juxtapositions such as "this is obviously a conflict between the principles of autonomy and beneficence," if doing so leads to a failure to explore the full details underlying a dilemma. These principles and other terms used in this article are defined in **Table 1**.

DECISION-MAKING STANDARDS IN PEDIATRICS

For competent adult patients, honoring the principle of autonomy means that the patient can decide whether to accept or refuse any proposed medical procedure, even if a physician or medical team thinks that the patient's decision is not the wisest choice. Particularly in the United States, a high value is placed on the choices of the individual patient, with the exception of unusual situations like public health emergencies, when certain choices might put others at risk.[10] When adult patients are not able to speak for themselves, family members or other authorized decision makers and the medical team attempt to decide what the patient would want, either by trying to understand the patient's prior wishes for treatment (expressed in conversations or in written documents such as advance directives) or by using the process of substituted judgment, in which an authorized representative attempts to determine what a patient would likely have wanted. When none of these options is available, the decision maker or the medical team attempt to decide by considering the patient's best interests, or what is believed by consensus to be what most individuals would consider best in the given situation (grounded in the principle of beneficence).[8,11]

For children who have not yet reached an age at which they are legally allowed to make their own decisions (typically 18 years old), autonomy is not an irrelevant concept; their opinions are still deserving of respect, even if they are not legally binding.[12] For this reason, clinicians may seek the assent of a child for treatments or procedures, whenever it is feasible and appropriate to do so, along with informed permission from the parent or other authorized decision maker. The assent/permission framework is usually more appropriate than the term informed consent when one is speaking of decisions being made for another.[13,14]

For children, the parent or parents are usually the appropriate surrogate decision maker.[15] Most institutions have policies consistent with the relevant state laws about who is the next appropriate surrogate if a parent is either unavailable or an inappropriate decision maker. Other possible surrogates include extended family or court-appointed guardians. Yet, even when the medical team believes that a parent may not be a reliable surrogate (eg, in cases of suspected child abuse), a specific legal process must be followed before that parent's decision-making rights can be terminated. The team should continue to keep a parent informed and included in decision making while any such legal process is under way.

However, parents do not have absolute decision-making authority for everything that happens regarding their children. Although parents are granted broad leeway in determining the upbringing, education, and medical care that their children receive, courts have determined that parents cannot make martyrs of their children,[16] and parental authority is sometimes overridden when there is a risk of immediate harm to a child. One example of parental authority being overridden is when a medical team obtains a court order to transfuse a child with blood against the wishes of a parent who is a Jehovah's Witness and who therefore objects to blood transfusion on religious grounds.[17] Overriding a parent in such a circumstance is often justified when the refusal of therapy would be highly likely to lead to significant harm or death and the provision of the therapy has clear benefit with only few or short-term burdens.

Table 1
Glossary of common ethical terms

Advance directive	A set of written instructions in which a competent adult specifies preferences for medical decisions in possible future circumstances in which they may not be able to communicate choices
Assent	Approval or agreement to a diagnostic test or medical intervention, usually expressed by a minor or other person lacking legal decision-making capacity
Autonomy	Moral principle stating that the patient has the right to refuse or choose treatment
Beneficence	Moral principle stating that a practitioner should act in the best interest of the patient
Organ donation after a circulatory determination of death (DCDD, formerly known as DCD or non–heart-beating donation)	A process by which life-sustaining medical therapies are discontinued and death declared by cardiopulmonary criteria, followed shortly thereafter by organ procurement
Dead-donor rule	The standard that a patient must be declared dead before the procurement of vital organs
DNAR order	*Do not attempt resuscitation*: a legal order signed by a physician to respect the wishes of a patient or of a surrogate decision maker to not undergo specified interventions (such as cardiopulmonary resuscitation) if the patient suffers a cardiac or respiratory arrest
DNI order	*Do not intubate*: a legal order signed by a physician to respect the wishes of a patient or of a surrogate decision maker to not undergo intubation
Informed consent	Permission obtained from a competent patient to perform a specific test or procedure. It implies understanding of the medical test or procedure (and of its alternatives) and autonomy in the decision-making process
Informed permission	Approval or agreement to a diagnostic test or medical intervention, usually expressed by a parent or proxy on behalf of a minor or other person lacking medical decision-making capacity
Justice	Moral principle concerning the distribution of scarce health resources, and the decision of who receives which treatment (fairness and equality)
Nonmaleficence	Moral principle stating that physicians must refrain from providing ineffective treatments or acting with malice toward patients (*Do no harm*)
Principle of double effect	Principle stating that an act causing both a good and a bad effect (eg, unintentionally hastening a patient's death with medications administered to relieve pain) can be justified if the intended effect is beneficial

(continued on next page)

Table 1 *(continued)*	
Substituted judgment	The concept that a surrogate decision maker can give consent for a procedure or treatment if the patient is unable (or unwilling) to give consent themselves, by attempting to determine what a patient would likely have wanted
Surrogate decision maker	A health care proxy who has decision-making capacity on behalf of a patient who is unable or unwilling to give consent themselves

Decisions become more complicated when the benefit is less certain or the therapy more prolonged.[18] The medical team can serve as a safeguard to verify that any decision that a parent is making falls within a range of acceptable options in similar cases. If the team and a parent agree that a decision is appropriate, there is generally no need for further review by an ethics committee or the courts.

Whereas many investigators state that parental decisions should adhere to the same best interests standard applied when an adult patient's wishes cannot be known,[11] some investigators argue that a parent is not compelled to choose a single best option when making a decision for a child and is legitimately allowed to choose from any number of acceptable options when balancing the competing interests of an entire family.[19] Along the same lines, others have outlined criteria for what degree of harm justifies the state's overriding a parental choice or refusal of therapy (**Box 1**).[20] Yet, until such a threshold is reached, any number of choices might be acceptable if harm to the child is avoided or the choice is consistent with the choice that a reasonable parent would make.[21] In practice, the parents and the medical team usually navigate these types of choices without explicitly considering what decision-making standards are being applied. Yet, when decisions are difficult, it can sometimes be helpful to take a step back and reassess which goals make sense in light of these

---

Box 1
Diekema's conditions for justifying state intervention based on risk of harm to child

1. By refusing to consent are the parents placing their child at significant risk of serious harm?

2. Is the harm imminent, requiring immediate action to prevent it?

3. Is the intervention that has been refused necessary to prevent the serious harm?

4. Is the intervention that has been refused of proven efficacy, and therefore, likely to prevent the harm?

5. Does the intervention that has been refused by the parents not also place the child at significant risk of serious harm, and do its projected benefits outweigh its projected burdens significantly more favorably than the option chosen by the parents?

6. Would any other option prevent serious harm to the child in a way that is less intrusive to parental autonomy and more acceptable to the parents?

7. Can the state intervention be generalized to all other similar situations?

8. Would most parents agree that the state intervention was reasonable?

Adapted from Diekema DS. Parental refusals of medical treatment: the harm principle as threshold for state intervention. Theor Med Bioeth 2004;25(4):243–64; with permission.

standards. Is a parent making a decision based on what the child would say if they could speak? Asking a parent to focus on what the child would want if that could be known may help assuage feelings of guilt or a desire to never give up. In most of these situations, parents struggle when they wonder whether they are caring for their child in the best way possible, and it can be helpful to offer support by emphasizing that the decisions that they make are loving decisions that other families would choose as well.

Decision making differs slightly when it concerns participation in research rather than choices in clinical care. More stringent criteria are applied when the research study being proposed does not offer the prospect of direct benefit to the child/research subject. Institutional review is necessary to determine that a research protocol carries minimal risk or only a minor increase above minimal risk.[22] In cases in which the research protocol is nontherapeutic, most institutions require the assent of children older than a certain age before participation. For some types of emergency research, exceptions to informed consent may be sought when the time frame in which a therapy needs to be applied makes it impossible to follow a standard consent procedure. Federal guidelines exist to ensure appropriate oversight of such protocols as well as community acceptance of the need for the research.[23] A thorough discussion of the ethics of pediatric research is beyond the scope of this article.

ISSUES SPECIFIC TO END-OF-LIFE CARE

Approximately 50,000 children die every year in the United States.[24,25] Although there is some evidence that more children may be going home to die, most of these deaths still occur in the hospital, and more often than not in the intensive care unit (ICU).[26,27] Managing pain and other symptoms at the end of life, as well as supporting patients and families emotionally throughout the dying process, are therefore core clinical skills for pediatric intensivists.

Over the past several decades, tremendous advances have been made in the ability to support failing organ systems in the ICU, sometimes for prolonged periods.[6] Mechanical ventilation, mechanical circulatory supports such as ventricular assist devices, and renal replacement therapies are all examples of interventions that can be life-saving. However, there are times when such therapies serve only to prolong the time that it takes to die.[28] It is also possible that even when such aggressive interventions are life-saving, the quality of life for the patient who is rescued is not believed to be worth the burdens of the therapies. Multiple court cases have upheld the right of competent adult patients or their appropriate surrogates to refuse life-sustaining therapies when such interventions are believed to be unlikely to lead to long-term survival or to maintain a good quality of life.[29] For children, it is also possible to withhold or withdraw life-sustaining measures such as cardiopulmonary resuscitation (CPR) or mechanical ventilation when the parents and medical team agree that the burdens of such therapies outweigh the possible benefits. Some evidence exists that most children dying in hospitals now do so with some sort of order limiting the escalation of life-sustaining measures in place.[30–32]

Do Not Attempt Resuscitation *Orders*

Do not attempt resuscitation (DNAR) orders are used when decisions are made not to pursue specified therapies.[33,34] DNAR has recently become a preferred term rather than *Do not resuscitate*, because including the word attempt is believed to be less likely to imply that resuscitation is always successful. Education regarding success rates of CPR in various scenarios may correct overly optimistic public expectations of success based on media exposures.[35] Some centers have gone even further and use the term *Allow natural death* rather than DNAR, with a goal of emphasizing the benefit of such orders rather than what will be withheld.[36,37]

When writing DNAR orders, it is important to be as specific as possible regarding which interventions are to be avoided. In some cases, the family and team may decide to limit cardiac interventions such as chest compressions, defibrillation, and medications if a full cardiopulmonary arrest occurs. In others, a decision may be made not to intubate if respiratory failure develops (sometimes abbreviated as DNI for Do not intubate). It is important in discussions with patients and families to focus on which goals one hopes to achieve by implementing or avoiding specific interventions, rather than presenting a list of possible therapies and asking for a yes/no decision about each one. However, the ICU physician needs to translate those overall goals into specific orders to give the team guidance on how to proceed.

It is generally accepted that any medical therapy that can be withheld may also appropriately be withdrawn in identical circumstances, and that just because a therapy is in place does not imply that there is an obligation to continue it.[38,39] However, for many patients, families, and some members of the medical team, there can be a significant psychological difference between deciding not to start a therapy and discontinuing it. Many families may therefore be more comfortable deciding to limit escalation of therapies rather than discontinuing them. In such cases, the passage of time may clarify the trajectory of the critical illness, and if it becomes apparent that suffering is present with little hope of a good outcome, the family may become more comfortable stopping.

The provision of artificial nutrition and hydration represents a special circumstance because it is a medical intervention, but is believed by many to be a normal part of caring for a patient, which should therefore not be withheld.[40–42] Children differ in many respects from adults when decisions are made about continuing nutrition, because many parents see providing nourishment to their child as one of the primary roles of a parent. Children also, in the normal course of development, depend on others to feed them, so having to do so via feeding tubes or formulas does not seem unusual. It is generally accepted that nutrition and hydration should be withheld only when a patient is actively dying or when providing the nutrition is worsening suffering. Examples of the latter are if new procedures are required to provide nutrition (such as placement of a feeding tube) or if feeding is causing intractable gastrointestinal distress or fluid overload. Discontinuing nutrition or hydration may also be justified in those who permanently lack consciousness (**Box 2**).[40] After a withdrawal of technology in

---

Box 2
Patients for whom it may be appropriate to consider withholding artificial nutrition and hydration per American Academy of Pediatrics guideline

1. Patients in the terminal stages of dying for whom artificial nutrition and hydration only prolong the process and may increase morbidity

2. Patients with severe life-limiting organ failure such as intestinal or cardiac failure, for whom the provision of artificial nutrition and hydration is shown to cause significantly more burden than benefit

3. Patients who permanently lack consciousness, such as patients in a persistent vegetative state

Adapted from Diekema DS, Botkin JR. Clinical report–forgoing medically provided nutrition and hydration in children. Pediatrics 2009;124(2):813–22; with permission.

the ICU, this question becomes important only if the patient survives for more than a few days after the withdrawal.

Managing Symptoms at the End of Life and the Principle of Double Effect

Dying patients frequently have pain or dyspnea that requires medical management.[43,44] Clinicians at the bedside sometimes worry that pharmacologic interventions intended to relieve such suffering may also hasten death, and such concerns may lead to the undertreatment of symptoms.[45] The principle of double effect justifies using whatever doses of medication are necessary to relieve such suffering, even if death is hastened[8(pp128-132)]. This principle distinguishes the intended effect of an action from the foreseeable but unintended negative effect. An act can be justified if:

1. The intended effect is beneficial (in this case, the relief of suffering)
2. Only the good effect is intended (the clinician's desire is to relieve suffering, not to hasten death)
3. The bad effect is not the means of achieving the good effect (eg, suffering is not relieved only by causing death)
4. The good effect must outweigh the bad effect (eg, hastening death may be justified to relieve suffering when death is imminent, but is not justified if death is not otherwise anticipated for many years)

In practice, it is difficult to judge intent, but medications that are titrated to effect can be justified even if very high doses of such medications are needed.[46] In most cases, doses of narcotics and benzodiazepines are not associated with time to death after the withdrawal of mechanical ventilation, if the amount given is targeted to the relief of suffering,[47,48] so clinicians should be reassured that it is rare for appropriate interventions to hasten death. For patients who have developed tolerance to these medications over time, large doses may be required to relieve pain or dyspnea, and doses may justifiably be escalated higher than the usual amounts when necessary.

The principle of double effect also clarifies why some medications are inappropriate at the end of life.[39,49] Neuromuscular blocking agents, for example, do not relieve suffering (and may interfere with the clinician's ability to detect the patient's suffering) and cause immediate death by paralyzing the respiratory muscles. Neuromuscular blockade should therefore never be administered as a ventilator is being withdrawn or to a spontaneously breathing patient at the end of life. Similarly, medications such as high-dose potassium chloride, the sole intent of administration of which is to hasten death rather than relieve suffering, is inappropriate.

Futility Disputes and Resolution of Conflict

When intensive care interventions are no longer expected to lead to prolonged survival or a good quality of life for a patient, such interventions are sometimes described as futile. Although it is generally accepted that there is no obligation for the health care team to provide therapies that are medically ineffective, reaching consensus about what defines futile or ineffective care has been elusive.[50-54] Some cases are clear: extracorporeal life support, operative procedures, or dialysis are not offered or even mentioned if they are not expected to benefit the patient. A physician is also able to make decisions regarding how long to continue resuscitative efforts; once it is reasonably certain that no return of spontaneous circulation will be achieved (the amount of time may vary depending on the patient and the circumstances), CPR can and should stop. However, conflict can arise when the medical team has become convinced that ongoing interventions will not achieve the desired goal, but the patient or family demand that everything be done.[28,55] In many cases, a determination of how likely a therapy is to succeed involves some sort of value judgment, either regarding how small a chance of success is worth pursuing, or what quality of life is worth living. A patient or family may therefore be willing to accept a smaller chance of success or a worse quality of life than clinicians believe is reasonable. Or it may be that the patient or family's trust in the medical team, or at least trust in the team's ability to prognosticate, has been lost.

Some states and institutions have tackled the difficulty with defining futility by establishing a procedural approach for resolving conflicts rather than trying to define what futile care is. The best-known example of such a procedural approach is the Texas Advance Directives Act.[56,57] This statute outlines a process that hospitals can follow if they believe that patients or families are demanding care that will be ineffective. When a medical team feels that interventions are ineffective but a patient or family asks that supportive measures continue, the team can request an institutional review (by an ethics committee or medical advisory committee). The patient/family must be notified that a review process has started. If the review committee agrees that ongoing therapy is not indicated, the patient/family is informed and a 10-day waiting period begins, during which the patient/family can seek options for transfer of care or go to court to ask for an extension of the waiting period. If the patient or family does not elect to pursue those options, then the life-sustaining therapies can be withdrawn at the end of the waiting period. If this process is followed, the statute grants the clinicians and institutions immunity from prosecution or civil suits regarding the withdrawal.

There is a small case series in the pediatric literature[58] describing the application of the Texas protocol in 5 patients at 2 hospitals. In some of the cases, the medical teams believed that the process helped the families accept that their child was dying without forcing them to be the ones to make a decision about withdrawal or DNAR. However, in 1 of the cases, transfer of care was sought and the patient lived for 2 more years. Although the fact that 1 child survived for some time shows how difficult it can be to know when medical interventions are ineffective,[59] a reasonable argument could also be made that the process worked in this circumstance.

In some cases, parents may understand that their child is dying but be unwilling to participate in a decision to stop interventions because doing so would feel like they are giving up on their child. It is possible in those circumstances to take an informed non-dissent approach, in which the clinician outlines a medically reasonable plan, states which interventions seem reasonable and which do not, and gives the family a chance to object to the plan but does not explicitly ask the family's permission to limit therapies.[60–62] An example of such a statement might be: "Considering that he is already on the maximal support we can provide with a ventilator and medications to help his blood pressure, if his heart stops at this point I do not expect that CPR or shocking him would be able to get him back. I'm therefore not planning to do those things that I don't think will help. Let me know if you have questions about that or would rather talk about it further. At the same time, we are doing everything we can think of that has a chance of helping him." Such an approach keeps the family informed and offers them the opportunity to object to the physician's recommendations, but does not ask them to be the ones to make a choice if they are uncomfortable doing so.

In cases in which a family believes strongly that full resuscitative efforts should be attempted, even if the medical team is convinced that doing so will be ineffective, proceeding with a short trial of resuscitative measures may be necessary. A time-limited trial of well-coordinated, vigorous CPR does more to maintain the skills of the medical team and trust of the family than a show code or slow code performed merely for the sake of appearances.[33,63,64] The medical team can decide how long it is appropriate to try; prolonged attempts at resuscitation are not always necessary to confirm for the team and family that the interventions will not be successful.[65]

Conflicts between a patient or family and the medical team can often be avoided by focusing on mutual goals rather than perseverating on particular decisions where disagreement exists.[66,67] Team discussions to make sure that a consistent message is being given to a family by all disciplines and specialties are important, and regular follow-up, with a consistent team representative whenever possible, can be helpful.[68] Bringing long-term subspecialists or primary physicians into a discussion can also be useful. Supporting a family by acknowledging that they are showing devotion to their child in a difficult situation can also help to build an alliance.[34,69] Hospital ethics committees may be able to help mediate conflicts. Social workers and hospital chaplains can offer additional support. The courts should be an option of last resort when the medical team believes that a family's decisions are reaching a point of being harmful to the child.

PEDIATRIC ORGAN DONATION AND TRANSPLANTATION

Advances in surgical technique, critical care, and immunologic therapies over the past 60 years have enabled organs obtained from both living and cadaveric organ donors to save or improve the lives of many patients with end-stage organ failure. Organ donation and transplantation raise innumerable ethical issues, ranging from what constitutes valid consent for donation, to concerns about the just distribution of scarce resources, to questions about how to define death.[70] In this section, primarily ethical issues that surround the procurement of organs from patients declared dead by neurologic or circulatory criteria are discussed. Although many issues of consent, coercion, and fair distribution are also raised by living donation,[71] a full discussion is beyond the scope of this article because it is rare for children to be suitable living donors (other than through minimal risk procedures such as bone marrow donation).

Procurement of organs from patients who have died generally follows 1 of 3 paths:

1. After a declaration of death by irreversible cessation of neurologic function
2. After a planned withdrawal of technological support (controlled organ donation after a circulatory determination of death [DCDD])
3. After a cardiac arrest, when return of spontaneous circulation cannot be achieved (uncontrolled DCDD; uncommon in the United States but frequent in some European countries)

The process of organ donation is different in donors who are declared dead by neurologic versus circulatory criteria. The differences and separate ethical challenges of each of these processes are described in the following section, but uncontrolled DCDD is not the focus.

THE DETERMINATION OF DEATH

Before the advent of modern critical care, there was some variability in the methods used to determine when death had occurred.[72] However, it was not until the development of mechanical ventilation that it became apparent that some patients could be maintained with artificial supports even after all detectable brain function had ceased. This situation was first described as *coma depassé* in the late 1950s in France.[73] The technological advances of critical care thus spurred a reexamination of what constitutes death and how it is best diagnosed. The concomitant refinement of organ transplantation techniques also led to a related need to come to a societal consensus on who was eligible to be an organ donor.

A President's Commission in the United States therefore developed guidelines for determining death, whether by cardiopulmonary or neurologic criteria. These efforts culminated in the Uniform Determination of Death Act,[74,75] a draft state law approved in 1981 by the National Conference of Commissioners on Uniform State Laws, in cooperation with the American Medical Association, the American Bar Association, and the President's Commission for the Study of Ethical Problems in Medicine and Biomedical and Behavioral Research, which states that:

An individual who has sustained either
(1) irreversible cessation of circulatory and respiratory functions, or
(2) irreversible cessation of all functions of the entire brain, including the brain stem, is dead
A determination of death must be made in accordance with accepted medical standards

The law was intentionally nonspecific about when these criteria had been met, and individual states and institutions set their own criteria for diagnosing when death has occurred.

Irreversible cessation of brain function, total brain failure,[76] or death determined by neurologic criteria are more appropriate terms than the commonly used brain death, because brain death implies to some that only the brain is dead, not the individual. A patient who has irreversible cessation of brain function is clinically and legally dead, even if some somatic functions are maintained by technological support. In the United States, declaration of death by neurologic criteria requires documentation over time of the absence of cortical and brainstem function, which can be determined clinically or by reliance on confirmatory tests, such as electroencephalography or brain flow isotope studies.[77]

Even within the medical community, the determination of death by neurologic criteria is not without controversy and misunderstandings.[78] Some argue that the concept of death by neurologic criteria is fundamentally flawed, because patients diagnosed with this condition have the capability to maintain an extensive range of integrative functioning of the organism as a whole, such as hemodynamic stability, maintenance of body temperature, the elimination of wastes, or maintenance of a pregnancy.[79,80] Some countries rely on brainstem criteria, rather than focusing on the function of the entire brain.[81] Some religious or cultural communities reject the concept of neurologic criteria altogether, and some states caution against or forbid overriding a family who has objections to diagnosing death in this way.[82] Conflict in such cases can be difficult for families and hospital staff, and early involvement of hospital administration, legal counsel, and religious leaders from the patient's community should usually be sought.

DEAD-DONOR RULE

The dead-donor rule is the concept that it is unethical to cause death by recovering organs and unethical for cadaveric organ procurement to precede death. It was formulated to preserve the principle of *Do no harm* in the face of an increasing need for organs for transplantation. Some have argued that the dead-donor rule should be abandoned,[83] and that it would be possible to set societally acceptable standards to allow someone who is not dead to become an organ donor (such as patients with such severe brain injury that they have an irreversible loss of consciousness and anticipated imminent death). Anencephalic infants are 1 category of patient who would become eligible organ donors by these criteria.[84] The difficulty with broadening the criteria is that the line between who is eligible to be a donor and who is not could become less distinct, and there is a risk that the desire to help those who need organ transplants would lead to overly aggressive attempts to identify donors and public distrust of the system.[76]

Current regulations and community agreement, as delineated in the Uniform Anatomic Gift Act (2006), require that potential donors be declared dead before organ procurement. This statute also regulates the maintenance and prioritization of waiting lists for potential organ recipients to ensure a fair and just process of allocation.

CONTROVERSIES OVER DCDD

DCDD is an increasingly common practice in US hospitals.[85] In cases in which a terminally ill or injured patient cannot be declared dead by neurologic criteria, this process may provide a patient and family with the opportunity to donate the vital organs. The typical scenario is a neurologically devastated patient for whom a family has made a decision to withdraw technological support. If the family chooses to donate organs, then the withdrawal is monitored in a controlled setting that allows a surgical team to procure organs shortly after the heart stops and death is declared. Death is determined by the traditional cardiopulmonary standard, but the timing and setting of declaration are affected by the organ procurement process, because prolonged periods of waiting between cessation of circulation and the declaration of death or between the declaration of death and arrival in the operating room lead to warm ischemic time, which could damage the organs. However, a brief waiting period between cessation of circulation and organ procurement is necessary to ensure that circulatory function does not return. There is variability in the required waiting period between institutions,[86] with the Institute of Medicine[87] initially recommending 5 minutes of observation, and the Society of Critical Care Medicine[88] and National Conference on Donation After Cardiac Death report,[89] later recommending that "not less than 2 minutes is acceptable and not more than 5 minutes is recommended."

There is debate about whether the timing of the process violates the dead-donor rule.[90] Critics argue that not enough time has passed to guarantee that the cessation of circulation is irreversible, because it would still be possible to restore the patient's cardiac function if resuscitation attempts were begun. Supporters argue that the objection is irrelevant because resuscitation is not going to be attempted, and that the state is therefore permanent.[91,92] It is important to separate discussions about withdrawal of technological support and organ donation, to avoid introducing organ procurement as the reason for the withdrawal of support.[93] In addition, there should be a clear separation between the surgical team who are going to procure organs and the team in the operating room who care for the patient and have responsibility for discontinuing therapies and providing appropriate end-of-life comfort measures. Many centers require the surgical team to stay in another room until death is declared to avoid any pressure on the clinicians caring for the patient to hasten the dying process. If death has not occurred within a certain time frame after withdrawal, typically an hour, plans for organ procurement are abandoned and the patient returns to the ICU for ongoing end-of-life care.

SUMMARY

Ethically charged situations are common in pediatric critical care.[38] Although most situations are managed with minimal controversy within the medical team or between the team and patients/families, it is important to practice with a continuing awareness of areas in which controversies can develop. Familiarity with institutional resources, such as hospital ethics committees, and national guidelines, such as publications from the American Academy of Pediatrics, American Medical Association, or the Society of Critical Care Medicine, are an essential part of the toolkit of any intensivist. Open discussion with colleagues and within the multidisciplinary team can also help ensure that when difficult situations arise, they are addressed in a proactive, evidence-based, and collegial manner.

REFERENCES

1. Code of Medical Ethics of the American Medical Association. Available at: http://www.ama-assn.org/resources/doc/ethics/1847code.pdf [Accessed October 20, 2012].
2. Beecher HK. Ethics and clinical research. N Engl J Med 1966;274(24):1354–60.
3. Caplan AL. Too hard to face. J Am Acad Psychiatry Law 2005;33(3):394–400.
4. Jonsen AR. A short history of medical ethics. New York: Oxford University Press; 2000.
5. Lo B. Resolving ethical dilemmas: a guide for clinicians. 2nd edition. Philadelphia: Lippincott Williams & Wilkins; 2000.
6. Namachivayam P, Shann F, Shekerdemian L, et al. Three decades of pediatric intensive care: who was admitted, what happened in intensive care, and what happened afterward. Pediatr Crit Care Med 2010;11(5):549–55.
7. Hawryluck L, Crippen D. Ethics and critical care in the new millennium. Crit Care 2002;6(1):1–2.
8. Beauchamp T, Childress JF. Principles of biomedical ethics. 5th edition. New York: Oxford University Press; 2001.
9. Brandt AM. Racism and research: the case of the Tuskegee Syphilis Study. Hastings Cent Rep 1978;8(6):21–9.
10. Snyder L. American College of Physicians ethics manual: sixth edition. Ann Intern Med 2012;156(1 Pt 2):73–104.
11. Kopelman LM. The best interests standard for incompetent or incapacitated persons of all ages. J Law Med Ethics 2007;35(1):187–96.
12. Informed consent, parental permission, and assent in pediatric practice. Committee on Bioethics, American Academy of Pediatrics. Pediatrics 1995; 95(2):314–7.
13. Morrison W, Feudtner C. The contested territory of medical decision-making for children. In: Ravistsky V, Fiester A, Caplan A, editors. Penn Center guide to bioethics. New York: Springer; 2009. p. 449.
14. Zawistowski CA, Frader JE. Ethical problems in pediatric critical care: consent. Crit Care Med 2003;31(Suppl 5):S407–10.
15. Arnold RM, Kellum J. Moral justifications for surrogate decision making in the intensive care unit: implications and limitations. Crit Care Med 2003;31(Suppl 5): S347–53.
16. Zelizer VA. Pricing the priceless child: the changing social value of children. Princeton (NJ): Princeton University Press; 1994.
17. Sheldon M. Ethical issues in the forced transfusion of Jehovah's Witness children. J Emerg Med 1996;14(2):251–7.
18. Feudtner C. Ethics in the midst of therapeutic evolution. Arch Pediatr Adolesc Med 2008;162(9):854–7.
19. Ross LF. Children, families, and health care decision making. Oxford (NY): Clarendon Press; 1998.
20. Diekema DS. Parental refusals of medical treatment: the harm principle as threshold for state intervention. Theor Med Bioeth 2004;25(4):243–64.

21. Cooper R, Koch KA. Neonatal and pediatric critical care: ethical decision making. Crit Care Clin 1996;12(1):149–64.
22. Ross LF. Informed consent in pediatric research. Camb Q Healthc Ethics 2004; 13(4):346–58.
23. Morris MC, Nadkarni VM, Ward FR, et al. Exception from informed consent for pediatric resuscitation research: community consultation for a trial of brain cooling after in-hospital cardiac arrest. Pediatrics 2004;114(3):776–81.
24. Kochanek KD, Kirmeyer SE, Martin JA, et al. Annual summary of vital statistics: 2009. Pediatrics 2012;129(2):338–48.
25. Minino AM, Murphy SL, Xu J, et al. Deaths: final data for 2008. Natl Vital Stat Rep 2011;59(10):1–126.
26. Feudtner C, Kang TI, Hexem KR, et al. Pediatric palliative care patients: a prospective multicenter cohort study. Pediatrics 2011;127(6):1094–101.
27. Ramnarayan P, Craig F, Petros A, et al. Characteristics of deaths occurring in hospitalised children: changing trends. J Med Ethics 2007;33(5):255–60.
28. Feudtner C, Morrison W. The darkening veil of "do everything". Arch Pediatr Adolesc Med 2012;166(8):694–5.
29. Gostin LO. Deciding life and death in the courtroom. From Quinlan to Cruzan, Glucksberg, and Vacco–a brief history and analysis of constitutional protection of the 'right to die'. JAMA 1997;278(18):1523–8.
30. Prendergast TJ, Puntillo KA. Withdrawal of life support: intensive caring at the end of life. JAMA 2002;288(21):2732–40.
31. Vernon DD, Dean JM, Timmons OD, et al. Modes of death in the pediatric intensive care unit: withdrawal and limitation of supportive care. Crit Care Med 1993; 21(11):1798–802.
32. Lee KJ, Tieves K, Scanlon MC. Alterations in end-of-life support in the pediatric intensive care unit. Pediatrics 2010;126(4):e859–64.
33. Burns JP, Edwards J, Johnson J, et al. Do-not-resuscitate order after 25 years. Crit Care Med 2003;31(5):1543–50.
34. Morrison W, Berkowitz I. Do not attempt resuscitation orders in pediatrics. Pediatr Clin North Am 2007;54(5):757–71, xi–xii.
35. Diem SJ, Lantos JD, Tulsky JA. Cardiopulmonary resuscitation on television. Miracles and misinformation. N Engl J Med 1996;334(24):1578–82.
36. Cohen RW. A tale of two conversations. Hastings Cent Rep 2004;34(3):49.
37. Knox C, Vereb JA. Allow natural death: a more humane approach to discussing end-of-life directives. J Emerg Nurs 2005;31(6):560–1.
38. Solomon MZ, Sellers DE, Heller KS, et al. New and lingering controversies in pediatric end-of-life care. Pediatrics 2005;116(4):872–83.
39. American Academy of Pediatrics Committee on Bioethics: guidelines on foregoing life-sustaining medical treatment. Pediatrics 1994;93(3):532–6.
40. Diekema DS, Botkin JR. Clinical report–forgoing medically provided nutrition and hydration in children. Pediatrics 2009;124(2):813–22.
41. Casarett D, Kapo J, Caplan A. Appropriate use of artificial nutrition and hydration–fundamental principles and recommendations. N Engl J Med 2005; 353(24):2607–12.
42. Carter BS, Leuthner SR. The ethics of withholding/withdrawing nutrition in the newborn. Semin Perinatol 2003;27(6):480–7.
43. Wolfe J, Grier HE, Klar N, et al. Symptoms and suffering at the end of life in children with cancer. N Engl J Med 2000;342(5):326–33.
44. Ullrich CK, Mayer OH. Assessment and management of fatigue and dyspnea in pediatric palliative care. Pediatr Clin North Am 2007;54(5):735–56, xi.

45. Truog RD, Brock DW, White DB. Should patients receive general anesthesia prior to extubation at the end of life? Crit Care Med 2012;40(2):631–3.
46. Zernikow B, Michel E, Craig F, et al. Pediatric palliative care: use of opioids for the management of pain. Paediatr Drugs 2009;11(2):129–51.
47. Chan JD, Treece PD, Engelberg RA, et al. Narcotic and benzodiazepine use after withdrawal of life support: association with time to death? Chest 2004;126(1): 286–93.
48. Partridge JC, Wall SN. Analgesia for dying infants whose life support is withdrawn or withheld. Pediatrics 1997;99(1):76–9.
49. Truog RD, Campbell ML, Curtis JR, et al. Recommendations for end-of-life care in the intensive care unit: a consensus statement by the American College [corrected] of Critical Care Medicine. Crit Care Med 2008;36(3):953–63.
50. Miles SH. Medical futility. Law Med Health Care 1992;20(4):310–5.
51. Baskett PJ, Steen PA, Bossaert L. European Resuscitation Council guidelines for resuscitation 2005. Section 8. The ethics of resuscitation and end-of-life decisions. Resuscitation 2005;67(Suppl 1):S171–80.
52. Medical futility in end-of-life care: report of the Council on Ethical and Judicial Affairs. JAMA 1999;281(10):937–41.
53. Schneiderman LJ, Jecker NS, Jonsen AR. Medical futility: its meaning and ethical implications. Ann Intern Med 1990;112(12):949–54.
54. Truog RD, Brett AS, Frader J. The problem with futility. N Engl J Med 1992; 326(23):1560–4.
55. Quill TE, Arnold R, Back AL. Discussing treatment preferences with patients who want "everything". Ann Intern Med 2009;151(5):345–9.
56. Fine RL, Mayo TW. Resolution of futility by due process: early experience with the Texas Advance Directives Act. Ann Intern Med 2003;138(9):743–6.
57. Truog RD. Tackling medical futility in Texas. N Engl J Med 2007;357(1):1–3.
58. Okhuysen-Cawley R, McPherson ML, Jefferson LS. Institutional policies on determination of medically inappropriate interventions: use in five pediatric patients*. Pediatr Crit Care Med 2007;8(3):225–30.
59. Frader J, Michelson K. Can policy spoil compassion? Pediatr Crit Care Med 2007; 8(3):293–4.
60. Kon AA. Informed nondissent rather than informed assent. Chest 2008;133(1): 320–1 [author reply: 321].
61. Kon AA. Informed non-dissent: a better option than slow codes when families cannot bear to say "let her die". Am J Bioeth 2011;11(11):22–3.
62. Morrison WE. Is that all you got? J Palliat Med 2010;13(11):1384–5.
63. Truog RD. Is it always wrong to perform futile CPR? N Engl J Med 2010;362(6): 477–9.
64. Morrison W, Feudtner C. Quick and limited is better than slow, sloppy, or sly. Am J Bioeth 2011;11(11):15–6.
65. Lantos JD, Meadow WL. Should the "slow code" be resuscitated? Am J Bioeth 2011;11(11):8–12.
66. Way J, Back AL, Curtis JR. Withdrawing life support and resolution of conflict with families. BMJ 2002;325(7376):1342–5.
67. Feudtner C. Tolerance and integrity. Arch Pediatr Adolesc Med 2005;159(1):8–9.
68. Michelson KN, Emanuel L, Carter A, et al. Pediatric intensive care unit family conferences: one mode of communication for discussing end-of-life care decisions. Pediatr Crit Care Med 2011;12(6):e336–43.
69. Back AL, Arnold RM, Baile WF, et al. When praise is worth considering in a difficult conversation. Lancet 2010;376(9744):866–7.

70. Evans DW. The American Academy of Pediatrics policy statement on organ donation. Pediatrics 2010;126(2):e491–2 [author reply: e492].
71. Brown-Saltzman K, Diamant A, Fineberg IC, et al. Surrogate consent for living related organ donation. JAMA 2004;291(6):728–31.
72. Farrell MM, Levin DL. Brain death in the pediatric patient: historical, sociological, medical, religious, cultural, legal, and ethical considerations. Crit Care Med 1993; 21(12):1951–65.
73. Mollaret P, Goulon M. [The depassed coma (preliminary memoir)]. Rev Neurol (Paris) 1959;101:3–15 [in French].
74. Determination of death (Uniform Determination of Death Act of 1981); natural death (Natural Death Act of 1981). Lexis DC Code DC 1982; Sect. 6.2401 6.2421 to 6.2430 amended Feb 1982:Unknown.
75. Bernat JL, Culver CM, Gert B. Defining death in theory and practice. Hastings Cent Rep 1982;12(1):5–8.
76. President's Council on Bioethics. Controversies in the determination of death. Washington, DC: President's Council on Bioethics; 2008.
77. Nakagawa TA, Ashwal S, Mathur M, et al. Guidelines for the determination of brain death in infants and children: an update of the 1987 Task Force recommendations. Crit Care Med 2011;39(9):2139–55.
78. Youngner SJ, Landefeld CS, Coulton CJ, et al. 'Brain death' and organ retrieval. A cross-sectional survey of knowledge and concepts among health professionals. JAMA 1989;261(15):2205–10.
79. Miller FG, Truog RD. Decapitation and the definition of death. J Med Ethics 2010; 36(10):632–4.
80. Truog RD. Is it time to abandon brain death? Hastings Cent Rep 1997;27(1):29–37.
81. Truog RD. Brain death–too flawed to endure, too ingrained to abandon. J Law Med Ethics 2007;35(2):273–81.
82. Olick RS. Brain death, religious freedom, and public policy: New Jersey's landmark legislative initiative. Kennedy Inst Ethics J 1991;1(4):275–92.
83. Truog RD, Miller FG. "Brain death" is a useful fiction. Crit Care Med 2012;40(4): 1393–4 [author reply: 1394].
84. Steinberg A, Katz E, Sprung CL. Use of anencephalic infants as organ donors. Crit Care Med 1993;21(11):1787–90.
85. Halpern SD, Barnes B, Hasz RD, et al. Estimated supply of organ donors after circulatory determination of death: a population-based cohort study. JAMA 2010;304(23):2592–4.
86. Antommaria AH, Trotochaud K, Kinlaw K, et al. Policies on donation after cardiac death at children's hospitals: a mixed-methods analysis of variation. JAMA 2009; 301(18):1902–8.
87. Institute of Medicine Division of Healthcare Services. Non-heart-beating organ transplantation: practice and protocols. Washington, DC: National Academies Press; 2000.
88. Ethics Committee, American College of Critical Care Medicine, Society of Critical Care Medicine. Recommendations for nonheartbeating organ donation. A position paper by the Ethics Committee, American College of Critical Care Medicine, Society of Critical Care Medicine. Crit Care Med 2001;29(9):1826–31.
89. Bernat JL, Capron AM, Bleck TP, et al. The circulatory-respiratory determination of death in organ donation. Crit Care Med 2010;38(3):963–70.
90. Carcillo JA, Orr R, Bell M, et al. A call for full public disclosure and moratorium on donation after cardiac death in children. Pediatr Crit Care Med 2010;11(5):641–3 [author reply: 643–5].

91. Halpern SD, Truog RD. Organ donors after circulatory determination of death: not necessarily dead, and it does not necessarily matter. Crit Care Med 2010;38(3): 1011–2.
92. Marquis D. Are DCD donors dead? Hastings Cent Rep 2010;40(3):24–31.
93. Aulisio MP, Devita M, Luebke D. Taking values seriously: ethical challenges in organ donation and transplantation for critical care professionals. Crit Care Med 2007;35(Suppl 2):S95–101.

Index

Note: Page numbers of article titles are in **boldface** type.

See Chronic kidney disease (CKD)

A

Acute disseminated encephalomyelitis (ADEM)
    pediatric acute encephalitis and, 272–273
Acute encephalitis
    pediatric, **259–277**. *See also* Encephalitis, acute, pediatric
Acute kidney injury (AKI)
    in PICU, 285–297
        CRRT for, 296–297
        hemodialysis for, 295
        peritoneal dialysis for, 295–296
        RRT for, 295–297
Acute lung injury (ALI)
    transfusion-related
        in critically ill pediatric patients, 308–309
Acute lung injury (ALI)/acute respiratory distress syndrome (ARDS)
    treatment of, 175–176
Acute normovolemic hemodilution
    for anemia and transfusion-related issues in critically ill pediatric patients, 312
Acute respiratory failure, **167–183**
    described, 167–168
    epidemiology of, 171–172
    monitoring of, 172–174
    outcome of, 178–179
    oxygenation and, 169–170
    prognosis of, 178–179
    treatment of, 174–175
        in ALI/ARDS, 175–176
        in asthma, 176–177
        in bronchiolitis, 178
        ECMO in, 178
    ventilation and, 170–171
ADEM. *See* Acute disseminated encephalomyelitis (ADEM)
Adrenal insufficiency
    in PICU, 348
Airway clearance techniques
    in pediatric status asthmaticus management, 162
AKI. *See* Acute kidney injury (AKI)
Albuterol
    in pediatric status asthmaticus management, 157–158
ALI/ARDS. *See* Acute lung injury (ALI)/acute respiratory distress syndrome (ARDS)
Alveolar gas equation, 169

Crit Care Clin 29 (2013) 377–391
http://dx.doi.org/10.1016/S0749-0704(13)00013-4   criticalcare.theclinics.com
0749-0704/13/$ – see front matter © 2013 Elsevier Inc. All rights reserved.

Moving?

Make sure your subscription moves with you!

To notify us of your new address, find your **Clinics Account Number** (located on your mailing label above your name), and contact customer service at:

Email: journalscustomerservice-usa@elsevier.com

800-654-2452 (subscribers in the U.S. & Canada)
314-447-8871 (subscribers outside of the U.S. & Canada)

Fax number: 314-447-8029

**Elsevier Health Sciences Division
Subscription Customer Service
3251 Riverport Lane
Maryland Heights, MO 63043**

To ensure uninterrupted delivery of your subscription, please notify us at least 4 weeks in advance of move.

Printed and bound by CPI Group (UK) Ltd, Croydon, CR0 4YY

03/10/2024

01040436-0005